Cranio-Orbital Mass Lesions

Giulio Bonavolontà · Francesco Maiuri
Giuseppe Mariniello

Editors

Cranio-Orbital Mass Lesions

Diagnosis and Management

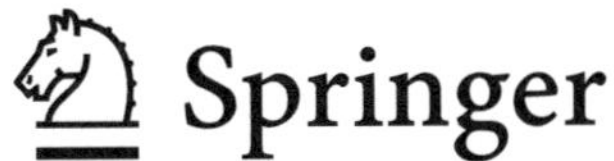

Springer

Editors
Giulio Bonavolontà
Dept. of Neuroscience
University of Naples Federico II
Naples, Italy

Francesco Maiuri
Dept. of Neuroscience
University of Naples Federico II
Naples, Italy

Giuseppe Mariniello
Dept. of Neuroscience
University of Naples Federico II
Naples, Italy

ISBN 978-3-031-35773-2   ISBN 978-3-031-35771-8   (eBook)
https://doi.org/10.1007/978-3-031-35771-8

This Springer imprint is published by the registered company Springer Nature Switzerland AG
The registered company address is: Gewerbestrasse 11, 6330 Cham, Switzerland

Preface

The contiguous intracranial and orbital compartments are often the site of mass lesions of different origin and histology, variably extending in both locations. Several previous books have discussed the tumors and nontumoral pathologies limited to the orbit and the best approaches according to the intraorbital location; on the other hand, no previous book is devoted to cranio-orbital pathologies.

This book arises from the large surgical experience of cranio-orbital mass lesions operated on by a multidisciplinary team of neurosurgeons and orbital surgeons in our university.

The cranio-orbital region, including the orbit and the contiguous anterior and middle cranial fossae, is anatomically complex. Many critical structures are involved during surgery of the cranio-orbital pathologies, including optic canal, superior and inferior orbital fissures, optic and oculomotor nerves, internal carotid and ophthalmic arteries, and cavernous sinus. The knowledge of these bone, nerve, and vascular structures and their variations is essential for planning the best surgical approach. Thus, the first part of this book is devoted to the surgical anatomy of the cranio-orbital region.

The management of intracranial tumors invading the orbit was a surgical challenge since the first years of the past century. Many surgeons have attempted to extend the frontal or pterional craniotomies to the orbital roof and rims. About 60 years ago Al Mefty introduced the supraorbital-pterional approach, which includes a pterional craniotomy and the resection of the superolateral orbital wall, allowing good exposure of even large cranio-orbital mass lesions.

The surgical treatment of cranio-orbital mass lesions can be challenging due to the involvement of critical structures and the consequent potential morbidity. Many surgical approaches (transcranial, transorbital, or combined) are available. Traditionally, neurosurgeons have been regarded as experts in exposing the superior and lateral surfaces of the orbit, whereas ophthalmologists are considered specialists in exposing the orbit through medial and transorbital routes. Thus, surgical procedures involving mass lesions in this region often require the collaboration of both neurosurgeons and ophthalmologists.

The choice of the most useful approach mainly depends on the location and extension of the lesion, its type and histology, the anatomical obstacles (mainly the position and relationship with the optic nerve), and the surgeon's expertise. Generally, the best route must avoid manipulation of the optic nerve and its vascular supply with the aim to preserve the vision. Although the classical more invasive approaches are still used mainly for large lesions, the more recently introduced less invasive endoscopic endonasal and transorbital approaches are widely employed. The indications, advantages, and limits of the various approaches are discussed in the third part of this book.

The last part is devoted to specific cranio-orbital mass lesions, both tumoral and nontumoral; their pathological and clinical aspects and their management options are discussed with the aid of the more recent contributions from the literature.

This book is useful not only for neurosurgeons and ophthalmologists, but also for otolaryngologists and maxillofacial surgeons, who often treat mass lesions contiguous to the cranial cavity and orbit. All these specialists will find important anatomical and surgical information useful in their surgical training and daily experience.

The authors invited to contribute to this topic have been carefully selected based on their extensive expertise in their respective areas. We thank all for their contributions which have significantly improved the quality of the book.

Naples, Italy	Giulio Bonavolontà
Naples, Italy	Francesco Maiuri
Naples, Italy	Giuseppe Mariniello

Contents

Part I

Surgical Anatomy of the Cranio-Orbital Region

Surgical Anatomy of the Orbit

1

Juan F. Villalonga, Matías Baldoncini,
Derek O. Pipolo, José Pailler,
Sebastian J. M. Giovannini, and Álvaro Campero

1.1 Introduction

The orbital region is a "crossroads" for various specialists: ophthalmologists, otorhinolaryngologists, maxillofacial, reconstructive surgeons, and neurosurgeons.

Surgical approaches to the orbit present significant difficulty to the general neurosurgeon due to several factors: its relatively small volume, four-sided irregular pyramidal shape, and location between the craniofacial structures and the brain [1].

The neurosurgeon who ventures into orbital surgery must possess extensive anatomical knowledge of this structure. Much of the literature on orbital anatomy describes in detail its complexity but fails to facilitate its comprehension [2].

Our team has set out to systematically illustrate the surgical anatomy of the orbit in this chapter.

1.2 Surgical Anatomy

The orbital cavities are located symmetrically on both sides of the nose. They present a four-sided pyramidal shape with a posterior apex, anterior base, and an axis set from the sagittal plane at a 20° angle. This simple architecture is key to human stereoscopic vision [3].

The curvilinear vertex, base, and walls present perforations and irregularities through which neurovascular bundles pass and muscles are inserted. In terms of thickness, the apex and base are made of thicker bone, while the walls contain a thinner width. Of the four walls, the lateral wall is the thickest while the medial is the thinnest. This osseous thickening at the apex and base helps protect the eye and nerves from possible injury. A distinctive feature of the orbit is that its elements are organized in groups of seven: seven bones, seven intraorbital extraocular muscles, and seven nerves [1].

1.2.1 Bones [1, 4–8]

The orbit is composed of seven bones: frontal, ethmoid, lacrimal, sphenoid, zygomatic, palatine, and maxilla. For its study, it is divided into a lateral wall, medial wall, roof, floor, base, and apex. The upper portion of the base is formed by the frontal bone and presents a notch through which the supraorbital nerve and vessels pass. The lateral wall comprises the zygomatic bone and the floor consists of the zygomatic bone laterally and maxilla medially. The internal wall is formed inferiorly by the frontal process of the maxilla and superiorly by the frontal bone. The frontal

J. F. Villalonga (✉) · M. Baldoncini · D. O. Pipolo
J. Pailler · S. J. M. Giovannini · Á. Campero
LINT, Facultad de Medicina, Universidad Nacional
de Tucumán, Tucumán, Argentina

G. Bonavolontà et al. (eds.), *Cranio-Orbital Mass Lesions*,
https://doi.org/10.1007/978-3-031-35771-8_1

sinus is found in the supero-medial region. From anterior to posterior, the medial wall is formed by the frontal process of the maxilla, the lacrimal bone, lamina papyracea of the ethmoid, forming the center of the medial wall and separating the orbit from the nasal cavity, and the sphenoid bone. The ethmoid bone articulates superiorly with the frontal bone (Fig. 1.1a). In between both bones, we find the anterior and posterior ethmoidal canals, which contain branches of the nasociliary nerve arising from the ophthalmic branch of the trigeminal nerve, branches of the ophthalmic artery, and the anterior and posterior ethmoidal arteries, respectively. The cranial openings of the ethmoidal canals are related to the anterior and posterior limits of the cribriform plate of the ethmoid and divide the orbit into bul-

bar and retrobulbar segments (Fig. 1.1b–d). The optic foramen is found between the sphenoid and ethmoid bones, through which the optic nerve and ophthalmic artery pass.

The thicker lateral wall separates the orbit from the temporal fossa at its anterior end and the middle cranial fossa at its posterior end. It is composed of the zygomatic bone, which has no contact with the brain, and forms the anterior limit of the temporal fossa through which the temporal muscle passes. In turn, it is continuous in depth with the greater wing of the sphenoid bone, which is the anterior limit of the middle cranial fossa in the endocranium. This disposition is the basis for lateral orbital approaches, by which a temporal craniotomy with a pure zygomatic osteotomy allows access to lesions without

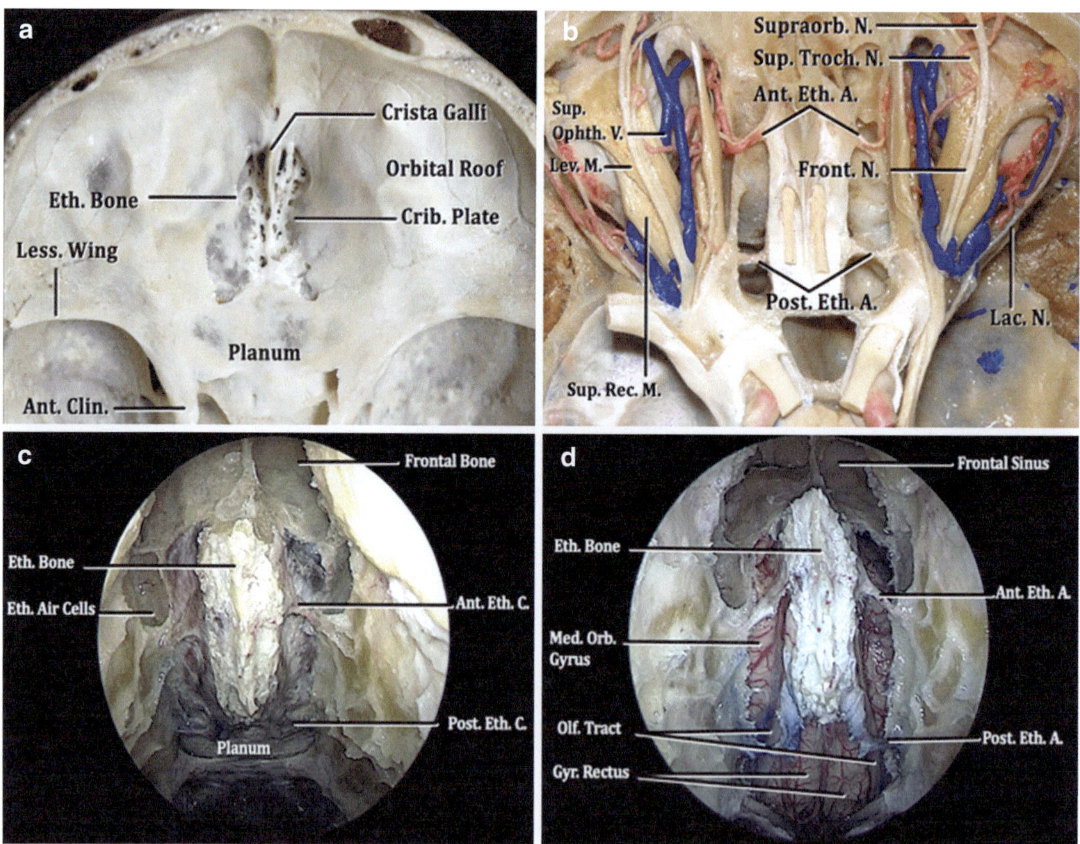

Fig. 1.1 360° anatomical dissection of the roof and medial wall of the orbit. (**a**) Superior aspect of the floor of the anterior cranial fossa that forms the roof of both orbits. (**b**) Superior aspect of both orbits; the periorbita and the orbital fat have been removed for anatomical exposure. (**c, d**) Endoscopic endonasal view of the roof of the nasal cavity and the medial wall of the orbit. Both arteries and ethmoidal canals can be seen. (**Original to the authors**)

the need for combined cranio-orbital approaches. At its anterior point, the lateral wall is continuous with the frontal bone of the orbital roof; however, at the posterior end, it is interrupted by the superior orbital fissure adjacent to the sphenoid bone. The lacrimal foramen, through which the recurrent meningeal branch of the ophthalmic artery passes, is anterior and superior to the superior orbital fissure.

The floor of the orbit is formed by the maxilla and zygomatic bone, which is continuous with the orbital process of the palatine bone posteriorly. The palatine bone contains two segments: a horizontal portion that forms the posterior segment of the hard palate and a vertical portion, with one process directed toward the sphenoid bone and the other toward the orbit. The floor separates the orbit from the maxillary sinus, located at the posterior end of the floor is the inferior orbital fissure; on the medial wall, the nasolacrimal duct is found. The inferior orbital fissure is an important surgical landmark as it communicates the orbit with the pterygopalatine fossa and consecutively with the nasal cavity. Through the external segment of the inferior orbital fissure, the orbit comes in contact with the temporal and infratemporal fossae.

The roof of the orbit is formed by the frontal bone that articulates in depth with the lesser wing of the sphenoid and ethmoid bones (Fig. 1.1a).

1.2.2 Muscles [1, 8]

There are seven extraocular muscles: four rectus, two oblique, and the levator palpebrae (Fig. 1.2). Only the inferior oblique muscle is attached to the medial wall of the orbit. The four rectus and the superior oblique muscle are indirectly attached to the apex of the orbit through a common annular fibrous tendon or annulus of Zinn. The superior orbital muscle passes through the trochlea, a rounded tendon attached to the frontal trochlear fovea located at the superomedial angle of the orbit (Fig. 1.2c).

The annulus of Zinn is inserted along the apex of the orbit, surrounding the opening of the optic canal and the central part of the superior orbital fissure. The contents encircled by the annulus include the optic nerve, ophthalmic artery, abducens or external oculomotor nerve, common oculomotor nerve, divided into its two upper and lower branches, and the ophthalmic branch of the trigeminal nerve. The trochlear nerve and the frontal and lacrimal branches of the trigeminal nerve are located outside the annulus.

1.2.3 Nerves [1, 8–10]

There are seven nerves within the orbit passing through the superior orbital fissure with exception of the optic nerve, which traverses the optic canal (Fig. 1.3a). The optic nerve innervates the retina, which is protected by dura and arachnoid in its intracanalicular and intraorbital course. Upon entry into the orbit through the optic foramen, the optic nerve crosses the medial sector of the annulus of Zinn along with the ophthalmic artery, directed toward the ocular globe. The ciliary ganglion is located on the lateral aspect of the optic nerve at the junction of its anterior 2/3 and posterior 1/3 (Fig. 1.3b–d).

The common oculomotor nerve innervates the extra orbital muscles except for the lateral rectus and superior oblique muscles. It enters through the orbital apex and divides into two branches: superior and inferior. Both branches cross the annulus of Zinn on its lateral aspect. At this point, the nasociliary nerve is located between the superior and inferior rami. Once within the orbit, the superior branch supplies innervation to the superior muscular complex (consisting of the levated palpebrae and superior rectus muscle). The inferior branch innervates the inferior rectus, medial rectus, and inferior oblique muscles. On its trajectory, an ascending collateral branch reaches the ciliary ganglion, responsible for parasympathetic innervation. These fibers synapse in the ciliary ganglion and continue as short ciliary nerves to the pupillary sphincter.

The external oculomotor nerve is formed by the union of several fibers within the cavernous sinus and is responsible for motor innervation of the lateral rectus muscle. Upon its entry into the orbit, it crosses the annulus of Zinn lateral to the

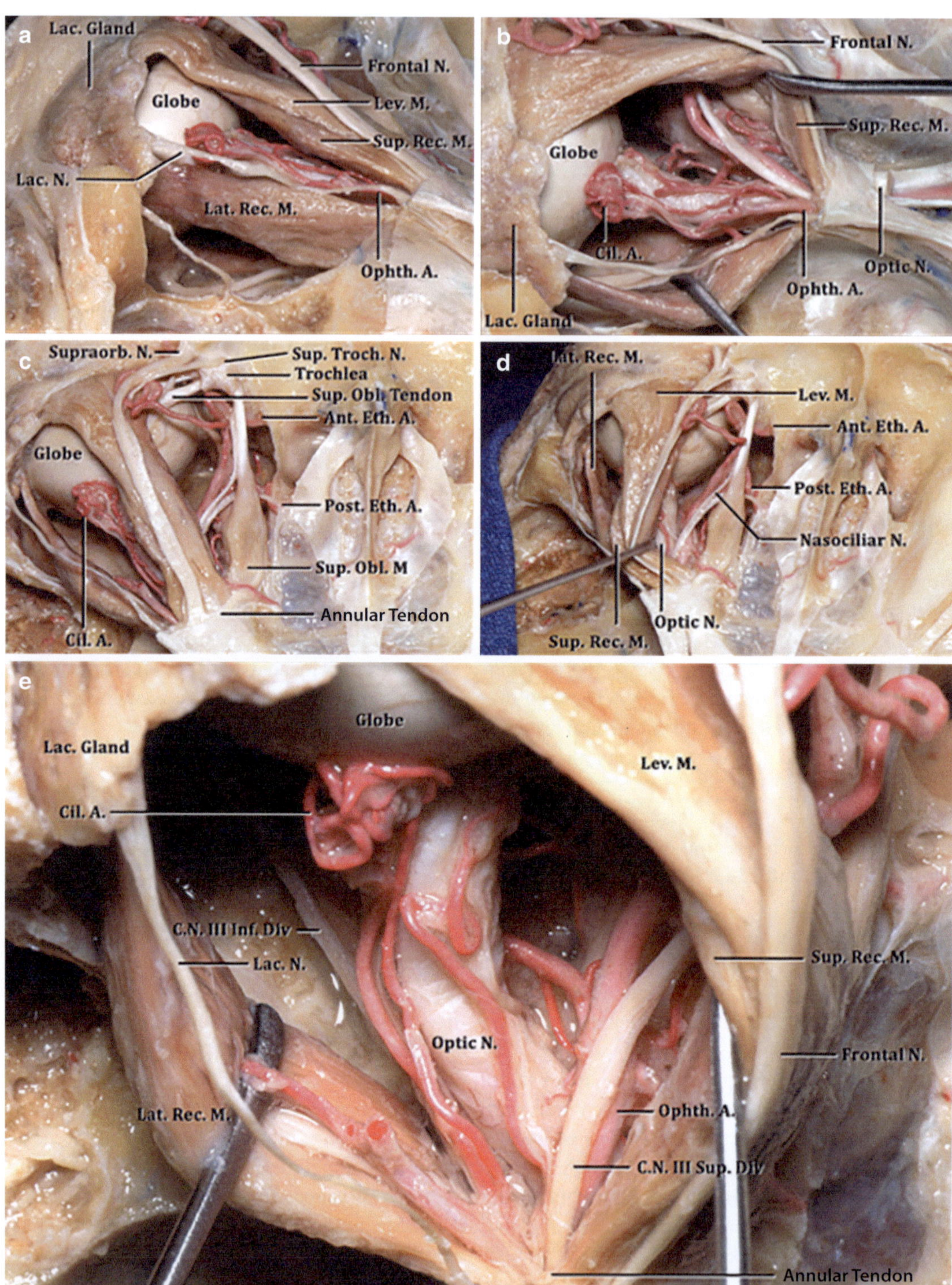

Fig. 1.2 Left orbit dissection. The periorbita and the orbital fat have been removed for anatomical exposure. (**a**) Left lateral view. (**b**) Left lateral view after muscle mobilization. (**c**) Superior view. (**d**) Superior view after muscle mobilization. (**e**) Enlarged view of the superior aspect of the orbit focused on the optic nerve. The lateral rectus and superior rectus muscles have been reflected. (**Original to the authors**)

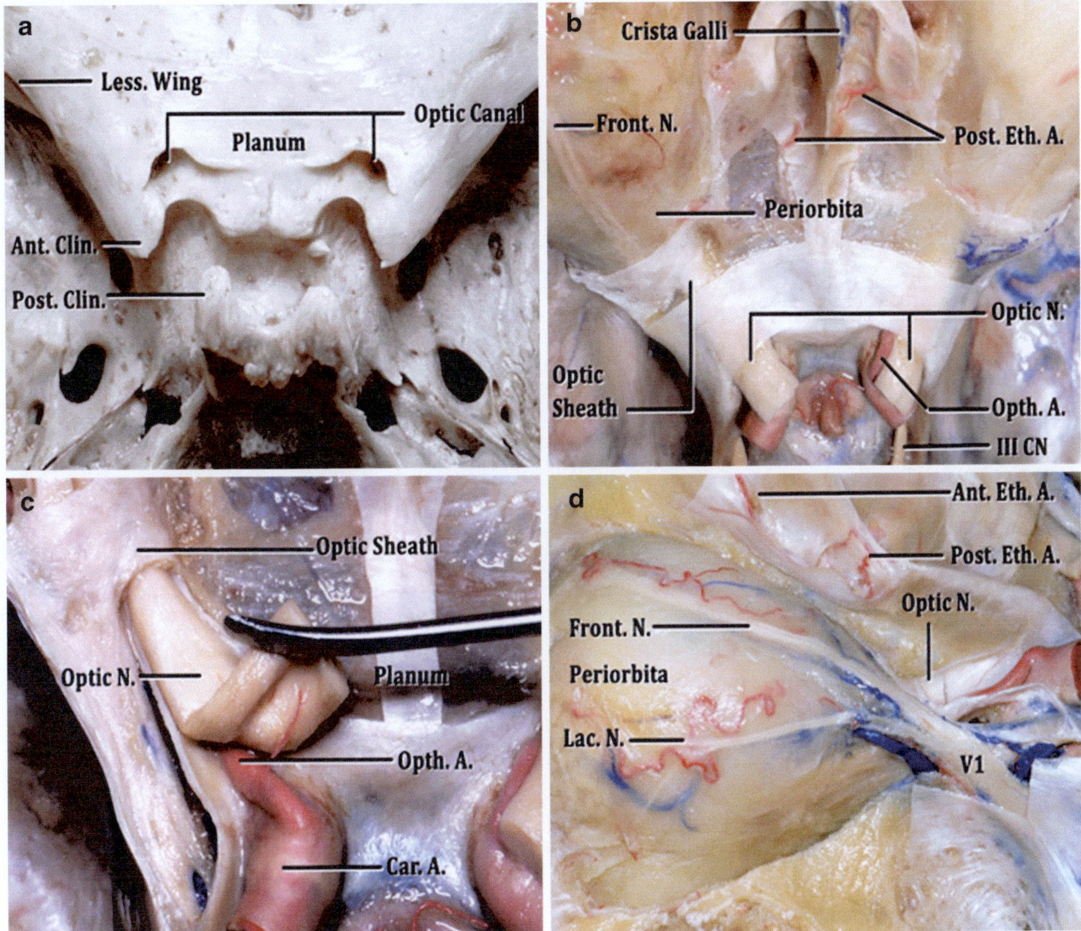

Fig. 1.3 Anatomical dissection focused in the apex of the orbit and optic canal. (**a**) Superior view of the sphenoid bone, both optic canals can be seen. (**b**) Superior aspect of both orbits. (**c**) Enlarged view of the optic canal; the falciform ligament has been removed. (**d**) Left lateral view of the periorbita. The anterior clinoid, lateral orbital wall, and roof have been removed. (**Original to the authors**)

fibers of the common oculomotor nerve and continues along the lateral aspect of the orbit until it reaches the lateral rectus muscle.

The trochlear nerve enters the orbit through the superior orbital fissure outside the annulus of Zinn, traversing near the medial wall until it reaches and innervates the superior oblique muscle.

The ophthalmic nerve (V1) is exclusively sensitive; its innervation territory includes the eyelids, forehead, ocular globe, cornea, and nasal cavities. The lacrimal secretion is ensured by the branch of the sphenopalatine ganglion and communicating branch of the maxillary nerve. The ophthalmic nerve presents three branches: lacrimal, frontal, and nasociliary (Fig. 1.2). After

entering the orbit outside the tendinous ring of Zinn, the lacrimal nerve follows the lateral wall and sends a branch communicating with the zygomatic nerve (branch of V2) for the lacrimal gland, and also a medial branch for the upper eyelid.

The frontal nerve enters outside the annulus of Zinn and follows the superior wall of the orbit. Upon reaching the orbital rim, it divides into two branches: medial (supratrochlear) and lateral (supraorbital) frontal nerves. The medial frontal nerve innervates the forehead, nose, and upper eyelid. The lateral frontal nerve passes through the supraorbital fissure and ascends beneath the forehead. The nasociliary nerve enters the orbit through the annulus of Zinn and contains several collateral branches: sensitive (toward the ciliary or ophthalmic ganglion), long ciliary nerve (to the ocular globe), and sphenoethmoidal branch (to the mucosa of the ethmoidal cells and sphenoid sinus). In the lateral wall of the orbit, it bifurcates giving the internal nasal nerve (i.e., anterior ethmoid nerve) and external nasal nerve (i.e., infratrochlear nerve). The internal nasal nerve passes through the cribriform plate and innervates the mucosa of the lateral walls, while the external nasal nerve innervates the mucosa of the lacrimal ducts.

1.2.4 Vascular Supply [4, 6, 8, 11]

The orbit, pertaining to both the endocranium and exocranium, is irrigated by the internal carotid artery, through the ophthalmic artery and by the external carotid artery via the infraorbital branch of the maxillary artery.

The ophthalmic artery is a branch of the supraclinoid segment of the internal carotid artery. The origin of the ophthalmic artery is usually medial to the anterior clinoid process, below the optic nerve (Fig. 1.3b–d). It enters the optic canal along with the optic nerve, located on the lateral and inferior face. Once it enters the orbital cavity, it remains on the lateral wall of the orbit and gives off dural branches. Subsequently the ophthalmic artery, accompanied by nasociliary nerve, crosses the optic nerve over its superior face (85% of cases) and ends parallel to the medial face of the orbit giving off its terminal branches of the supratrochlear and angular arteries. It is important to mention that in 15% of individual, the ophthalmic artery crosses the optic nerve over its inferior face. The knowledge of the anatomical trajectory of the ophthalmic artery is relevant during the opening of the falciform ligament, to avoid its injury. The ophthalmic artery gives rise to the central retinal, supraorbital, palpebral, lacrimal, short ciliary, long ciliary, infratrochlear, supratrochlear, and dorsal nasal arteries. In addition, it also emits dural branches and therefore can be compromised in skull base injuries.

The principal drainage route of the orbit is through the superior ophthalmic vein, formed by inflows from the supero-medial sector of the orbit. In addition, the inferior ophthalmic vein arises via inflows from the inferior-lateral aspect of the orbit. These veins are connected to each other on the superficial wall of the orbit by anastomoses formed by the facial and angular veins. The inferior ophthalmic vein can drain directly into the cavernous sinus but commonly joins the superior ophthalmic vein forming a common trunk, with the latter draining into the cavernous sinus.

1.3 Surgical Approaches According to Anatomy [12–17]

Among the various approaches to the orbit, we can include the following:

1. Transcranial approaches. Within this group, we recognize two large sub-groups:
   (a) Intracranial approaches: fronto-orbital and orbito-zygomatic.
   (b) Exocranial approaches: lateral orbitotomy.
2. Endoscopic approaches.
3. Transconjunctival approaches. These are specifically the domain of the ophthalmologist.

During multidisciplinary meetings, the neurosurgeon will have to determine whether a patient is candidate for surgery and the best approach. It is often difficult to determine the type of approach; our team follows the guidelines proposed by the School of Pittsburgh [18, 19]. According to these guidelines, each approach offers a certain surgical corridor corresponding to a time range of an analog clock:

- Lateral orbitotomy from 08:00 to 10:00 o'clock.
- Orbito-zygomatic craniotomy from 06:00 to 01:00 o'clock.
- Endonasal endoscopic approach from 01:00 to 07:00 o'clock.

Figure 1.4 illustrates the well-known concept of "around the clock" with cadaveric preparations.

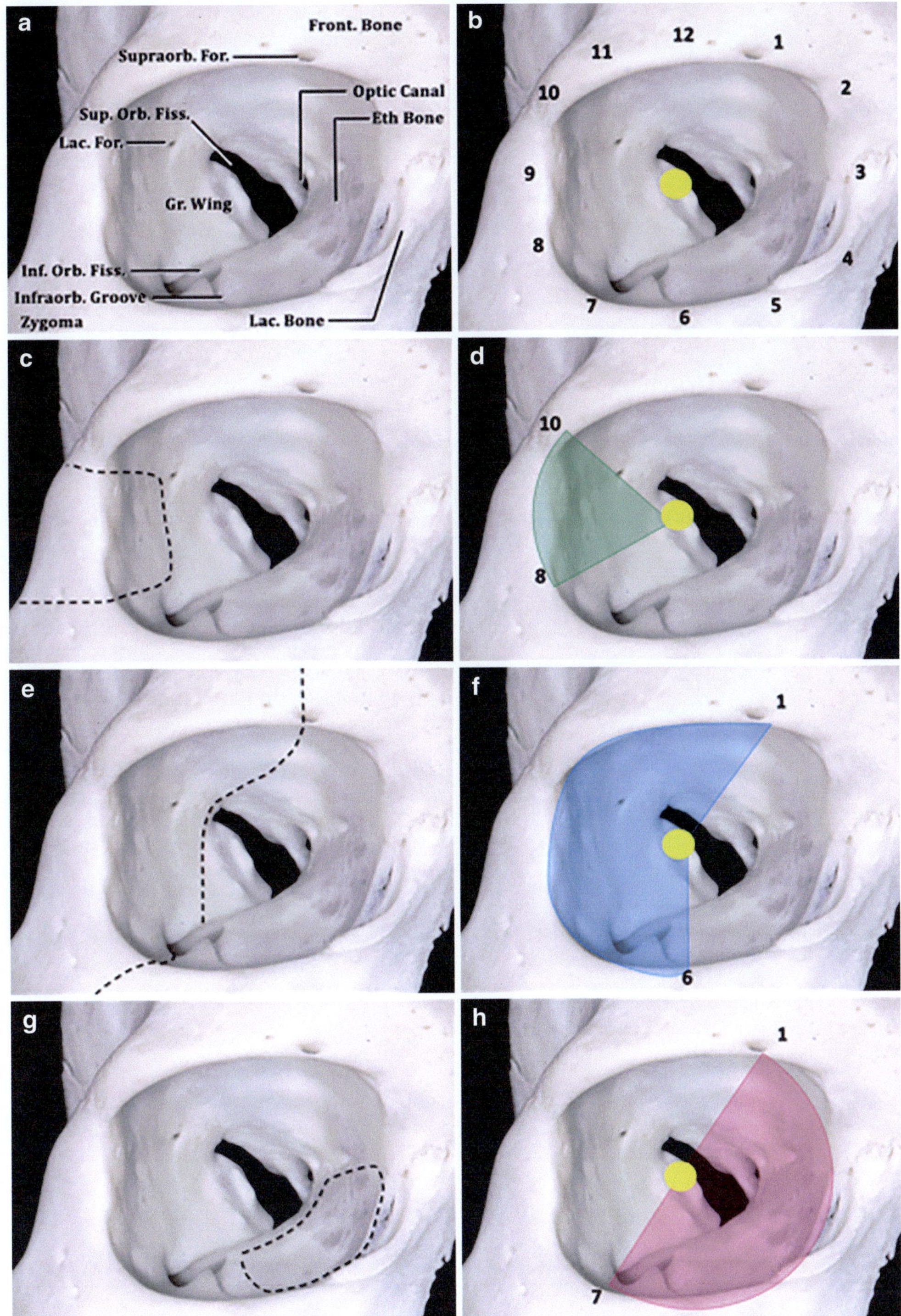

Fig. 1.4 The right orbit is used for demonstration of the clock model. (**a**) Right orbit with its anatomical landmarks. (**b**) "Around the clock model". (**c**, **d**) Lateral orbitotomy enables access to the orbit from 08:00 to 10:00 o'clock. (**e**, **f**) An orbito-zygomatic craniotomy gives orbital access from 06:00 to 01:00 o'clock. (**g**, **h**) An endoscopic endonasal approach gives access to the orbit between 01:00 and 07:00 o'clock. (**Original to the authors**)

References

1. Martins C, Costa ESIE, Campero A, Yasuda A, Aguiar LR, Tatagiba M, et al. Microsurgical anatomy of the orbit: the rule of seven. Anat Res Int. 2011;2011:468727. https://doi.org/10.1155/2011/468727.
2. Villalonga JF, Saenz A, Revuelta Barbero JM, Calandri I, Campero A. Surgical anatomy of the orbit. A systematic and clear study of a complex structure. Neurocirugia (Astur: Engl Ed). 2019;30(6):259–67. https://doi.org/10.1016/j.neucir.2019.04.003.
3. Rhoton AL Jr. The orbit. Neurosurgery. 2002;51(4 Suppl):S303–34.
4. Martins C, Yasuda A, Campero A, Ulm AJ, Tanriover N, Rhoton A Jr. Microsurgical anatomy of the dural arteries. Neurosurgery. 2005;56(2 Suppl):211–51. https://doi.org/10.1227/01.neu.0000144823.94402.3d; discussion 51.
5. Natori Y, Rhoton AL Jr. Microsurgical anatomy of the superior orbital fissure. Neurosurgery. 1995;36(4):762–75. https://doi.org/10.1227/00006123-199504000-00018.
6. Bernardo A, Evins AI, Mattogno PP, Quiroga M, Zacharia BE. The orbit as seen through different surgical windows: extensive anatomosurgical study. World Neurosurg. 2017;106:1030–46. https://doi.org/10.1016/j.wneu.2017.06.158.
7. Di Somma A, Andaluz N, Cavallo LM, Keller JT, Solari D, Zimmer LA, et al. Supraorbital vs endo-orbital routes to the lateral skull base: a quantitative and qualitative anatomic study. Oper Neurosurg (Hagerstown). 2018;15(5):567–76. https://doi.org/10.1093/ons/opx256.
8. Testut L, Latarjet A. Tratado de Anatomía Humana. 9th ed. Barcelona: Salvat; 1968.
9. Latarjet M, Ruiz Liard A. Anatomía Humana. Buenos Aires: Médica Panamericana; 1983.
10. Kuntz C. The autonomic nervous system. 4th ed. Philadelphia: Lea & Febiger; 1953.
11. Vural A, Carobbio ALC, Ferrari M, Rampinelli V, Schreiber A, Mattavelli D, et al. Transorbital endo-scopic approaches to the skull base: a systematic literature review and anatomical description. Neurosurg Rev. 2021;44(5):2857–78. https://doi.org/10.1007/s10143-020-01470-5.
12. Castelnuovo P, Turri-Zanoni M, Battaglia P, Locatelli D, Dallan I. Endoscopic endonasal management of orbital pathologies. Neurosurg Clin N Am. 2015;26(3):463–72. https://doi.org/10.1016/j.nec.2015.03.001.
13. Di Somma A, Kong DS, de Notaris M, Moe KS, Sanchez Espana JC, Schwartz TH, et al. Endoscopic transorbital surgery levels of difficulty. J Neurosurg. 2022;137:1187. https://doi.org/10.3171/2022.3.JNS212699.
14. Di Somma A, Guizzardi G, Valls Cusine C, Hoyos J, Ferres A, Topczewski TE, et al. Combined endoscopic endonasal and transorbital approach to skull base tumors: a systematic literature review. J Neurosurg Sci. 2021;66:406. https://doi.org/10.23736/S0390-5616.21.05401-1.
15. Schwartz TH, Henderson F Jr, Di Somma A, Kong DS, de Notaris M, Ensenat J, et al. Endoscopic transorbital surgery: another leap of faith? World Neurosurg. 2022;159:54–5. https://doi.org/10.1016/j.wneu.2021.12.081.
16. Yoo J, Park HH, Yun IS, Hong CK. Clinical applications of the endoscopic transorbital approach for various lesions. Acta Neurochir. 2021;163(8):2269–77. https://doi.org/10.1007/s00701-020-04694-y.
17. Rhoton AL Jr, Natori Y. The orbit and sellar region: microsurgical anatomy and operative approaches. New York: Thieme Medical; 1996.
18. Paluzzi A, Gardner PA, Fernandez-Miranda JC, Tormenti MJ, Stefko ST, Snyderman CH, et al. "Round-the-clock" surgical access to the orbit. J Neurol Surg B Skull Base. 2015;76(1):12–24. https://doi.org/10.1055/s-0033-1360580.
19. Abussuud Z, Ahmed S, Paluzzi A. Surgical approaches to the orbit: a neurosurgical perspective. J Neurol Surg B Skull Base. 2020;81(4):385–408. https://doi.org/10.1055/s-0040-1713941.

Optic Canal, Optic Strut, and Optic Nerve

Paolo Palmisciano, Yara AlFawares, Norberto Andaluz, Jeffrey T. Keller, and Mario Zuccarello

2.1 Introduction

Detailed knowledge and understanding of the surgical anatomy of the optic canal, optic nerve, and optic strut is of particular importance in skull base surgery. The proximity of these structures with critical neurovascular structures (i.e., the internal carotid artery and cavernous sinus) requires the surgeon to mentally visualize these relationships as one plan which approach will be applied [1]. This is particularly true in the current surgical era, which is characterized by the continuous development of open and endoscopic approaches to select different regions of the optic canal [2].

This chapter describes the detailed surgical anatomy of the optic canal, optic strut, and optic nerve to further improve understanding and visualization of their relationship with adjacent critical structures. Ultimately, the purpose is to assist skull base surgeons in planning optimal approaches tailored to each different lesion involving this region. In addition, embryological development and common anatomical variants are summarized with their important surgical implications.

2.2 Embryological Development

Lang [3] identified 10 ossification sites in the sphenoid bone and stated that the complexity of the ossification process contributes to normal anatomical variants. The embryological development of the optic canal starts at the third gestation month and can be divided into three stages: (1) cartilaginous formation of the optic foramen, (2) ossification of the cartilaginous optic foramen, and (3) formation of the optic canal. The cartilaginous optic foramen is formed from the cartilaginous lesser wing of the sphenoid, with progressive chondrification from posterolateral to superomedial [4]. The ossification of the cartilaginous optic foramen occurs around the 12th–17th gestational week from the sphenoid's lesser wing and presphenoid ossification centers, which outline the superolateral and medial margins [5]. The bony optic foramen takes a "keyhole" appearance with the inferolateral border formed by bony bridge joining the center of the lesser sphenoid wing to the postsphenoid center, delineating the anteroinferior segment of the optic strut. The transformation of the bony optic foramen into the bony optic canal begins at the fifth gestation month, with the intracranial ophthalmic

P. Palmisciano · N. Andaluz · J. T. Keller
M. Zuccarello (✉)
Department of Neurosurgery, University of Cincinnati College of Medicine, Cincinnati, OH, USA
e-mail: zuccarm@ucmail.uc.edu

Y. AlFawares
University of Cincinnati College of Medicine, Cincinnati, OH, USA

G. Bonavolontà et al. (eds.), *Cranio-Orbital Mass Lesions*,
https://doi.org/10.1007/978-3-031-35771-8_2

artery initially located more inferiorly [5]. The posterosuperior segment of the optic strut develops as single bony ridge from the center of the lesser sphenoid wing to the presphenoid center or as two bony ridges originating separately from the two centers and growing toward one another. This optic strut segment transforms the optic foramen into the bony optic canal with the cranial opening of horizontal-oval shape and the orbital opening of vertical-oval shape [6]. The intracranial ophthalmic artery relocates occupying a more superior position. The two segments of the optic strut are initially separated by a nonfunctional foramen, which obliterates during the last two fetal months leading to the physiological fusion of the two segments and the formation of a single optic strut. Regarding the optic nerve, it appears around the fourth to seventh gestational week from the retinal nerve fibers of the optic stalk, which is the embryological structure connecting the optic cup to the brain [7].

2.3 Surgical Technique

Several skull base pathologies, including traumatic, neoplastic, and vascular, often involve the optic canal, optic strut, and optic nerve, requiring surgeons to gain a keen understanding of such complex spaces to avoid potentially devastating complications. The identification of definite anatomical landmarks is essential for guiding the surgery. Also, anatomical variants need to be considered and investigated during pre-operative imaging planning, to familiarize with the individual anatomy of each patient during surgery. A wide range of intracranial and endoscopic surgical windows have been investigated to safely expose the optic nerve, ophthalmic artery, and internal carotid artery [2]. The selection of an optimal approach should be modified on a case-by-case basis, governed by the extension of the pathology, the surgical goal, and the surgeon's preference, including the expected risks of complications.

The orbital apex defines the region that connects the orbit with the intracranial space, housing the optic canal, the optic strut, and the

superior and inferior orbital fissures. Most commonly, the optic canal constitutes a single bony opening in the sphenoid bone containing the optic nerve, ophthalmic artery, and postganglionic sympathetic nerves. In rare cases, the optic canal cranial opening may be duplicated, with the lower canal containing the ophthalmic artery and the upper canal containing the optic nerve [8]. Moving from posterior (intracranial) to anterior (intraorbital), Slavin et al. [9] divided the optic canal into three functional portions. The first, horizontal-oval portion opens into the middle cranial fossa, bounded superiorly by the falciform ligament and laterally by the anterior clinoid process. The cavernous sinus lies inferiorly with the cavernous (C4) segment of the internal carotid artery and cranial nerves IV, V1, V2, and VI, and the clinoid (C5) carotid segment turns superolaterally into the ophthalmic (C6) carotid segment that gives origin to the ophthalmic artery, which enters the optic canal below the optic nerve [10]. Similarly, in cases where the ophthalmic artery originates from the A1 segment of anterior cerebral artery, it also enters the optic canal below the optic nerve [11]. The ophthalmic artery may also originate from the middle meningeal artery [12] and then enter the orbit through the superior orbital fissure [13] or by penetrating the optic strut [14]. The second, round portion of the optic canal includes the canal itself, walled by two roots of the lesser wing of the sphenoid, from supero-medial-posterior to infero-lateral-anterior, at a 30° angle. Absence of the medial wall of the optic canal leads to a direct connection between the ethmoid sinus and the optic nerve, favoring the extension of infective agents [15]. The third, vertical-oval portion of the optic canal, known as optic foramen, involves the intraorbital opening, which can be identified immediately posterior to the optic tubercle creating a transorbital view. The optic canal is covered internally by two fused dural layers that continue from the intracranial dural lining and contain the optic nerve and ophthalmic artery [16]. While the dural covering of the optic canal's floor continues to the anterior margin of the distal dural ring, the dural lining of the optic canal's roof forms the falciform ligament from the base of the anterior clinoid process to the dura of the planum sphenoidale, and the dural layer of the optic canal's medial wall fuses with the diaphragm sellae.

The optic strut defines the bony bridge of the lesser wing of the sphenoid located between the anterior clinoid process and the body of the sphenoid, forming the inferolateral wall of the optic canal, and separating it from the superior orbital fissure [17]. The optic strut has a triangular-shaped or wing-shaped appearance, delineating the anterior limit of the clinoid (C5) segment of the internal carotid artery [18] and the dorsal extent of the distal dural ring [19]. The base of the optic strut may be identified via the transsphenoidal endonasal endoscopic view as the "lateral optic-carotid recess," which is a bony depression located between the optic nerve and internal carotid protuberances on the lateral wall of the sphenoid sinus [2]. Kerr et al. [20] identified four anatomical variants of the optic strut position in relation to the prechiasmatic sulcus: (1) sulcal or adjacent to the prechiasmatic sulcus; (2) postsulcal, when located posteriorly to the prechiasmatic sulcus; (3) asymmetric; and (4) presulcal, when located anteriorly to the prechiasmatic sulcus. The optic strut may be duplicated when the posterosuperior segment develops above the ophthalmic artery, forming two separate optic strut cranial openings with the optic nerve coursing through superior opening [5]. The optic strut may also assume a "keyhole" radiological appearance when its posterosuperior segment is absent or present only in a rudimentary form. In rare cases, the optic strut may be totally absent, with the optic canal and superior orbital fissure forming a single cranial opening [21].

The optic nerve is contained within the optic canal and borders inferiorly the optic strut, coursing from the optic chiasm to the eye bulb. Engin et al. [8] divided the optic nerve into four segments from posterior to anterior: (1) intracranial, (2) intracanalicular, (3) intraorbital, and (4) intraocular. The intracranial optic nerve segment lies inferior to the gyrus rectus and olfactory tract, coursing through the subarachnoid space intersecting the anterior cerebral artery and anterior communicating artery complex in the cistern of the lamina terminalis. While the anterior clinoid process is located laterally, proximal to the two dural rings that mark the transition from the cavernous (C4) carotid segment to the clinoidal (C5) segment, the tuberculum sellae and the middle clinoid process are located medially. The optic nerve enters the optic canal below the falciform ligament, forming the intracanalicular optic nerve segment that courses in an anterolateral direction, superomedially to the optic strut. The inferior surface of the intracanalicular ON segment forms a protuberance on the upper part of the sphenoid sinus, located anterolaterally to the sellar floor [10]. After endoscopic endonasal sphenoidotomy, the ON protuberance can be easily identified superiorly to ipsilateral carotid protuberance, which is located laterally to the sellar floor and corresponds to the cavernous (C4) internal carotid segment [10]. The lateral optic-carotid recess is sited between these two bony protuberances and can be used to detect the intracranial optic canal opening superomedially, the clinoid internal carotid segment inferomedially, the superior orbital fissure inferolaterally, and the orbital apex laterally [2]. From an endoscopic view, the intracanalicular optic nerve segment may be also identified using a vertical line touching the medial border of the anterior ascending cavernous (C4) internal carotid artery segment [22]. After entering the muscle cone within the orbital apex, the intraorbital optic nerve segment extends in the globe with a S-shape to allow the mobility of the globe within the orbit [15]. Both the intracanalicular and intraorbital segments are surrounded by the optic nerve sheath.

2.4 Operative Nuances

Surgical exposure of the optic canal is required to resect tumors extending into the optic canal from the orbital or intracranial compartments and to relieve compression of the edematous optic nerve in case of craniofacial trauma or pseudotumor cerebri [23]. Historically, ophthalmologists approached orbital apex lesions from a lateral orbitotomy corridor, which was introduced by Krönlein in 1889 [24]. In 1922, Dandy was the first to use the transcranial approach to operate on a patient with bilateral optic canal meningiomas, concluding to have obtained better optic canal exposure compared to the traditional lateral access [25]. From that point in time, multiple surgical windows, first open and then endoscopic, have been investigated to access the optic canal region [2]. Open surgical corridors, including the pterional, frontotemporal-orbital, supraorbital, and subfrontal, offer maximal exposure of the superior and lateral surfaces of the intracanalicular optic nerve segment. Transcranial routes to approach the optic canal can be extradural or intradural, with the use of either route depending on the surgeon's preference and expertise [26]. Based on our experience, we prefer to access the optic canal extradurally by removing the anterior clinoid process, sectioning the falciform ligament, and unroofing the optic canal with optic strut removal to increase the decompression of the optic nerve. Such step, coupled with the distal dural ring excision particularly in cases of aneurysms, allow for the mobilization of the optic nerve and internal carotid artery creating an additional corridor in the optic-carotid space. This favors proximal control of the internal carotid artery, avoiding excessive traction of the optic nerve responsible for irreversible injury and offering safe dissection of the tumor from the optic nerve [27]. All these maneuvers reduce the risk of injuring the optic nerve. However, in cases of meningiomas, the surrounding dura should not be resected since its coagulation may compromise the optic nerve's blood flow and impairing visual function by causing optic neuropathy [27]. An anterior clinoidectomy may also be performed with an intradural technique, but it may increase the risks of injuring the surrounding vasculature. We have recently used the ultrasonic bone curette (SONOPET®, Stryker, Kalamazoo, MI, USA) to reduce the risks of optic nerve and vascular injury, which may occur during bone drilling [28]. Any potential risk of thermal injury to the optic nerve associated with the use of ultrasonic bone curettes may be avoided by operating the SONOPET® at low power settings. In some cases, the anterior clinoid process may be pneumatized, or it can be fused with the middle cli-

noid process, forming the "caroticoclinoid foramen", or with the posterior clinoid process, forming the "interclinoid bridge" [8, 29, 30]. These anatomical variations should be carefully evaluated at pre-operative CT scans, and, if present, an intradural clinoidectomy is recommended to avoid any injury to the internal carotid or ophthalmic artery. The main limitation of open transcranial approaches consists in the difficulty to safely expose the inferior and medial surfaces of the optic nerve without risking injury of the internal carotid artery and/or the cavernous sinus. Some authors suggest the use of contralateral transcranial approaches to access the optic canal and treat medially projecting aneurysms of the ophthalmic (C6) internal carotid artery segment [31].

The endoscopic transsphenoidal route provides an optimal surgical corridor for accessing lesions originating from the sphenoid wing, cavernous sinus, or tuberculum sellae and displacing the optic nerve superiorly and laterally [2]. Using the lateral optic-carotid recess as a landmark to identify the optic nerve, internal carotid artery, and ophthalmic artery, the bone overlying the tuberculum and planum sellae can be removed to access the optic chiasms and the inferomedial quadrant of the intracanalicular optic nerve segment. Navigation and micro-doppler may assist in identifying the internal carotid artery, especially in cases with tortuous "kissing ICA" where the ophthalmic internal carotid artery segment needs to be mobilized laterally or inferiorly to expose the inferior quadrant of the intracranial optic nerve segment. Bone removal may also be extended laterally to the tuberculum sellae (i.e., trans-medial optic-carotid recess) to access the distal intracranial optic nerve segment and the superomedial surface of the clinoid (C5) and ophthalmic (C6) carotid segments [2]. Abhinav et al. [32] reported the feasibility to decompress up to 270° of the optic canal using the endonasal endoscopic approach, but this technique requires extensive intracranial extension with delicate manipulation of the optic nerve and leads to high risks of causing cerebrospinal fluid leakage. Although the endonasal endoscopic corridor requires no brain retraction, the main limitation is the inability to expose the superior surface of the intracanalicular optic nerve segment and transection of the falciform ligament to free the optic nerve without opening the subarachnoid space and causing cerebrospinal fluid leakage. In addition, pneumatization of the sphenoid sinus plays a big role in determining the surgical access through the transsphenoidal route, expecting unfavorable outcomes in patients with poorly pneumatized sinuses, which require prolonged drilling and thermal injury to the optic nerve [33].

Although several studies have demonstrated that the transcranial approaches provide greater circumferential decompression and exposure of the optic nerve with minimal risk of cerebrospinal fluid leakage, the selection of the best surgical approach should be tailored on each patient's anatomy, pathology, and clinical scenario [2, 22]. The pterional approach may be preferred to achieve a wide optic canal decompression or to access the superior and lateral surfaces of the intracranial optic nerve segment. The frontotemporal-orbital approach is indicated in treating lesions that extend into the lateral orbit. The subfrontal approach offers better inferomedial exposure of the distal intracranial optic nerve segment. The endoscopic endonasal transsphenoidal route provides the best access to the inferior and medial quadrants of the intracanalicular optic nerve, allowing expanded exposure of the intraorbital and intracranial segments using the transplanum trans-tuberculum, trans-medial optic-carotid recess, and transcanalicular approaches. The transcranial and endoscopic corridors should be considered as complementary options for accessing the optic canal, optic strut, and optic nerve regions, and not as mutually exclusive.

2.5 Conclusions

Knowledge of the surgical anatomy of the optic canal, optic strut, and optic nerve is necessary for skull base surgeons involved in the treatment of traumatic, oncological, and vascular pathologies to minimize the surgical morbidity and achieve optimal outcomes. Although some anatomical variants and abnormalities may be detected in several cases, the overall persistency of definite anatomical landmarks allows effective surgical planning. Open transcranial and endoscopic endonasal surgical approaches should be tailored on a case-by-case basis with relation to the individual patient's anatomy, pathology, and clinical scenario.

References

1. Demartini Z, Zanine SC. Microanatomic study of the optic canal. World Neurosurg. 2021;155:e792–6. https://doi.org/10.1016/j.wneu.2021.08.144.
2. Caporlingua A, Prior A, Cavagnaro MJ, et al. The intracranial and intracanalicular optic nerve as seen through different surgical windows: endoscopic versus transcranial. World Neurosurg. 2019;124:522–38. https://doi.org/10.1016/j.wneu.2019.01.122.
3. Lang J. Surgery of the cranial base tumors. In: Clinical anatomy of the head: neurocranium, orbit, craniocervical regions. Berlin: Springer-Verlag; 1983. p. 99–121.
4. Fawcett. Notes on the development of the human sphenoid. J Anat Physiol. 1910;44(Pt 3):207–22.
5. Kier EL. Embryology of the normal optic canal and its anomalies an anatomic and roentgenographic study. Investig Radiol. 1966;1(5):346–62. https://doi.org/10.1097/00004424-196609000-00023.
6. Duke-Elder S, Wybar KC. The anatomy of the visual system. In: System of ophthalmology, volume 2. London: H. Kimpton; 1958.
7. Lee AG, Morgan ML, Palau AEB, et al. Anatomy of the optic nerve and visual pathway. In: Nerves and nerve injuries. Amsterdam: Elsevier; 2015. p. 277–303. https://doi.org/10.1016/B978-0-12-410390-0.00020-2.
8. Engin Ö, Adriaensen GFJPM, Hoefnagels FWA, Saeed P. A systematic review of the surgical anatomy of the orbital apex. Surg Radiol Anat. 2021;43(2):169–78. https://doi.org/10.1007/s00276-020-02573-w.
9. Slavin KV, Dujovny M, Soeira G, Ausman JI. Optic canal: microanatomic study. Skull Base. 1994;4(3):136–44. https://doi.org/10.1055/s-2008-1058965.
10. Bouthillier A, van Loveren HR, Keller JT. Segments of the internal carotid artery: a new classification. Neurosurgery. 1996;38(3):425–33. https://doi.org/10.1097/00006123-199603000-00001.
11. Hassler W, Zentner J, Voigt K. Abnormal origin of the ophthalmic artery from the anterior cerebral artery: neuroradiological and intraoperative findings. Neuroradiology. 1989;31(1):85–7. https://doi.org/10.1007/BF00342037.
12. Hayreh SS, Dass R. The ophthalmic artery: I. Origin and intra-cranial and intra-canalicular course.

Br J Ophthalmol. 1962;46(2):65–98. https://doi.org/10.1136/bjo.46.2.65.

13. Regoli M, Bertelli E. The revised anatomy of the canals connecting the orbit with the cranial cavity. Orbit. 2017;36(2):110–7. https://doi.org/10.1080/01676830.2017.1279662.

14. Hokama M, Hongo K, Gibo H, Kyoshima K, Kobayashi S. Microsurgical anatomy of the ophthalmic artery and the distal dural ring for the juxta–dural ring aneurysms via the pterional approach. Neurol Res. 2001;23(4):331–5. https://doi.org/10.1179/016164101101198703.

15. Selhorst J, Chen Y. The optic nerve. Semin Neurol. 2009;29(1):29–35. https://doi.org/10.1055/s-0028-1124020.

16. Meyer F. Zur Anatomie der Orbitalarterien. Morphol Jahr. 1887;12:414–58.

17. Curragh DS, Valentine R, Selva D. Optic strut terminology. Ophthalmic Plast Reconstr Surg. 2019;35(4):407–8. https://doi.org/10.1097/IOP.0000000000001394.

18. Seoane E, Rhoton AL, de Oliveira E. Microsurgical anatomy of the dural collar (carotid collar) and rings around the clinoid segment of the internal carotid artery. Neurosurgery. 1998;42(4):869–84. https://doi.org/10.1097/00006123-199804000-00108.

19. Beretta F, Sepahi AN, Zuccarello M, Tomsick TA, Keller JT. Radiographic imaging of the distal dural ring for determining the intradural or extradural location of aneurysms. Skull Base. 2005;15(4):253–62. https://doi.org/10.1055/s-2005-918886.

20. Kerr R, Tobler W, Leach J, et al. Anatomic variation of the optic strut: classification schema, radiologic evaluation, and surgical relevance. J Neurol Surg B Skull Base. 2012;73(6):424–9. https://doi.org/10.1055/s-0032-1329626.

21. Le Double A. Traite Des Variations Des Os Du Crane de l'Homme, vol. 1. Paris: Vigot Freres; 1903.

22. Gogela SL, Zimmer LA, Keller JT, Andaluz N. Refining operative strategies for optic nerve decompression: a morphometric analysis of transcranial and endoscopic endonasal techniques using clinical parameters. Oper Neurosurg. 2018;14(3):295–302. https://doi.org/10.1093/ons/opx093.

23. Maurer J, Hinni M, Mann W, Pfeiffer N. Optic nerve decompression in trauma and tumor patients. Eur Arch Otorhinolaryngol. 1999;256(7):341–5. https://doi.org/10.1007/s004050050160.

24. Krönlein R. Pathologie and operativen Behandlung der Dermoidcysten der Orbita. Beitr z Klin Chir Tubing. 1889;4:149–63.

25. Dandy WE. Prechiasmal intracranial tumors of the optic nerves. Am J Ophthalmol. 1922;5(3):169–88. https://doi.org/10.1016/S0002-9394(22)90261-2.

26. Hassler W, Eggert HR. Extradural and intradural microsurgical approaches to lesions of the optic canal and the superior orbital fissure. Acta Neurochir. 1985;74(3–4):87–93. https://doi.org/10.1007/BF01418794.

27. Andaluz N, Beretta F, Bernucci C, Keller JT, Zuccarello M. Evidence for the improved exposure of the ophthalmic segment of the internal carotid artery after anterior clinoidectomy: morphometric analysis. Acta Neurochir. 2006;148(9):971–6. https://doi.org/10.1007/s00701-006-0862-x.

28. Spektor S, Dotan S, Mizrahi CJ. Safety of drilling for clinoidectomy and optic canal unroofing in anterior skull base surgery. Acta Neurochir. 2013;155(6):1017–24. https://doi.org/10.1007/s00701-013-1704-2.

29. Mikami T, Minamida Y, Koyanagi I, Baba T, Houkin K. Anatomical variations in pneumatization of the anterior clinoid process. J Neurosurg. 2007;106(1):170–4. https://doi.org/10.3171/jns.2007.106.1.170.

30. Kim JM, Romano A, Sanan A, van Loveren HR, Keller JT. Microsurgical anatomic features and nomenclature of the paraclinoid region. Neurosurgery. 2000;46(3):670–82. https://doi.org/10.1097/00006123-200003000-00029.

31. Andrade-Barazarte H, Kivelev J, Goehre F, et al. Contralateral approach to internal carotid artery ophthalmic segment aneurysms. Neurosurgery. 2015;77(1):104–12. https://doi.org/10.1227/NEU.0000000000000742.

32. Abhinav K, Acosta Y, Wang WH, et al. Endoscopic endonasal approach to the optic canal. Oper Neurosurg. 2015;11(3):431–46. https://doi.org/10.1227/NEU.0000000000000900.

33. Di Somma A, Cavallo LM, de Notaris M, et al. Endoscopic endonasal medial-to-lateral and transorbital lateral-to-medial optic nerve decompression: an anatomical study with surgical implications. J Neurosurg. 2017;127(1):199–208. https://doi.org/10.3171/2016.8.JNS16566.

Microsurgical Anatomy of the Superior and Inferior Orbital Fissures

3

Antonio Bernardo, Alexander I. Evins, and Sergio Corvino

3.1 Introduction

The orbit is a natural bony cavity communicating with extracranial and intracranial spaces through three openings: the superior orbital fissure (SOF), which connects the orbit with the middle cranial fossa; the inferior orbital fissure (IOF), which connects the orbit with the pterygopalatine, infra-temporal, and temporal fossae; and the optic canal (OC), which connects the orbit with the supratentorial intradural space (Fig. 3.1) [1]. A detailed knowledge of the microsurgical anatomy of these bony openings, their contents, and the anatomical relationships of the encased structures is necessary for safe surgery, whether to or through the orbit.

A. Bernardo (✉) · A. I. Evins
Weill Cornell Medicine, Neurological Surgery, New York, NY, USA
e-mail: nitc@med.cornell.edu

S. Corvino
Weill Cornell Medicine, Neurological Surgery, New York, NY, USA

Division of Neurosurgery, Department of Neurosciences, Reproductive and Odontostomatological Sciences, University of Naples "Federico II", Naples, Italy

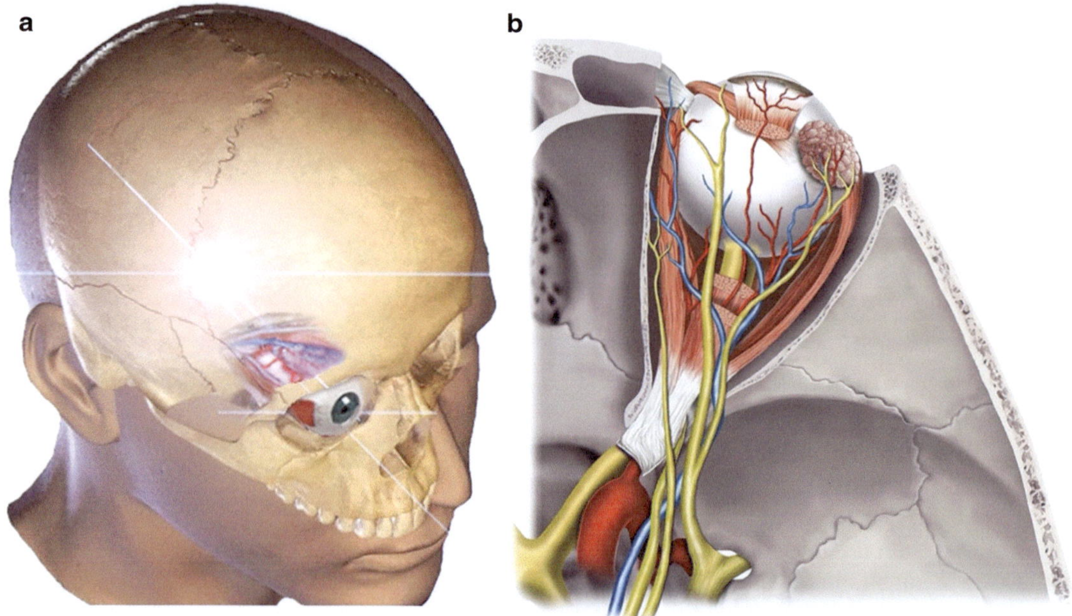

Fig. 3.1 Superolateral view of the right side of the skull. (**a**) The right orbit can be seen together with some of the intraorbital contents. (**b**) Superior view of the right orbit. The resection of the superior rectus muscle reveals the intraorbital intraconal structures. The extra-annular struc-tures (CN IV, frontal nerve, lacrimal nerve, and superior ophthalmic vein) are clearly seen running outside the annulus of Zinn. (Copyright 2023 Antonio Bernardo; published with permission)

3.2 Surgical Anatomy

3.2.1 Superior Orbital Fissure

The SOF is a narrow three-dimensional cleft located between the lesser and greater wings and the body of the sphenoid bone. It separates the lateral wall from the roof of the orbit and provides a direct and short communication between the contents of the orbital apex, anteriorly, and the cavernous sinus, posteriorly [2]. It has a triangular shape, oriented from posterior-to-anterior, medial-to-lateral, and inferior-to-superior direction, with a base, an apex, four margins (superior, lateral, medial, and inferior), and a roof. The base is located medially on the sphenoid body and the apex is located laterally between the greater and lesser sphenoid wings. The roof is represented by the intraorbital surface of the lesser sphenoid wing and the anterior clinoid process, while inferiorly the SOF blends into the inferior orbital fissure. The lateral border is formed by the greater sphenoid wing and has a course that is more horizontal in the superior half and more vertical in the inferior half. The medial margin is represented by the lateral aspect of the optic strut and the sphenoid body. The inferior border divides the SOF from the foramen rotundum and is represented by a bony bridge known as the maxillary strut.

At the SOF, the dura of the middle fossa and of the cavernous sinus joint the periorbita and the annular tendon (annulus of Zinn). A dural bridge, known as the meningo-orbital band (MOB) that tethers the fronto-temporal dura to the periorbita, is present at the lateral edge of the fissure [3–7]. The annular tendon gives rise to the extraocular muscles and is attached to the superior, medial, and inferior edges of the optic canal and to the lateral margin of the SOF. The SOF can be divided into three compartments: lateral, central, and inferior. The lateral sector hosts the neuro-vascular structures outside and superolaterally to the annulus and includes the trochlear, frontal, and lacrimal nerves and the superior ophthalmic vein (SOV). The lacrimal nerve is the most lateral nerve in the SOF, the frontal nerve is immediately medial to it, and the fourth cranial nerve is inferior and medial to the frontal nerve. The SOV lies inferomedially to the lacrimal nerve.

The central sector of the SOF, also referred to as the oculomotor foramen, hosts the structures crossing the annulus, namely the oculomotor, the nasociliary, and abducens nerves, and the sensory and sympathetic fibers of the ciliary ganglion and the inferior ophthalmic vein (IOV) (Fig. 3.2). Cranial nerve III, at the posterior margin of the SOF, splits into superior and inferior divisions which course into the central sector of the fissure.

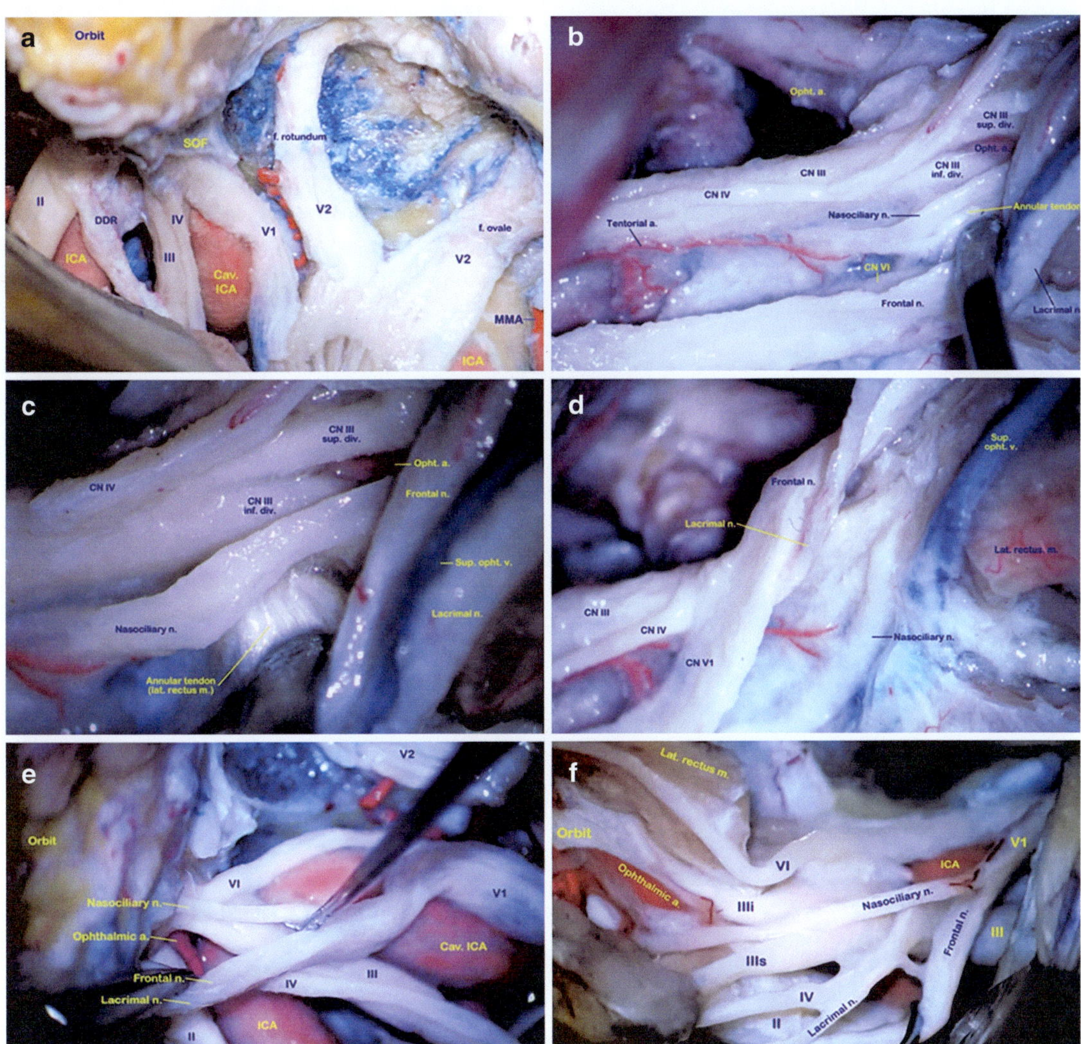

Fig. 3.2 Superior orbital fissure. (a) Unroofing and unlocking of the superior orbital fissure expands the working corridor to the orbit in transcranial approaches. (b–d) Loosening the extra-annular structures and opening the annulus of Zinn releases the dense anatomy of the orbital apex. (b, c) Lacrimal nerve, frontal nerve, trochlear nerve, and superior ophthalmic vein are clearly seen outside the annulus of Zinn. (d, e) Opening the annulus of Zinn via medial displacement of the extra-annular structures exposes the nasociliary and oculomotor nerves as they enter the orbit, (f) allowing for mobilization of both nerves and access to the medial superior orbital fissure and proximal contents of the orbit. a., artery; Cav., cavernous; CN, cranial nerve; DDR, distal dural ring; div., division; ICA, internal carotid artery; III, oculomotor nerve; IIIi, inferior division of the oculomotor nerve; IIIs, superior division of the oculomotor nerve; inf., inferior; lat., lateral; m., muscle; n., nerve; opht., ophthalmic; SOF, superior orbital fissure; Sup., superior; v, vein; V1, ophthalmic nerve; V2, maxillary nerve; V3, mandibular nerve. (Copyright 2023 Antonio Bernardo; published with permission)

The nasociliary nerve and the sympathetic fibers within the fissure run between the inferior division of the oculomotor nerve medially and the abducens nerve laterally. The IOV usually meets the SOV laterally to the annular tendon at the superior orbital fissure.

Finally, the inferior sector, which is below and outside the annulus, hosts orbital fat and orbital smooth muscle (Muller's muscle).

3.2.2 Inferior Orbital Fissure (IOF)

The IOF, also known as the sphenomaxillary fissure, is located in the orbital floor and separates it from the lateral wall (Fig. 3.3). It is oriented in an anterolateral direction from the maxillary strut to the zygomatic bone and has long anterior and posterior borders, represented by the intraorbital surface of the maxillary bone and the greater sphenoid wing, respectively, and short medial and lateral borders, represented by the sphenoid body and the zygomatic bone, respectively.

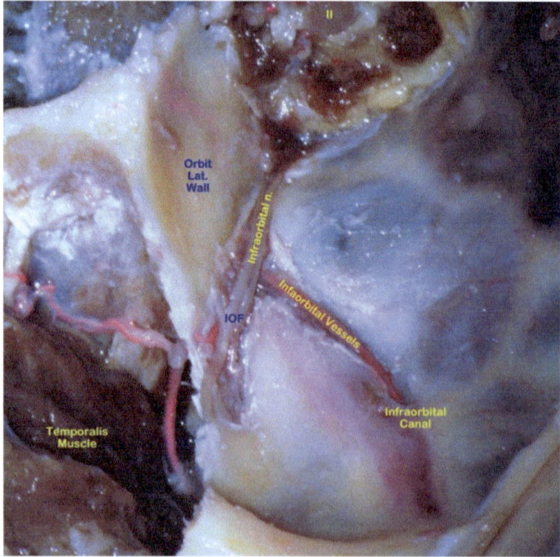

Fig. 3.3 Inferior orbital fissure. Anterosuperior view of the left orbit with the intraconal contents and the extraocular muscles removed. The lateral wall of the orbit has been drilled. The infraorbital nerve is seen traveling along the inferior orbital fissure and the infraorbital vessels are observed along the infraorbital groove, entering the infraorbital canal, en route to the infraorbital foramen. II, optic nerve; IOF, inferior orbital fissure; Lat., lateral. (Copyright 2023 Antonio Bernardo; published with permission)

It can be divided into three parts based on its communication with three different underlying areas [8, 9]: the anterolateral part communicates with the temporal fossa, the middle part with the infratemporal fossa and the posteromedial part with the pterygopalatine fossa. A bony ridge on the exocranial surface of the greater sphenoid wing, the infratemporal crest, separates the anterolateral and the middle parts of the IOF, and thus the temporal and the infratemporal fossae. The posteromedial portion of the inferior orbital fissure meets the medial part of the superior orbital fissure.

The Muller's muscle lies on the floor of the entire fissure, forming a bridge and separating the orbital content above from the pterygopalatine, infratemporal, and temporal fossae below.

The structures crossing the IOF include the zygomatic and infraorbital branches of the maxillary nerve, branches of the internal maxillary artery, and branches of the ophthalmic vein. The maxillary nerve enters the infraorbital groove with the infraorbital artery at the middle portion of the fissure to become the infraorbital nerve. The zygomatic nerve crosses the posterior margin of Muller's muscle in the middle portion of the fissure to run upward toward the lacrimal gland inside the periorbita. Anastomotic veins between the inferior ophthalmic vein and the pterygoid plexus cross the posteromedial part of the IOF.

3.3 Surgical Considerations

3.3.1 Superior Orbital Fissure

The SOF is a complex anatomical structure located at the junction of two complex surgical areas, the anterior cavernous sinus and orbital apex. Its intricate anatomy includes multiple neurovascular structures that change in the confined space as they pass from one compartment to another. The SOF can be directly affected by lesions or used as a surgical route to access the orbit from intracranial or intraorbital corridors and can be used to enhance surgical corridors to the parasellar region and cavernous sinus.

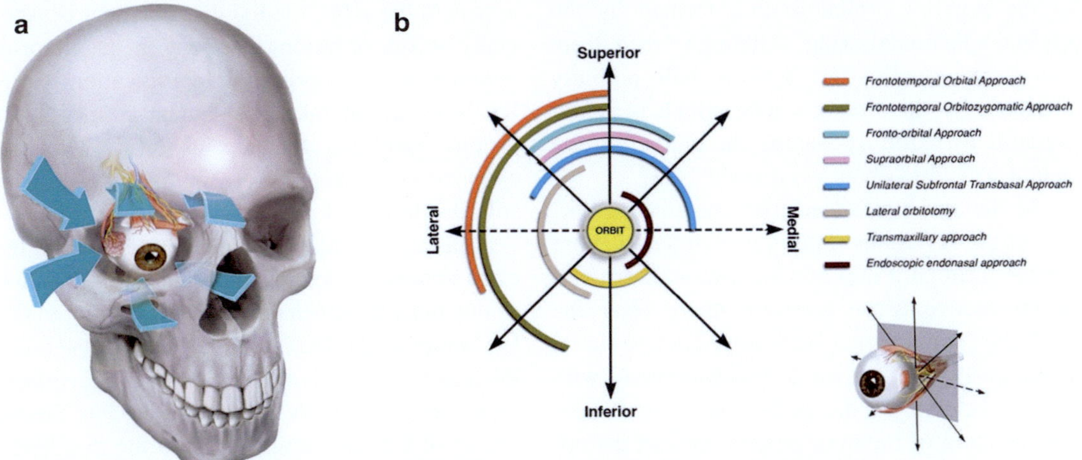

Fig. 3.4 Surgical corridors to the orbit. (**a**) Frontotemporal orbital approach, frontotemporal orbitozygomatic approach (superolateral arrow), fronto-orbital approach, supraorbital approach (superior arrow), unilateral subfrontal transbasal approach (superomedial arrow), transmaxillary approach (transmaxillary arrow), endoscopic endonasal approach (transnasal arrow), and a lateral orbitotomy (lateral arrow). (**b**) Orbital exposure by approach. The frontotemporal orbital and frontotemporal orbitozygomatic approaches expose the superolateral and superomedial quadrants. The frontotemporal orbitozygomatic approach extends that exposure to most of the inferolateral quadrant. The fronto-orbital and the supraorbital approaches expose portions of the superior quadrants. The unilateral subfrontal transbasal approach exposes the inferomedial and a portion of the superolateral quadrant. The lateral orbitotomy provides good access to most of both lateral quadrants. The transmaxillary approach allows for good exposure of portions of the inferior quadrants. The endoscopic endonasal approach provides access to most of both medial quadrants. (Copyright 2023 Antonio Bernardo; published with permission)

Many surgical approaches are available for accessing the orbit, sellar, and parasellar regions, including the pterional, fronto-orbitozygomatic, and subfrontal (Fig. 3.4). The structures of the SOF take on different spatial relationships depending on the surgical perspective of the various approaches. A simple pterional approach in combination with anterior clinoidectomy, unroofing of the optic nerve canal, and extensive removal of the lesser and greater sphenoid wings leads to excellent extradural visualization of the SOF's contents and related topography—anterior cavernous sinus and orbital apex. However, if circumstances dictate a different surgical perspective, thorough knowledge of the neural topography of the region is essential to enable safe and efficacious choices, such as the lateral orbitotomy, endoscopic endonasal approach, or endoscopic transorbital approach. Other approaches, such as the medial orbitotomy and anterior medial micro-orbitotomy, do not necessarily involve exposure of the SOF.

The pterional approach is one of the most widely used neurosurgical approaches, and the SOF serves as an important anatomical landmark whether the SOF is the target or encountered en route to the target.

The spatial relationships of the various components of the SOF and of the surrounding structures as they are encountered by the surgeon performing a pterional approach are of utmost importance, and appropriate sequential surgical steps need to be taken to expose the region fully via this approach. To adequately expose the SOF, the bony anterior clinoidal process, located between the superior orbital fissure laterally and the optic canal medially, needs to be removed. The optic strut, which connects the anterior clinoidal process with the lateral aspect of the body of the sphenoidal bone, needs to be carefully removed. In order to adequately expose the extrannular components of the SOF, the remainder of the lesser sphenoidal wing, the posterior orbital roof, is removed as well as the lateral wall of the superior orbital fissure, formed by the greater sphenoidal wing. Although freed from bony containment, the SOF is still partially obscured by the temporal lobe which is gently elevated by carefully peeling the dura from the neural structures about to cross the SOF.

As the dura is elevated from the anterior portion of the cavernous sinus, the cranial nerves are visible through a thin and semi-transparent veil of connective tissue covering them. Near the SOF, the cranial nerves are wrapped in a common meningeal sheath, which, as it is continuous with the periosteum of the orbit anteriorly, allows mobilization of the dura propria without disruption of the venous channels of the cavernous sinus. Once the SOF is fully exposed, the nerve structures that pass through it to enter the orbit become clearly visible. In order to widen the surgical corridors to the cavernous sinus and orbit, these structures must be identified, isolated, and unlocked. The most lateral nerve in the SOF, and therefore the first one encountered in the pterional approach, is the lacrimal nerve; the frontal nerve is immediately medial and the trochlear nerve is inferior and medial. The superior ophthalmic vein lies inferomedially to the lacrimal nerve.

When the goals of surgery include access to the cavernous sinus or orbit, it is extremely important to free the contents of the SOF [10]. The most lateral aspect of the SOF contains the extra-annular structures—CN IV, the frontal nerve, the lacrimal nerve, and the superior ophthalmic vein. Of these, CN IV is the most medial and the lacrimal nerve the most lateral, with the frontal nerve in the middle. The extra-annular structures can be displaced laterally, medially, or split depending on the target area of exposure. Split displacement of the extra-annular structures allows for the enlargement of the space between CN IV and CN V1 (Parkinson's/infratrochlear triangle)—the main access point to the body of the cavernous sinus. Medial and lateral displacement of the extra-annular structures, including mobilization of the lacrimal and frontal nerves, allows for the unlocking of CN IV and exposure of the annulus of Zinn, facilitating subsequent

access to the orbit. Medial displacement is especially useful for lesions involving the lateral orbit and/or lesions necessitating identification of CN VI, whereas lateral displacement is useful for lesions involving the medial orbit. Maximal exposure of the annulus of Zinn is achieved with split displacement.

Lateral, medial, or split displacement of the extra-annular structures is based on the location of the incision, which can be either medial to CN IV, lateral to the lacrimal nerve, or between CN IV and the frontal nerve. For lateral displacement, an incision is placed along the medial aspect of CN IV, continuing into the periorbita, just distal to the SOF. The extra-annular bundle, comprising CN IV, the frontal nerve, and the lacrimal nerve, is then displaced laterally, exposing the annulus of Zinn and its contents. For split displacement, an incision is placed between CN IV and the lacrimal nerve, continuing into the periorbita. CN IV is carefully displaced medially, and the frontal and lacrimal nerve bundle is displaced laterally. For medial displacement, an incision is made lateral to the frontal nerve, continuing into the periorbita, and the extra-annular bundle is displaced medially.

In order to expose the SOF and its contents, the temporal dura must be peeled off and elevated. Since CN III, IV, and V1 run in the inner dural layer of the lateral wall of the cavernous sinus, they can be safely exposed extradurally through the peeling of the temporal dura after cutting the meningo-orbital band. For this purpose, the MOB represents a valid landmark for the interperiosteal-dural dissection of the lateral wall of the cavernous sinus and the subsequent extradural clinoidectomy [3–6]. Cutting the MOB provides a well-defined cleavage plane between the endosteal and meningeal layers, which allows for the cranial nerves coursing in the inner layer of the lateral wall of the cavernous sinus and entering the SOF to be seen wrapped by a common meningeal sheath. Exposure of CN IV is riskier because it runs inside the sinus, covered by V1 and adjacent to the horizontal segment of the cavernous internal carotid artery, and thus requires violation of the venous space.

3.3.2 Inferior Orbital Fissure

The anterolateral third of the IOF has been used as a landmark for lateral and antero-lateral approaches to the orbit such as lateral orbitotomy and fronto-orbito-zygomatic approach [11]. The IOF can also be used as landmarks for endoscopic approaches to the anterolateral skull base.

The IOF in an important landmark in the lateral orbitotomy and both one- and two-piece orbitozygomatic osteotomies. In the one-piece orbitozygomatic approach, after detaching the posterior root of the zygoma, a cut is placed to connect McCarty's keyhole to the IOF. In the two-piece orbitozygomatic approach, the zygomatic bone is divided just above the level of the malar eminence after detaching the posterior aspect zygomatic arch. A cut is initiated on the inferior margin of the zygomatic bone proceeding superiorly until halfway across the bone, the globe is retracted medially, and the IOF is identified within the orbit and used as a landmark for placing a cut from the superior margin of the zygomatic bone to the IOF, connecting with the previous cut. After freeing the superior orbital rim and roof medially and posteriorly, the final cut proceeds across the lateral wall of the orbit until reaching the most lateral aspect of the inferior orbital fissure.

In the endoscopic transorbital approaches, the IOF serves as the inferior limit of intraorbital bone removal [12]. Following skeletonization of the orbital rim, subperiosteal dissection of the periorbita from the lateral wall of the orbit is performed until the superior and inferior orbital fissures are visualized and bone is drilled between the IOF and SOF depending on the surgical target [13, 14].

The IOF is also encountered or traversed in endoscopic transnasal approaches to the pterygopalatine fossa and transmaxillary approaches to the orbit or middle cranial fossa [15, 16]. In endoscopic endonasal approaches, the IOF provides access to the temporal fossa via its anterior third, to the infratemporal fossa via its middle third, and to the pterygopalatine fossa via its posteromedial third. Total maxillary antrostomy and ethmoidectomy expose the posterior aspect of the IOF, after removal of the posterior wall of maxillary antrum and ascending process of the palatine and provides access to the foramen rotundum and pterygopalatine fossa. Access to the middle third and partial access to the anterior third of the IOF can be achieved following a modified medial maxillectomy and removal of the posterior two-thirds of the inferior turbinate. This approach affords additional access to the pterygomaxillary fissure and infratemporal fossa. Exposure of the anteromedial aspect of the IOF can be improved by adding an anterior transmaxillary corridor through a sublabial incision. Proper combination of these transnasal and transmaxillary endoscopic approaches can ensure sufficient exposure of the anterior skull base regions through the IOF.

3.4 Conclusion

Comprehensive knowledge of the surgical anatomy and thorough familiarity with complex surgical techniques used in various approaches allows for a broader surgical armamentarium. Each approach must be tailored to provide the best access to a particular intraorbital or intracranial region and afford optimal control of the neurovasculature, whether the orbit is the main surgical target or is used as a corridor to intracranial lesions.

References

1. Rhoton AL. The orbit. Neurosurgery. 2002;51(4 Suppl):S303–34.
2. Ammirati M, Bernardo A. Anatomical study of the superior orbital fissure as seen during a pterional approach. J Neurosurg. 2007;106(1):151–6. https://doi.org/10.3171/jns.2007.106.1.151.
3. Fukuda H, Evins AI, Burrell JC, Iwasaki K, Stieg PE, Bernardo A. The meningo-orbital band: microsurgical anatomy and surgical detachment of the membranous structures through a frontotemporal craniotomy with removal of the anterior clinoid process. J Neurol Surg B Skull Base. 2014;75(2):125–32. https://doi.org/10.1055/s-0033-1359302.
4. Froelich SC, Aziz KM, Levine NB, Theodosopoulos PV, van Loveren HR, Keller JT. Refinement of the extradural anterior clinoidectomy: surgi-

cal anatomy of the orbitotemporal periosteal fold. Neurosurgery. 2007;61(5 Suppl 2):179–85. https://doi.org/10.1227/01.neu.0000303215.76477.cd; discussion 85–6.

5. Coscarella E, Başkaya MK, Morcos JJ. An alternative extradural exposure to the anterior clinoid process: the superior orbital fissure as a surgical corridor. Neurosurgery. 2003;53(1):162–6; discussion 6–7. https://doi.org/10.1227/01.neu.0000068866.22176.07.

6. Saenz A, Villalonga JF, Solari D, Baldoncini M, Mantese B, Lopez-Elizalde R, et al. Meningo-orbital band detachment: a key step for the extradural exposure of the cavernous sinus and anterior clinoid process. J Clin Neurosci. 2020;81:367–77. https://doi.org/10.1016/j.jocn.2020.09.055.

7. Bernardo A, Evins AI, Mattogno PP, Quiroga M, Zacharia BE. The orbit as seen through different surgical windows: extensive anatomosurgical study. World Neurosurg. 2017;106:1030–46. https://doi.org/10.1016/j.wneu.2017.06.158.

8. Shimizu S, Tanriover N, Rhoton AL, Yoshioka N, Fujii K. MacCarty keyhole and inferior orbital fissure in orbitozygomatic craniotomy. Neurosurgery. 2005;57(1 Suppl):152–9; discussion 9. https://doi.org/10.1227/01.neu.0000163600.31460.d8.

9. Aziz KM, Froelich SC, Cohen PL, Sanan A, Keller JT, van Loveren HR. The one-piece orbitozygomatic approach: the MacCarty burr hole and the inferior orbital fissure as keys to technique and application. Acta Neurochir. 2002;144(1):15–24. https://doi.org/10.1007/s701-002-8270-1.

10. Bernardo A, Evins AI. Anterolateral routes to the skull base-the frontotemporal approaches and exposure of the sellar and parasellar regions. World Neurosurg. 2023;172:131–45. https://doi.org/10.1016/j.wneu.2022.11.055.

11. De Battista JC, Zimmer LA, Theodosopoulos PV, Froelich SC, Keller JT. Anatomy of the inferior orbital fissure: implications for endoscopic cranial base surgery. J Neurol Surg B Skull Base. 2012;73(2):132–8. https://doi.org/10.1055/s-0032-1301398.

12. Chen HI, Bohman LE, Emery L, et al. Lateral transorbital endoscopic access to the hippocampus, amygdala, and entorhinal cortex: initial clinical experience. ORL. 2015;77(6):321–32. https://doi.org/10.1159/000438762.

13. Locatelli D, Restelli F, Alfiero T, et al. The role of the transorbital superior eyelid approach in the management of selected spheno-orbital meningiomas: in-depth analysis of indications, technique, and outcomes from the study of a cohort of 35 patients. J Neurol Surg B Skull Base. 2022;83(2):145–58. https://doi.org/10.1055/s-0040-1718914.

14. Di Somma A, Andaluz N, Cavallo LM, de Notaris M, Dallan I, Solari D, Zimmer LA, Keller JT, Zuccarello M, Prats-Galino A, Cappabianca P. Endoscopic transorbital superior eyelid approach: anatomical study from a neurosurgical perspective. J Neurosurg. 2018;129(5):1203–16. https://doi.org/10.3171/2017.4.JNS162749. PMID: 29243982.

15. DelGaudio JM. Endoscopic transnasal approach to the pterygopalatine fossa. Arch Otolaryngol Head Neck Surg. 2003;129(4):441. https://doi.org/10.1001/archotol.129.4.441.

16. Zhang X, Tabani H, El-Sayed I, Russell M, Feng X, Benet A. The endoscopic endonasal transmaxillary approach to meckel's cave through the inferior orbital fissure. Oper Surg. 2017;13(3):367–73. https://doi.org/10.1093/ons/opx009.

Part II

General Clinics and Imaging of Cranio-Orbital Mass Lesions

Clinical and Opthalmological Evaluation

4

Lucia Ambrosio, Gaetano Fioretto, and Ciro Costagliola

4.1 Introduction

The clinical evaluation of patients with suspected or diagnosed orbital or cranio-orbital mass lesions is based on several important steps; these include the careful anamnesis and clinical history, the inspection of the eye and adnexa to evidence proptosis, eyelid and eye surface abnormalities, the functional evaluation of the visual acuity, visual field, ocular motility, and eye fundus. The optical coherence tomography (OCT) and ophthalmic ultrasonography are important complementary studies to the diagnosis. All these diagnostic steps are discussed in this chapter.

4.2 History

4.2.1 Family and Patient History

The remote anamnesis should investigate possible congenital diseases potentially associated with orbital mass lesions, such as neurofibromatosis [1, 2], Von Hippel-Lindau disease [3], familial cavernous malformations [4, 5]. Previous surgical procedures for oncological diseases, such as breast or prostatic cancer, must suggest the possibility of an orbital metastasis [6, 7]. Previous nasal and maxillary surgery may presage a mucocele [8] or a carcinoma with secondary invasion of the orbit. Several patients with ophthalmological problems underwent a neurosurgical procedure for skull base tumors, mainly of the suprasellar and parasellar regions; in such cases, a late orbital involvement due to tumor progression or recurrence must be suspected [9, 10]. In patients with previous diagnosis of orbital pathology and previous orbital surgery, clinical presentation, surgical description and histological diagnosis must carefully be reviewed.

4.2.2 First Complaints and Symptoms

Most patients with cranio-orbital mass lesions seek ocular consultation for proptosis, eventually associated with pressure sensation and orbital pain. Decrease of vision and diplopia may occur later [9, 10].

The pressure sensation is probably due to increasing orbital pressure secondary to slow expanding tumors or cysts. It has also been observed in patients with decompensation of the

L. Ambrosio · C. Costagliola (✉)
Division of Ophthalmology, Department of
Neurosciences and Reproductive and
Odontostomatological Science, University Federico
II, Naples, Italy
e-mail: Ciro.costagliola@unina.it

G. Fioretto
Department of Neuroscience, University of Naples
Federico II, Naples, Italy

orbital apparatus after a long-standing inflammatory tumor [11].

Pain is a frequent symptom of orbital lesions. It may be continuous or episodic, sometimes nocturnal, and is often severe. The referred site of pain may be related to the location of the mass lesion. Pain located to the deep orbit may be referred to an orbital apex lesion, mainly if associated with ocular motility disturbance. If the pain is more intense in the infero-medial orbital compartment, it should suggest a malignant tumor of the ethmoid or maxillary sinus. If pain is referred to the lateral orbital compartment, a malignant neoplasm or an inflammatory process of the lacrimal gland may be present.

Headache is a less frequent symptom which may accompany inflammatory and vasculitic diseases, cranio-orbital meningiomas and secondary orbital invasion by malignant tumors. The head noise may be referred in patients with orbital vascular malformations or less frequently with intracranial vascular lesions contiguous to the orbit. It is more frequently of pulsating type and synchronous with the heartbeat.

4.2.3 Chronology of the Evolution Before Diagnosis

The length of the clinical history, the type of onset, and the rate of progression of the symptoms are very important for the diagnosis, although they are often difficult to define.

The period of onset is mostly referred for more relevant symptoms, such as visual impairment and diplopia; on the other hand, dating the onset of the proptosis is more difficult. In many cases, prior photographs may show that slight proptosis was already present many years before [11]. Lesions with a long interval time from the presentation are usually benign.

The onset of symptoms may be slow or acute. A slow clinical onset should suggest a benign mass lesion; an acute onset of symptoms is more typical for malignant and inflammatory mass lesions [12, 13]. However, this is not always true. A hemorrhage within an asymptomatic benign cranio-orbital cyst may cause acute symptoms;

otherwise, a malignant mass lesion may initially present with slow symptoms. Thus, the rate of symptom progression is more relevant.

An indolent course with isolated proptosis for several years suggests a cyst or a benign tumor [14]. In this context, sudden increase of the proptosis should suggest malignant degeneration. The rapid evolution of symptoms after the onset may be referred to as malignant tumor, but it is also more typical of an inflammatory lesion.

4.3 Inspection of the Eye and Adnexa

Inspection of the eye and adnexal structures should include the assessment of the proptosis, the state of the eyelids, and the surface of the eye.

4.3.1 Assessment of Proptosis

Proptosis, or forward protrusion of the eye globe, is an almost constant sign of orbital mass lesions [11, 15, 16]. It may be evidenced with a front view (Fig. 4.1), but the patient observation from above the eyebrow allows to better define the different globe position between the affected and the normal side.

The degree of globe displacement as compared to the contralateral is quantified in millimeters with the Hertel exophthalmometer, eventually with Krahn modification. The normal values derived with the Krahn device ranges from 14 to 21 mm in adults. Values <14 mm are considered

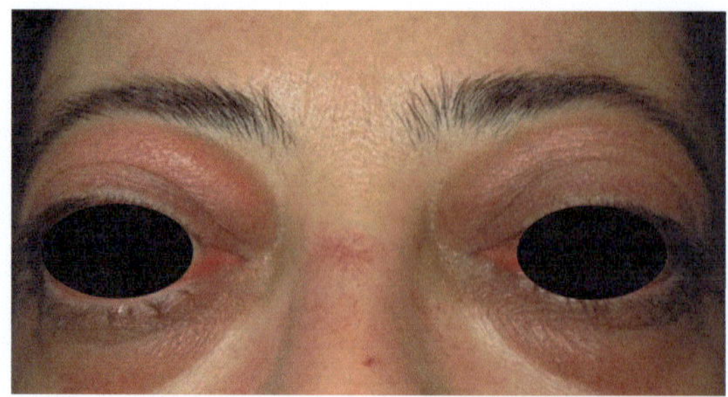

Fig. 4.1 Bilateral proptosis. (Image courtesy of Prof. Diego Strianese, Oculoplastic Unit University of Naples Federico II)

diagnostic for enophthalmos. Values >21 mm, although sometimes found in individuals as an ereditary tendency, may be diagnostic of proptosis, mainly when the difference between the two eyes is >2 mm.

Proptosis is associated with displacement of the eye in about of 80% of orbital mass lesions [11]. The type of displacement may be correlated with the tumor location. Superolateral and lacrimal gland mass lesions cause infero-medial displacement; medial and inferior lesions mainly cause eye displacement superiorly and laterally. Apical or intracranial lesions present with axial proptosis. The presence of eye displacement without proptosis is a rare event which may be observed for tumors arising from the eyelid and invading the orbit.

Although proptosis from orbital mass lesions is almost always unilateral, bilateral proptosis may be observed for several malignant lymphomas, metastatic carcinomas, or dural arteriovenous malformations; more often an unilateral orbital tumor may extend to the contralateral eye during its course.

Palpation of the proptotic eye may elicit tenderness, as for intraorbital mucoceles and cystic lesions. Pulsation synchrone with the arterial pulse is typical of the carotid-cavernous fistula. However, the pulsation may rarely be observed for some high vascular tumors and cavernous malformations.

4.3.2 Eyelids

Several eyelid abnormalities may be observed in patients with cranio-orbital mass lesions, including retraction, edema, rubor, ecchymosis.

The most accurate means to detect eyelid retraction is measurement of the distance between the margin of the upper eyelid and the superior orbital fold. When eyelid retraction occurs, the superior palpebral fold deepens, and the interval between palpebral fold and lid margin is shortened. Thus, the fold-lid margin ratio is a more reliable marker of eyelid retraction.

Orbit neoplasms with rapid growth may cause severe proptosis so that the eye is pushed out of a protective cover of the eyelid, thus mimicking an eyelid retraction. The true eyelid retraction with increased fold-lid margin ratio may occur for some slowly growing neoplasms.

Edema of the eyelid without erythema or other inflammatory signs may be associated with vascular and neurogenic tumors, probably secondary to long-standing venous stasis. Edema with inflammatory signs, such as hyperemia and/or tenderness is commonly associated with thyroid eye disease and orbital inflammatory syndromes, both infectious and non-infectious. Mild edema of the superior eyelid may occur for tumors located in the superior areas of the orbit. Edema of the nasal portion of the upper eyelid suggests a mucocele of the frontal sinus. Some degree of eyelid edema is also associated with orbital carcinomas. Finally, bilateral edema of all four eyelids is a frequent finding of orbital lymphomas.

Eyelid hyperemia and rubor may accompany fast-growing neoplasms and acute inflammatory mass lesions located in the anterior orbital areas, such as rhabdomyosarcoma and leukemia [12].

Ecchymosis of the eyelid may be associated with hematoma, metastatic neuroblastoma, but also to amyloidosis, plasmacytoma, and leukemia infiltrates.

4.3.3 Surface of the Eye

Several changes of the eye surface may be observed in patients with orbital mass lesions. Dilated, tortuous, reddish-purple vessels are diagnostic of vascular malformations or shunts. Episodes of subconjunctival hemorrhage may be a presenting sign of orbital mass lesions, mainly cavernous hemangiomas and lymphangiomas.

The epibulbar discoloration, defined salmon-hued lesion, is an objective sign typical of orbital lymphoma [13]. The painless and slowly growing mass of salmon color appears along the surface of the eye in a superior location. It results from forward extension of the orbital mass.

Epibulbar melanotic spots are signs of an intraocular melanoma or primary melanoma of the conjunctive.

4.3.4 External Mass

An external mass in the anterior orbit can sometimes be present. The mass must be evaluated for mobility, consistency (solid versus cystic), relationships with the orbital bones and underlying soft tissues. Mass lesions which may more frequently present with an external palpable mass include lacrimal gland tumors, dermoid cyst, and mucocele.

4.4 Functional Evaluation of the Eye

Determining the ocular function is a fundamental step in the diagnosis of patients with orbital mass lesions. In fact, the preservation of the visual function is the most important aim of surgery of orbital tumors.

The ocular function may be affected by an orbital mass in different ways: dislocation of the eye and optic nerve, anatomic contact between tumor and eye, infiltration of the nerves and muscles, damage to the blood supply to the eye.

4.4.1 Visual Acuity

The visual acuity should be measured at distance in Slenner or LogMAR notations. Near vision may also be measured but it does not replace the determination of distance acuity.

In many cases of orbital mass lesions, there is no correlation between visual acuity and entity of proptosis. Even gliomas arising from the optic nerve may remain asymptomatic or may present with proptosis and normal vision for a long time [17, 18].

4.4.2 Visual Field

The perimetry, or visual field analysis, is realized by quantitative static methods, such as Humphrey's 24-2 or 30-2, but may also be performed by other means, such as Goldman perimetry and Octopus perimetry.

The role of the perimetry is to record the degree of pretreatment visual loss, with the aim to decide the surgical resection. Besides, the preoperative visual field is important to define the functional outcome of the treatment [11].

4.4.3 Ocular Motility

The impairment of the ocular motility is an important clinical finding of patients with cranio-orbital mass lesions. It occurs with different mechanisms and often depends on the intraorbital location and size of the lesion itself. A mass lesion confined to one sector or quadrant of the orbit may cause diplopia only when the ocular rotation occurs into the area occupied by the mass. However, very large tumors may be associated with diplopia in all directions.

Apical mass lesions cause diplopia early in the eye movement, because of the early impairment of the oculomotor nerves at the superior orbital fissure.

Apical and medial orbital masses may sometimes cause transient diplopia and obfuscation of the vision during the forced eye excursion in the direction of the impaired extraocular muscles; this is due to transient compression to the vascular supply of the orbital portion of the optic nerve [11].

Besides the compression mechanism, diplopia from orbital mass lesions may be secondary to edema, inflammation, or infiltrations of the affected muscle. The muscle infiltration mainly occurs in orbital metastatic carcinomas and often evolves in muscular contracture and eye deviation.

Diplopia is usually the first symptom of schwannomas of the oculomotor nerves, in association with functional impairment of the involved nerve [19, 20]. However, nerve-related symptoms and signs may be absent [17].

4.4.4 Ophthalmoscopy

The ophthalmoscopic study is not highly relevant in the diagnosis of orbital mass lesions.

Indentations of the eye wall and choroidal folds are mainly observed in tumors of the anterior portion of the orbit.

Pallor of the optic disc and less frequently hyperemia, edema, or optic disc elevation are associated with optic nerve tumors (meningioma or glioma) or to retinoblastoma [11].

4.4.5　Intraocular Pressure

An increase in the intraocular pressure is associated with orbital vascular pathologies, including carotid-cavernous fistulas, arteriovenous malformations of the posterior orbit, dural vascular shunts. All these conditions cause rise of the orbital venous pressure. The increase of the intraocular pressure is resistant to medical therapy, but it is associated with scarce or no visual impairment.

4.4.6　Auscultation

In patient with suspected orbital mass lesions, the discovery of the bruit is suggestive of a vascular malformation of the orbit or contiguous intracranial compartment. This finding is evident in arteriovenous fistulas but not in the venous malformations, and thus it results from the arterial flow. Although the bruit is usually evidenced in the affected orbit, it may also be present at the frontal and temporal region.

4.4.7　Optical Coherence Tomography (OCT)

OCT is a helpful ancillary test [21–23]. It is typically performed for quantitative measurement of retinal nerve fiber layer (RNFL) thickness, retinal ganglion cell (RGC) layer thickness, and qualitative and quantitative assessment of macular health. In the presence of optic nerve damage, the RNFL and RGC layers are thinned; the quantitative measurement is a reliable indicator of stability or progression of damage over time. In the presence of orbital diseases, the RGC layer thickness is a more reliable indicator than RNFL thickness because the RNFL thickness may be increased by venous congestion (Fig. 4.2). Thus, increasing RNFL thickness over time may be considered an objective measurement of increasing venous congestion and/or a sign of optic nerve head inflammation, infiltration, or ischemia. The OCT is more sensitive in the assessment of change over time than ophthalmoscopy, serial fundus photography, or magnetic resonance (MR).

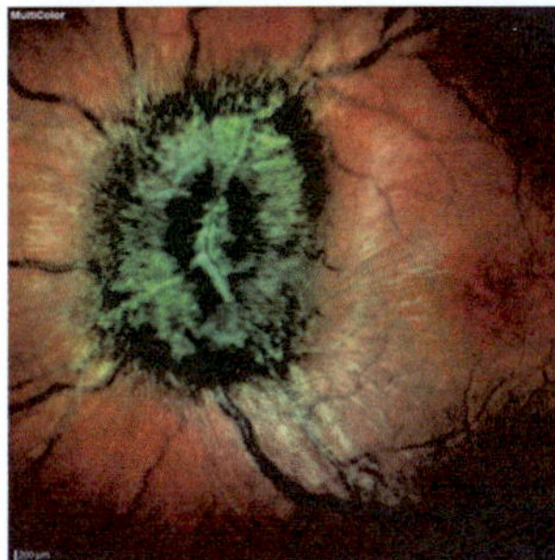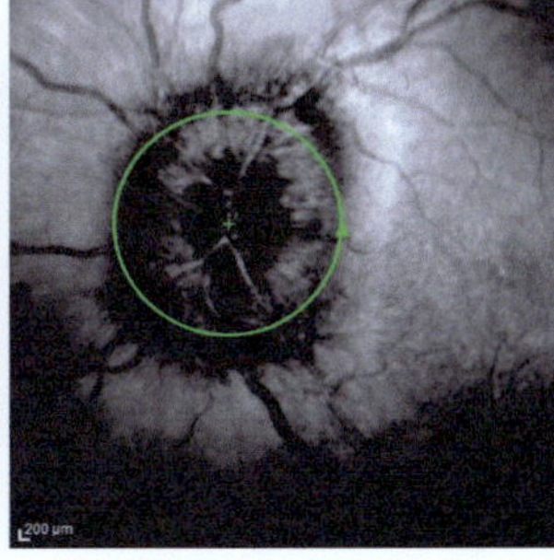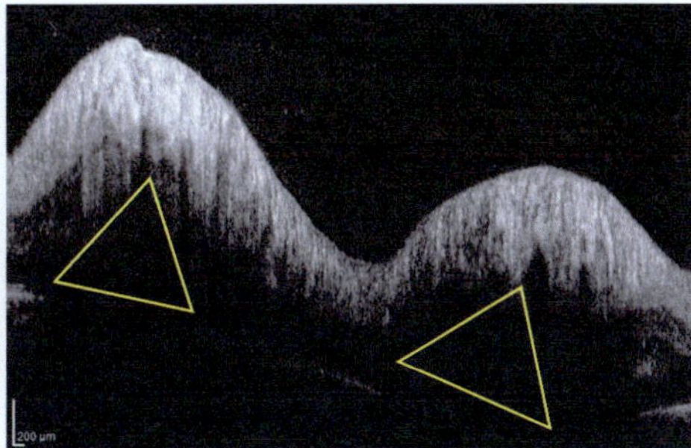

Fig. 4.2 Papilledema. The OCT scan of the optic nerve head shows the triangular subretinal hyporeflective space (in yellow) in papilledema. (Image courtesy of Dr. Gilda Cennamo, University of Naples Federico II)

4.5 Ophthalmic Ultrasonography

The ophthalmic ultrasonography, performed by a skilled echographer, is a very useful test [24]. It is more sensitive than computed tomography (CT) or MR in the assessment of intraocular, retinal, or subretinal diseases and is helpful to CT or MR in the characterization of orbital mass lesions (Figs. 4.3 and 4.4). If CT and MR have been used in the initial evaluation of an orbital abscess or mid- or anterior orbital inflammatory disease, such as posterior scleritis, serial B-mode ultrasound is adequate in monitoring the response to treatment, thus minimizing the need for several neuroradiological studies. If CT and MR have evidenced a mid or anterior orbital tumor or an infiltrative process, the echography is helpful in assessing the internal acoustic characteristics of the lesion.

Lymphoma, melanoma, and cysts have no or low internal reflectivity; other mass lesions have mid- (such as schwannoma) to high internal reflectivity (such as many carcinomas or cavern-

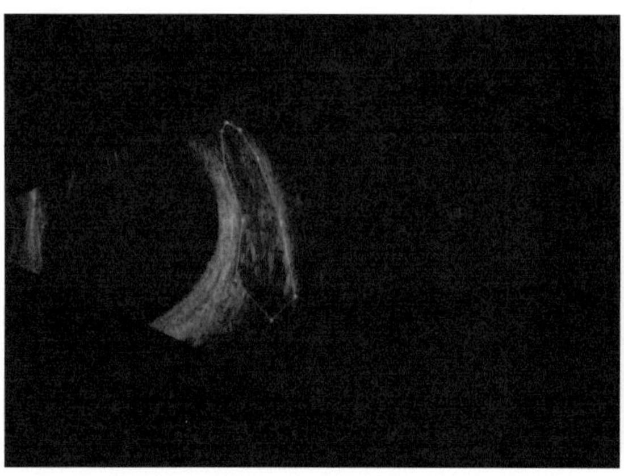

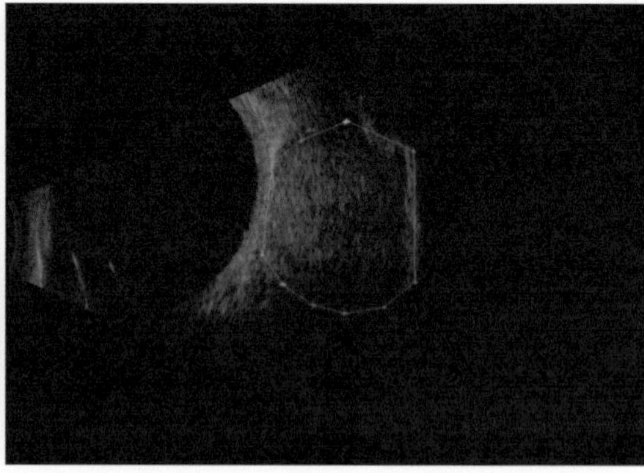

Fig. 4.3 The ultrasound b-scan picture is compatible with a lymphangioma-type pathology located in the superior-medial angle of the orbit. The lesion is bounded by green lines; and it shows a decreased volume after compression, this is a typical phenomenon of cystic tumors. (Image courtesy of Dr. Maria Angelica Breve, University of Naples Federico II)

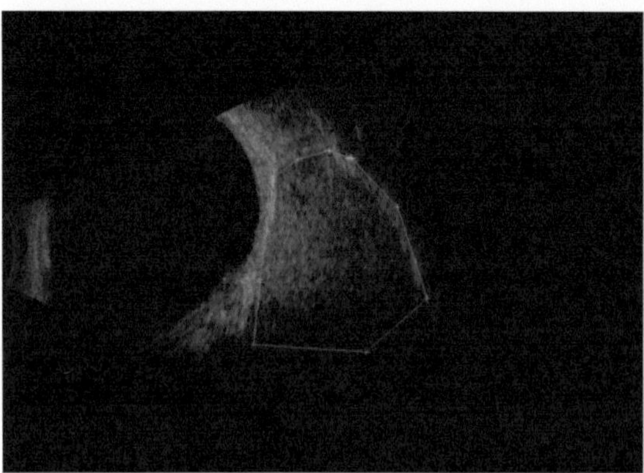
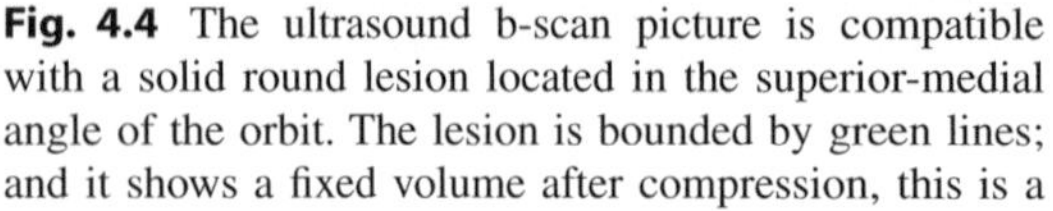

Fig. 4.4 The ultrasound b-scan picture is compatible with a solid round lesion located in the superior-medial angle of the orbit. The lesion is bounded by green lines; and it shows a fixed volume after compression, this is a typical phenomenon of solid tumors. (Image courtesy of Dr. Maria Angelica Breve, University of Naples Federico II)

ous hemangioma). Ultrasonography also allows real-time dynamic assessment of tumor adherence or infiltration to adjacent tissues [25–28].

The B-mode echography is also an useful tool for image-guided fine needle aspiration biopsy (FNAB) of orbital tumors. This scarcely invasive diagnostic technique is mostly performed for the identification of metastatic tumors, allowing definitive diagnosis without necessity of open biopsy. It also aids in the cytopathologic diagnosis of lacrimal gland mass inflammations, lymphoma, pleomorphic adenoma, or carcinoma.

Ultrasonography can be done quickly in the clinic at a low cost. It is the unique imaging technique able to reveal dynamic changes such as compressibility and internal reflectivity, as well as the cystic nature of lesions. Doppler imaging provides information regarding vascular flow characteristics within a lesion. This modality is typically applicable to anteriorly located mass lesions.

Thus, ultrasonography is an important complementary imaging technique to CT and MR for defining the orbital mass lesions.

References

1. Beres SJ, Avery RA. Optic pathway gliomas secondary to neurofibromatosis type 1. Semin Pediatr Neurol. 2017;24(2):92–9. https://doi.org/10.1016/j.spen.2017.04.006.
2. Rasool N, Odel JG, Kazim M. Optic pathway glioma of childhood. Curr Opin Ophthalmol. 2017;28(3):289–95. https://doi.org/10.1097/ICU.0000000000000370.
3. McGrath LA, Mudhar HS, Salvi SM. Hemangioblastoma of the optic nerve. Surv Ophthalmol. 2019;64(2):175–84. https://doi.org/10.1016/j.survophthal.2018.10.002.
4. Strianese D, Bonavolontà G, Iuliano A, Mariniello G, Elefante A, Liuzzi R. Risks and benefits of surgical excision of orbital cavernous venous malformations (so-called cavernous hemangioma): factors influencing the outcome. Ophthalmic Plast Reconstr Surg. 2021;37(3):248–54. https://doi.org/10.1097/IOP.0000000000001767.
5. Maiuri F, Mariniello G, Corvino S, et al. Cavernous malformations to be investigated for familiarity: the role of Ki67 MIB1. World Neurosurg. 2021;155:e75–82. https://doi.org/10.1016/j.wneu.2021.08.008.
6. Magliozzi P, Strianese D, Bonavolontà P, et al. Orbital metastases in Italy. Int J Ophthalmol. 2015;8(5):1018. https://doi.org/10.3980/J.ISSN.2222-3959.2015.05.30.
7. Allen R. Orbital metastases: when to suspect? When to biopsy? Middle East Afr J Ophthalmol. 2018;25(2):60. https://doi.org/10.4103/MEAJO.MEAJO_93_18.
8. Plantier D, Neto D, Pinna F, Voegels R. Mucocele: clinical characteristics and outcomes in 46 operated patients. Int Arch Otorhinolaryngol. 2019;23:88–91. https://doi.org/10.1055/s-0038-1668126.
9. Scarone P, Lecherq D, Hèron F, Robert G. Long-term results of exophthalmos in a surgical series of 30 spheno-orbital meningiomas. Clinical article. J Neurosurg. 2009;111:1069–77.
10. Mariniello G, de Divitiis O, Corvino S, et al. Recurrences of spheno-orbital meningiomas: risk factors and management. World Neurosurg. 2022;161:e514–22. https://doi.org/10.1016/j.wneu.2022.02.048.
11. Rootman J. Disease of the orbit. A multidisciplinary approach. 2th ed. Philadelphia: Lippincott Williams and Wilkins; 2002.
12. Garrity JA, Henderson JW. Henderson's orbital tumors. 4th ed. Philadelphia: Lippincott Williams and Wilkins; 2007.
13. Bonavolontà G, Strianese D, Grassi P, et al. An analysis of 2,480 space-occupying lesions of the orbit from 1976 to 2011. Ophthalmic Plast Reconstr Surg. 2013;29(2):79–86. https://doi.org/10.1097/IOP.0B013E31827A7622.
14. Jurdy L, Merks JHM, Pieters BR, et al. Orbital rhabdomyosarcomas: a review. Saudi J Ophthalmol. 2013;27(3):167–75. https://doi.org/10.1016/J.SJOPT.2013.06.004.
15. Diagnosis and management of orbital lymphoma. American Academy of Ophthalmology. https://www.aao.org/eyenet/article/diagnosis-management-of-orbital-lymphoma. Accessed 6 Dec 2022.
16. Shields JA, Shields CL. Orbital cysts of childhood - classification, clinical features, and management. Surv Ophthalmol. 2004;49(3):281–99. https://doi.org/10.1016/j.survophthal.2004.02.001.
17. Wladis EJ, Adamo MA, Weintraub L. Optic nerve gliomas. J Neurol Surg B Skull Base. 2021;82(1):91–5. https://doi.org/10.1055/s-0040-1722634.
18. Huang M, Patel J. Optic nerve glioma. StatPearls. Treasure Island, FL: StatPearls Publishing; 2022. https://www.ncbi.nlm.nih.gov/books/NBK557878/.
19. Bullock JD, Bartley GB. Dynamic proptosis. Am J Ophthalmol. 1986;102(1):104–10. https://doi.org/10.1016/0002-9394(86)90218-7.
20. Goto H. Review of ocular tumor in practical ophthalmology, vol. 24. Tokyo: Bunkodo; 2008.
21. Fard MA, Fakhree S, Eshraghi B. Correlation of optical coherence tomography parameters with clinical and radiological progression in patients with symptomatic optic pathway gliomas. Graefes Arch Clin Exp Ophthalmol. 2013;251(10):2429–36. https://doi.org/10.1007/s00417-013-2394-4.

22. Chan NCY, Chan CKM. The role of optical coherence tomography in the acute management of neuro-ophthalmic diseases. Asia Pac J Ophthalmol (Phila). 2018;7:265–70.

23. Areas LM, Lavinsky F, Lavinsky D, Lindenmeyer RL, et al. Swept source optical coherence tomography documenting optic nerve involvement in an aggressive T-cell lymphoma. Neuro-Ophthalmology. 2021;45:189–92.

24. Nasr AM, Chacra GIA. Ultrasonography in orbital differential diagnosis. In: Karcioglu Z, editor. Orbital tumors. Berlin: Springer; 2015.

25. Douglas VP, Flores C, Douglas KA, Strominger MB, Kasper E, Torun N. Oculomotor nerve schwannoma: case series and literature review. Surv Ophthalmol. 2022;67(4):1160–74. https://doi.org/10.1016/J.SURVOPHTHAL.2021.11.008.

26. Ozoner B, Gungor A, Ture H, Ture U. Surgical treatment of trochlear nerve schwannomas: case series and systematic review. World Neurosurg. 2022;162:e288–300. https://doi.org/10.1016/J.WNEU.2022.03.006.

27. Nakamizo A, Matsuo S, Amano T. Abducens nerve schwannoma: a case report and literature review. World Neurosurg. 2019;125:49–54. https://doi.org/10.1016/J.WNEU.2019.01.123.

28. Katoh M, Kawamoto T, Ohnishi K, Sawamura Y, Abe H. Asymptomatic schwannoma of the oculomotor nerve: case report. J Clin Neurosci. 2000;7(5):458–60. https://doi.org/10.1054/JOCN.1999.0240.

Renata Conforti, Donatella Franco,
Francesco Briganti, and Ferdinando Caranci

5.1 Introduction

Cranio-orbital masses in adults include a broad spectrum of non-tumoral and tumoral benign and malignant pathologies. Imaging allows in some cases to define these lesions and to evaluate their location and real extension, but only few may specifically be characterized by imaging.

In this chapter, we focus on magnetic resonance imaging (MRI) and computed tomography (CT) features of the most common cranio-orbital tumors. Noninvasive MRI thin fat signal intensity suppression (FS) sequences without and with intravenous contrast injection allows the best orbital tissue characterization.

CT is the gold standard diagnostic method in case of osseous lesions (orbital, sinuses); it can detect any possible widening or erosions of orbital bony structures and the eventual presence of calcifications within the lesion.

Moreover, MRI and CT studies are particularly useful for tumors that extend toward the orbit and which do not originate from structures contained therein.

The diagnostic study of the orbit should imply the knowledge of the complex anatomy of this narrow region [1, 2], that is packed with multiple different structures: eye globe, muscles, nerves, arteries and veins, fat, lacrimal gland, meninges.

Bilateral symmetry is essential for the detection of orbital lesions; any asymmetry of these structures must be considered and detailed with contrast enhanced studies that are particularly advantageous for detecting small lesions by merely looking for asymmetric signal or contrast enhancement [1].

A trick to facilitate the radiological diagnosis of the cranio-orbital lesions is to narrow the differential diagnosis by localizing the lesion into an orbital compartment and ascertain the structure of origin (Fig. 5.1).

The orbit can be subdivided into the preseptal and postseptal compartments by the septum [3]. The postseptal orbit is subdivided by the cone of extraocular muscles, which separate the extraconal and intraconal compartments [3] (Figs. 5.1, 5.2, and 5.3).

In general, five anatomical orbital imaging patterns can be identified, based on the division of the orbit into compartments: intraconal, optic nerve sheath complex, extraconal, orbital apex and cavernous sinus, extraocular muscle and diffuse (involving any orbital structure). Lesions may either be located to a single compartment or

R. Conforti · D. Franco · F. Caranci (✉)
Medicine of Precision Department, University of
Campania "Luigi Vanvitelli", Naples, Italy
e-mail: ferdinando.caranci@unicampania.it

F. Briganti
Department of Neurosciences and Reproductive and
Odontostomatological Sciences, Service of
Neuroradiology, "Federico II" University,
Naples, Italy

Fig. 5.1 Orbital compartments. Each compartment is characterized by different colors (intraconal brown, muscles yellow, extraconal red). (**Original to the authors**)

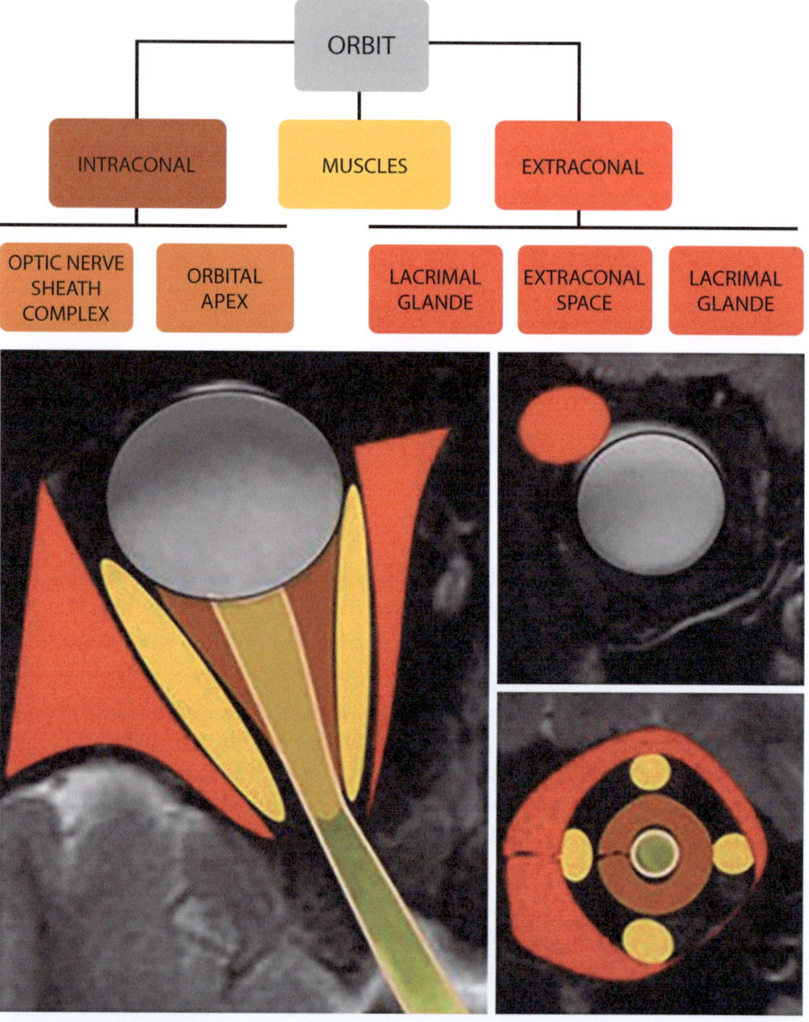

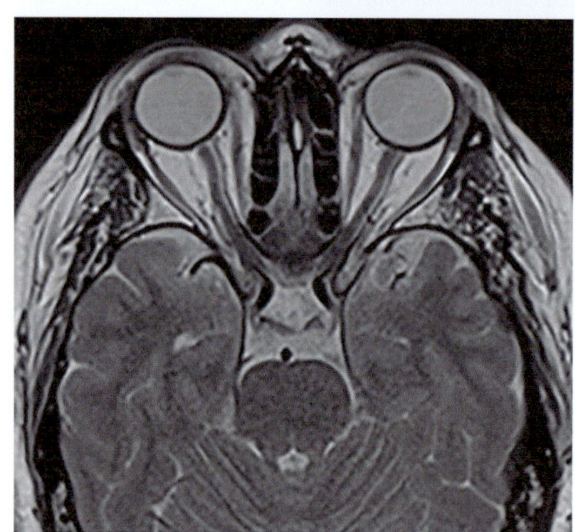

Fig. 5.2 MR orbital anatomy (T2 weighted axial section). (**Original to the authors**)

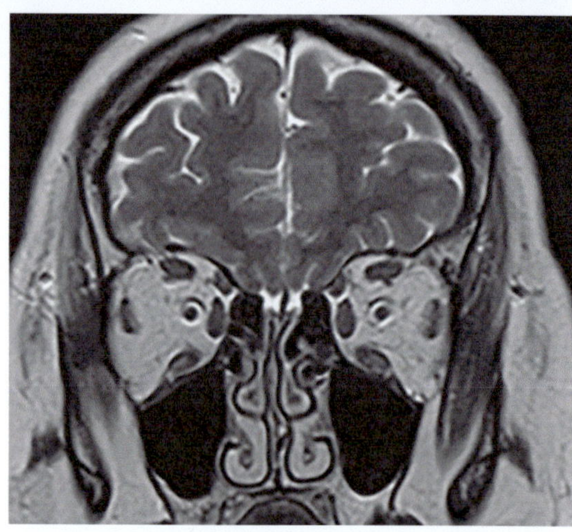

Fig. 5.3 MR orbital anatomy (T2 weighted coronal section). (**Original to the authors**)

be multicompartmental [3]; cross-sectional imaging allows to delineate specific patterns of compartmental involvement [3, 4].

Characterization of the lesion with clinical correlation leads to a probable diagnosis [1]. A basic depiction of anatomical structures within the orbit on T1- and T2-w images is mostly important; besides location and extension (extra- and intraorbital), assessment of signal intensity (on T1- and T2-w images), mass effect [1] and enhancement patterns of the lesion are fundamental for the diagnosis [1, 5, 6].

We will review the most frequent lesions of the cranio-orbital region with emphasis on their typical appearances and key imaging features that can help in the differential diagnosis.

5.2 Imaging

The diagnosis of cranio-orbital mass lesion is suggested by the clinical symptoms and signs. Imaging plays an important role to confirm the diagnosis and characterize and assess the extent of the lesion and the involvement of the adjacent structures [7].

5.2.1 Magnetic Resonance Imaging

MRI is the preferred imaging method. Standard MRI study of the orbit would include thin sections (usually 2–3 mm thickness and interslice gap of 0–1 mm) with sequences acquired in the axial, coronal, and sagittal planes [1, 2].

The protocol for MR imaging of the orbit and cranio-orbital structures includes: in the axial plane T1-, T2- and fat sat T2-w sequences, furthermore volumetric highly T2-w images (CISS, DRIVE, FIESTA, SPACE); in the sagittal plane (including along the course of the optic nerve) T1- and fat sat T2-w sequences; in the coronal plane T1-, fat sat T2-w, and short tau inversion recovery (STIR) sequences.

While most lesions are easily detectable, small lesions may often be missed; a few general rules may aid in reducing the false-negative rate [1].

High-spatial resolution, contrast-enhanced, and fat-saturated sequences are essential for evaluating the small anatomic spaces of the orbit [2, 5, 6]. Volumetric 3D isometric sequences allow thinner slice and reconstructions along the oblique directions of the optic nerve, with pure anatomical detail.

MRI can differentiate the structure of pathologic tissues basing on the signal intensity characteristics (solid, cystic degeneration/necrosis, fat, blood), thus defining internal architecture of the lesions (homogenous or heterogeneous) [7]; moreover, it may show the eventual presence of flow voids within the lesion [5] and its grade of enhancement and vascularization when completed by intravenous paramagnetic contrast material [1].

The shape of the lesion and its margins (well-defined, ill-defined, infiltrative), will orient toward an aggressive or benign growth pattern. In general, benign orbital lesions are more often both round or oval shaped and hyperintense on T2-w images, encroaching and deforming the adjacent structures, sometimes with hyperostosis; malignant tumors are characterized by irregular shape, molding around neighboring bone and intraorbital structures, with bony erosion and perineural involvement [4]. None of the imaging features have so high a sensitivity to distinguish in every case malignant and benign tumors; however, lowest sensitivity and positive predictive value for the inflammatory lesions is evidenced [4].

MRI evaluates the extent of the lesion and the invasion of adjacent critical structures (paranasal sinuses, maxillo-facial, and intracranial regions), defining the mass effect due to compression or invasion [1].

Diffusion-weighted imaging (DWI) is useful in case of infiltrative orbital masses [1]. Malignant tumors, especially orbital lymphomas, show visually and quantitatively lower apparent diffusion coefficient (ADC) values as compared to benign lesions, due to their higher cellularity; ADC values of $1.0–1.15 \times 10^{-3}$ mm^2/s represent, for some authors, an optimal threshold for predicting malignancy [11]. Moreover, DWI can help to localize a malignant component in a background of non-specific inflammation and to guide biopsy or intervention [8].

The combined use of DWI and dynamic contrast-enhanced MRI can aid to distinguishing malignant from benign lesions, in particular high-grade lymphoma from inflammation and reactive lymphoid hyperplasia [4].

Arterial spin labeling MRI can provide important perfusion characteristics [5].

Diffusion tensor imaging can be used to map optic nerve fibers when involved by cranio-orbital masses, thus detecting displacement or infiltration of the nerve itself. The antero-posterior orientation and large size of the optic nerve and tracts are radiological findings suggesting the tractography in a clinical setting [8]; it is useful to plane surgery, although the region of the orbital apex is still a weakness for this type of study [8].

Imaging at 3 T MRI, scanners as compared with 1.5 T, offers a superior signal-to-noise ratio as well as higher resolution in evaluating both orbital structures and intracranial pathologies; moreover, thin-section 3 T study depicts the optic nerves and orbital anatomy much better than 1.5 T scanner [2].

5.2.2 Computerized Tomography

CT compares negatively with MRI, due to its worse soft tissue contrast and spatial resolution [9], but it is the modality of choice for characterizing bone orbital lesions and evaluating calcifications [5, 8].

Bony orbit should routinely be examined in an evaluation of orbital soft tissue masses [10]. An osseous remodeling generally suggests the diagnosis of a slow-growing lesion, whereas bone erosion is more suggestive of an aggressive lesion [10]. In addition, CT study provides great details about the bony foramina, namely, the optic canal, superior orbital fissure, and infraorbital canal, along which perineural spread or intracranial extension may occur [10].

Thin-slice high resolution multidetector CT provides quick volumetric acquisitions and pre-cise depiction of the globe, optic nerve, intraconal, extraconal spaces, and intracranial compartments; CT studies are usually performed using 0.6–1 mm thin slices after intravenous injection of iodinated contrast material. Standard coronal and sagittal reconstructions are routinely obtained with bone and soft tissue settings, but every type of plane reconstruction can be obtained in post-processing procedures [8].

5.3 Epidemiology of Cranio-Orbital Mass Lesions

The incidence of different orbital mass lesions varies among large series, which report about 60% benign and 40% malignant pathologies in adults [11]. The frequency of malignancies is about 20% among young patients aged 1–18 years and increases with age, especially for the higher prevalence of lymphomas and metastatic tumors [11]. The most frequent primary orbital tumors in adults are lymphoproliferative lesions and cavernous malformations [11]. The radiological aspects of the most frequent cranio-orbital mass lesions of each compartment (intraconal and extraconal) will be described.

5.4 Intraconal Compartment

From a radiological point of view, the intraconal compartment includes three segments: (a) the globe; (b) the retrobulbar space-optic nerve sheath complex; and (c) the orbital apex and cavernous sinus, these last are in contiguity [3].

The following structures are evidenced: optic nerve-sheath complex, ophthalmic artery, common oculomotor nerve, abducens nerve, nasociliary branch of the ophthalmic nerve (cranial nerve V_1) [3].

5.4.1 Optic Nerve Sheath Complex

The optic nerve is an extension of the central nervous system, and hence, it is myelinated by oligodendrocytes and ensheathed by the meninges extending from the brain and in continuity with it [2].

A perivascular transport system inside the optic nerve parenchyma allows cerebrospinal fluid and interstitial fluid communications between the optic nerve and brain parenchyma through subarachnoid space, perivascular space, and lymphatic system [12–14].

The optic nerve consists of four segments in an antero-posterior direction: the optic nerve head, intraorbital, intracanalicular, and intracranial; it normally shows progressive tapering of width posteriorly.

MRI is superior to CT in demonstrating the optic nerve anatomy, particularly in the optic canal and intracranial segments where bone-related artifacts reduce the image definition on CT [6]. The course of the optic nerve is better demonstrated on oblique sagittal T2-w sequences that show the optic nerve throughout its length; intrinsic optic nerve signal abnormalities are best delineated on coronal T2-w FS sequences. Contrast enhancement requires comparing both pre- and postcontrast T1-weighted FS sequences.

The optic nerve sheath complex may be affected by a variety of neoplastic lesions of vascular, lymphoproliferative, or neurogenic origin [9].

5.4.1.1 Optic Nerve and Pathway Gliomas

Optic nerve and pathway gliomas (ONG) are the most common primary tumor of the nerve [5, 10]; they may occur anywhere along the optic pathway (25–48% in the intra-orbital segment) [10].

Nearly all ONGs are juvenile pilocytic astrocytomas (WHO grade 1) [13]; pilomyxoid astrocytoma is a rare variant [5]. ONG may occur isolated or as a manifestation of neurofibromatosis (NF) 1 [3, 5]; children with NF1 often show bilateral nerves involvement [10]. In NF1 patients, the orbital segment is the most common site, whereas most non-NF1 patients have intracranial tumors [2, 5]. Low-grade ONGs commonly occur in the pediatric age group [10]; rare higher grade, more aggressive ONGs (anaplastic astrocytomas or glioblastomas) occur in adults with no NF [3, 10].

ONGs may be asymptomatic and discovered incidentally in patients with NF1; symptomatic cases may present visual field deficit, vision loss, strabismus, or relative afferent pupillary defect [10].

MRI is the modality of choice to assess the intra-orbital and intracranial extension of the tumor [3, 10]. It shows fusiform expansion and tortuosity of the optic nerve that appears T1 iso-hypointense and T2 hyperintense, with variable contrast enhancement [3, 5, 10]; the nerve itself cannot be distinguished from the tumor, an useful characteristic for differentiating ONG from meningioma [10] (Fig. 5.4).

In the initial stages, the tumor may present on the coronal plane as asymmetric prominence of the perioptic CSF spaces on the involved side [3]. Cystic areas may be seen, while calcifications are rare [10].

On coronal plane, a rim of T2 hyperintensity is often observed at the periphery of the tumor [3], mimicking an expanded subarachnoid space while corresponding to leptomeningeal infiltration and proliferation (so-called arachnoidal gliomatosis) [10].

The contrast enhancement of ONG may suggest a more aggressive tumor [3], but it may be wax and wane; moreover, a decreased enhancement without change in size is often seen during chemotherapy (and it is more pronounced with some molecular targeted agents, such as *MEK* inhibitors and *BRAF* inhibitors) [5]. Therefore, increased size and extent of the tumor is more indicative of tumor progression, than the contrast enhancement degree [5].

The perineural arachnoidal gliomatosis may enhance after gadolinium per venam administration [2].

ONGs show increased diffusion on DWI (high ADC), and low fractional anisotropy (FA) values, attributed to low cellularity and low proliferative indices [8].

DTI tractography can be used in the presurgical evaluation by demonstrating integrity of the optic nerve in patients with resectable lesions [8].

CT is complementary to depict the optic canal widening and aids in differentiating from meningioma [6].

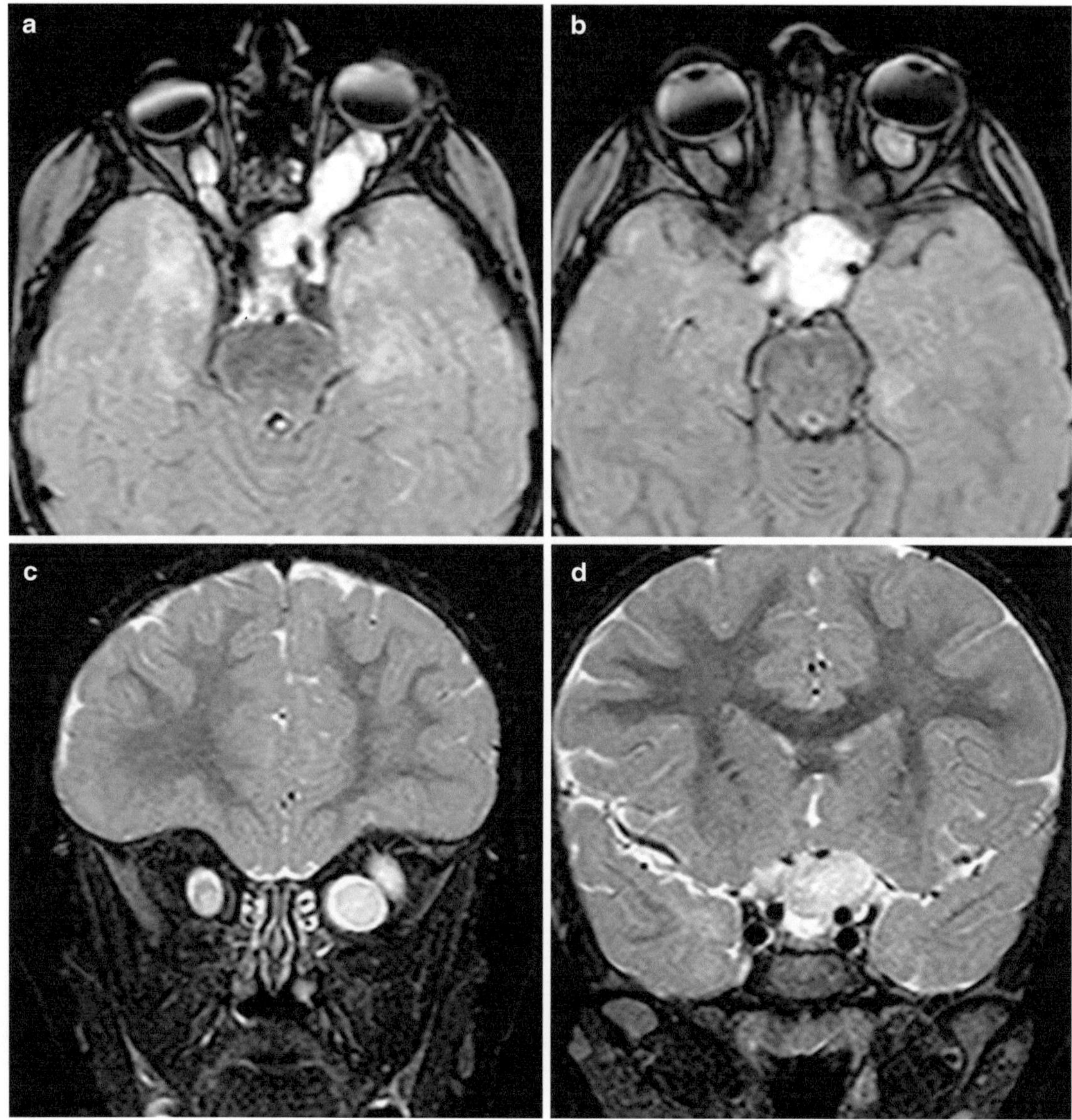

Fig. 5.4 Optic pathway glioma. (**a, b**) Flair sections on axial plane; (**c, d**) STIR sections on coronal plane. Fusiform expansion and tortuosity of the optic nerve with involvement of the optic chiasm (NF 1 patient). (**Original to the authors**)

If imaging features are typical, the diagnosis is presumed and biopsy is not usually required [2].

5.4.1.2 Optic Nerve Sheath Meningioma

Optic nerve sheath meningioma is the second most common optic nerve tumor, accounting for 2% of the orbital space-occupying masses sometimes in association with N.F [10]. It may be primary or secondary to perineural extension of intracranial sellar and parasellar meningiomas [3]. Primary optic nerve sheath meningiomas arise from meningoepithelial cap cells along the optic nerve from the globe to the prechiasmatic segment [2, 10]. Meningiomas secondarily extending into the orbit [5, 10] are more frequent and may originate from many intracranial structures: cavernous sinus, clinoid process, tuberculum sellae, planum sphenoidale.

The clinical presentation includes painless and slowly progressive loss of vision, due to insidious tumor growth [2, 5]. Optic nerve atrophy, compared to the contralateral nerve, is rare due to its compression [3, 5]. The long-term compression of the central retinal vein due to the meningioma is also responsible for optociliary shunt vessels [10].

As for ONGs, MRI cross-sectional features are characteristic of optic nerve meningioma [13] mainly for determining the tumor extent [10]. The tumor expands the nerve sheath, usually in a tubular fashion [5, 10]; unlike ONGs, the optic nerve can be separated from the meningioma.

The tumor growth patterns may be tubular, globular, fusiform, focal, and eccentric to the nerve [3, 10]. MRI well demonstrates all these growth patterns of enlargement of the optic nerve sheath [5] and the separation of the tumor from the underlying optic nerve [3, 10].

Optic nerve sheath meningioma is T1 and T2 hypointense and shows moderate to intense enhancement in T1-w post-contrast MRI images with fat suppression in a "tram-track" (axial) or "doughnut/target" pattern [3, 10], as the normal optic nerve surrounded by the enhancing nerve sheath tumor [6]. Other conditions showing tram-track sign include sarcoidosis, perioptic neuritis, orbital pseudotumor, perioptic hemorrhage, metastases, leukemia/lymphoma, and Erdheim–Chester disease [2].

Because of its hypercellularity nature, the optic nerve sheath meningioma often shows restricted diffusion with low ADC values [8].

It is important to define the portions of the optic nerve involved by the tumor (intraorbital, intracanalicular, and intracranial) [10]. While these meningiomas are generally slow growing, they may be aggressive in children [10]; thus, the radiological observation of the extent of involvement is mandatory. If the tumor tends to spread towards the optic chiasm, surgical intervention may be warranted to prevent extension to the contralateral side [10].

Noncontrast CT is optimal for depicting bone hyperostosis and tram-track calcifications (20–50% of cases [13]), which may be subtle or undetectable on MRI [3, 5].

Among meningiomas secondarily extending to the orbit, those spheno-orbital are the most frequent and insidious because of their infiltrative nature. They are characterized by two components: intraosseous and orbital/periorbital [15]. The bony involvement is characterized by hyperostosis of the sphenoid wing, orbital roof, superior orbital fissure, and optic canal; the orbital component can vary from a small intraorbital nodule to extensive periorbital and intraconal tumor mass. The dural component causes carpet-like extensions along the sphenoid wing and orbit [15] (Fig. 5.5).

5.4.1.3 Optic Nerve Secondary Tumors

Some tumors may secondarily involve the optic nerve as results of direct extension. These mostly include retinoblastoma and infiltrating orbital tumors, less frequently lymphoproliferative disorders and metastases.

These tumors are difficult to differentiate radiologically and may mimic optic neuritis. T2-w hypointense optic nerve thickening with diffuse enhancement and sheath thickening demonstrating tram-track appearance on postcontrast T1-w imaging may be seen in optic nerve lymphomas [3, 10].

5.4.2 Retrobulbar Lesions

The retrobulbar compartment predominantly consists of the orbital fat through which the cranial nerves and vessels pass within the annulus of Zinn at the orbital apex [3]. The superior and inferior ophthalmic veins span both the extraconal and intraconal spaces. The structure of origin of lesions that arise within this space can be deduced from their relationship to the adjacent structures [3].

5.4.2.1 Cavernous Hemangioma

The cavernous hemangioma (or cavernous malformation) is the most common benign vasculoproliferative orbital lesion in adults [3, 10].

Progressive painless proptosis is the most common clinical sign at presentation [10]; visual field deficits, and monocular vision loss most

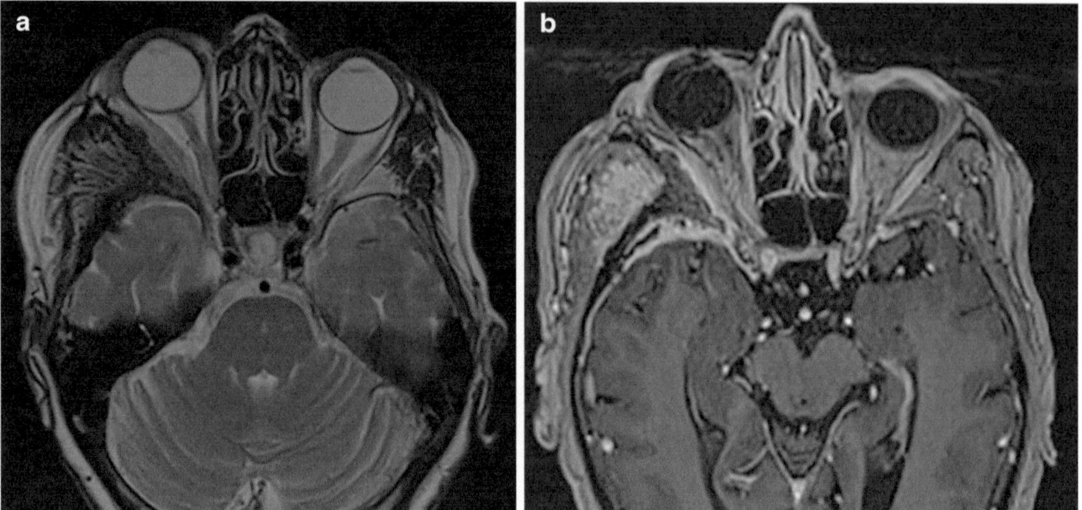

Fig. 5.5 Spheno-orbital meningioma. (**a**) T2-weighted section on axial plane; (**b**) post-contrast T1-weighted section on axial plane. Presence of a right dural enhancing mass, involving the lateral extraconal orbital compart-ment, the intracranial surface of the sphenoid wing, and the infratemporal fossa, associated with hyperostosis of the sphenoid wing. (**Original to the authors**)

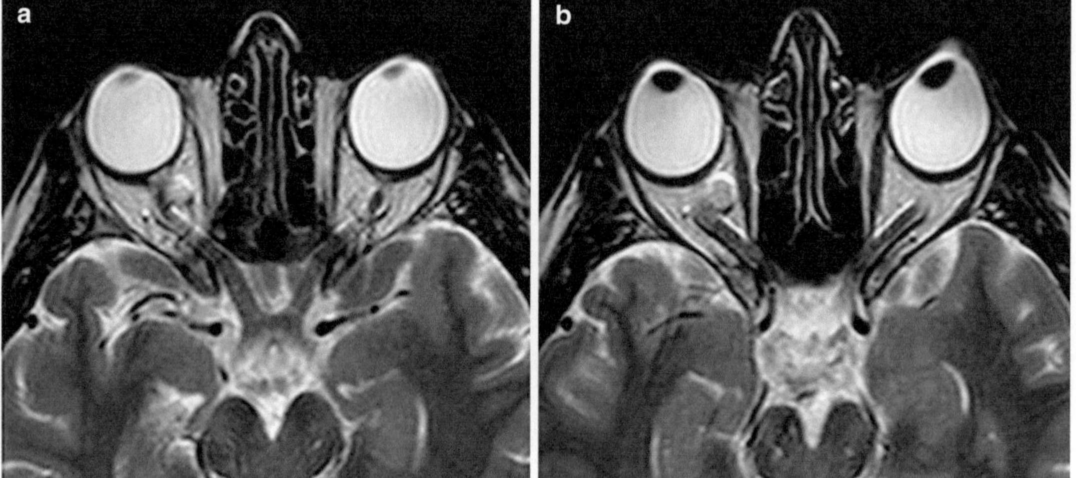

Fig. 5.6 Cavernous hemangioma. (**a**, **b**) T2-weighted sections on axial plane. Presence of an intraconal hyperintense lesion contiguous to the optic nerve. (**Original to the authors**)

often due to mass effect on the optic nerve are often present. Pain, eyelid swelling, diplopia, and a palpabe lump are less common [10].

Cavernous hemangiomas consist of dilated cavernous spaces with interspersed septae and fibrous pseudocapsule. They are located laterally in the intraconal space and are round, well-circumscribed and homogeneous [3, 10];

extraconal locations are rare. Cavernous malformations tend to displace and surrounding adjacent structures (extraconal muscles and the optic nerve) and may cause osseous remodeling (better seen on CT). At MRI, cavernous hemangiomas are isointense on T1-w relative to muscle and uniformly hyperintense on T2-wimages, with no flow voids [3, 10] (Fig. 5.6). Internal septations may be identified as linear hypointense bands within the lesion [3, 10], that appear bright on DW images [8]. At multiphase imaging, the contrast enhancement is poor on early arterial phase, owing to the scant arterial supply in these lesions; peripheral enhancement on arterial phase images with progressive centripetal fill in delayed venous phases, and progressive filling of the mass from periphery to center, with complete filling within 30 min, are evident [3, 10]. This enhancement pattern allows distinguishing cavernous hemangioma from other vascular lesions with rich arterial supply such as capillary hemangioma, hemangiopericytoma, and arteriovenous malformations [10]. These lesions rarely show calcifications, phleboliths, or hemorrhagic areas [6].

5.4.2.2 Solitary Fibrous Tumor

Orbital solitary fibrous tumor is a neoplastic lesion that originates, like the hemangiopericytoma, from vascular pericytes; these two tumors are considered an unique pathological entity in the World Health Organization classification of the central nervous system tumors because of their identical immunohistochemical profiles.

Primary solitary fibrous tumors of the orbit are rare, accounting for 1% of all orbital tumors [10]; they occur within the intraconal space [3]. Tumors of the paranasal sinuses may extent into the extraconal orbital space. Low-grade masses are usually lobulated and well circumscribed [3, 10]. Aggressive lesions have infiltrative borders with possible bone erosion [3, 10].

These tumors present with proptosis and palpable mass, while pain, diplopia, and decreased visual acuity are less common signs [10].

Unlike cavernous hemangioma, the orbital solitary fibrous tumor tends to be isointense relative to gray matter on T1-w and T2-w images and shows marked arterial phase enhancement with progressive washout on delayed phases [3, 10]. Calcifications are rare.

5.4.2.3 Extraocular Muscles Lesions

The extraocular muscles form the muscular cone extending from the superior orbital fissure to the posterior aspect of the globe and enclose the retrobulbar intraconal space [3]. They show an isointense signal intensity on both T1- and T2-w imaging compared to the temporal muscle [3] and moderate homogeneous contrast enhancement of their bellies. Pathological involvement of the extraocular muscles may result in focal or diffuse enlargement or atrophy, with or without associated signal abnormality [6]. Neoplastic lesions that involve the extraocular muscles include lymphomas and metastases, generally invading both the intraconal and extraconal compartments (see after).

5.4.3 Orbital Apex and Cavernous Sinus Lesions

The orbital apex disorders present in three clinical variants: orbital apex syndrome (OAS), superior orbital fissure syndrome (SOFS), and cavernous sinus syndrome (CSS) [3]. OAS consists of visual impairment and dyplopia due to involvement of the optic nerve and III, IV, VI, and V1 cranial nerves; SOFS presents with deficit of the III. IV, VI, and V1 nerve involvement; CSS shows additional involvement of the V2 nerve and sympathetic system (Horner's syndrome) [3]. Due to close relationship of these anatomical areas, they share many common pathologies, and one syndrome can evolve into other as the disease progresses.

OAS can develop due to compression by different tumors in the orbital apex, such as meningiomas, schwannomas, and neurofibromas; other involved neoplasms include head and neck tumors, hematologic cancers, and metastatic lesions [16]. Moreover, several inflammatory disorders such as idiopathic orbital inflammatory disease, sarcoidosis, and granulomatosis with angiitis (Wegener's granulomatosis) can involve the orbital apex [3].

Idiopathic orbital inflammatory disease, also known as orbit pseudotumor, is a nonspecific, noninfectious, non-neoplastic, inflammatory process of the orbit that manifests with many variants [5]. Any area of the orbit may be involved, mostly the extraocular muscles and lacrimal gland in both adults and children [5]; according to the location, it may be classified as myositic, perineural, lacrimal, orbital apex, and diffuse forms [3].

The myositic form involves the muscle bellies and tendons of extraocular muscles; optic perineuritis involves the optic nerve sheath with inflammatory soft tissue infiltrating the adjacent fat; idiopathic orbital inflammatory disease appears as ill-defined, diffuse mass like, and infiltrative soft tissue within the orbit [5].

The Tolosa Hunt syndrome is characterized by an inflammatory soft tissue involving the orbital apex, superior orbital fissure, optic canal, and cavernous sinus [2, 3], sometimes extending to the tentorial margins; it may evolve in sclerosis with chronic progressive fibrosis.

A high index of clinical suspicion is necessary to detect asymmetric appearance of the cavernous sinus or orbital apex in subtle cases of idiopathic orbital inflammatory disease [3]. Infiltrates are typically hypointense on T1-w images with variable signal intensity on T2-w images, commonly appearing as hypointense orbital mass-like [2, 3, 5], with homogeneous postcontrast enhancement (Fig. 5.7).

Imaging features of idiopathic orbital inflammatory disease may overlap with those of other entities (lymphoproliferative disorders and orbital cellulitis), thus making this condition a diagnosis of exclusion and requiring a biopsy [5]. The dramatic improvement with corticosteroids is the hallmark of orbital inflammatory syndrome [2].

Various tumors may originate by cavernous sinus wall, with the most common being the meningioma. It appears as a well-defined lesion usually hypo- to isointense on all sequences (due to its dense fibrous-cellular content) with intense postcontrast enhancement and a characteristic dural tail (Fig. 5.8).

Other neoplasms which may secondarily involve the cavernous sinus are bony lesions such as chordomas (related to the spheno-occipital synchondrosis) and chondrosarcomas (related to petroclival synchondrosis). They appear as areas of bony destruction with variable calcification, hyperintense on T2-w images and with heterogeneous postcontrast enhancement [3].

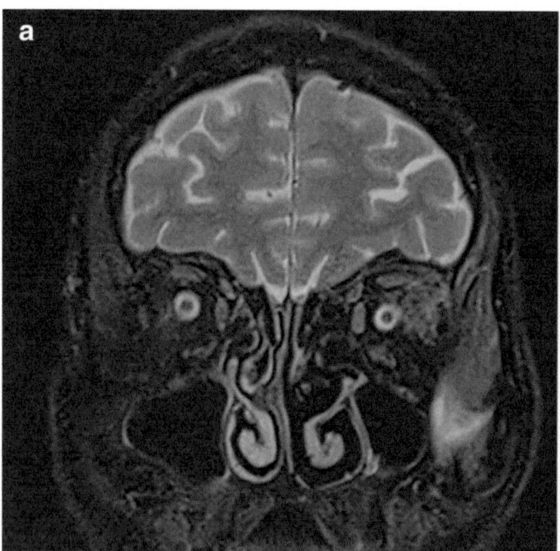
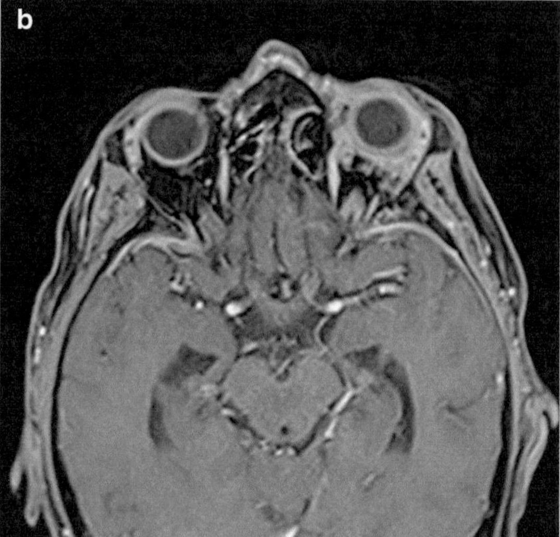
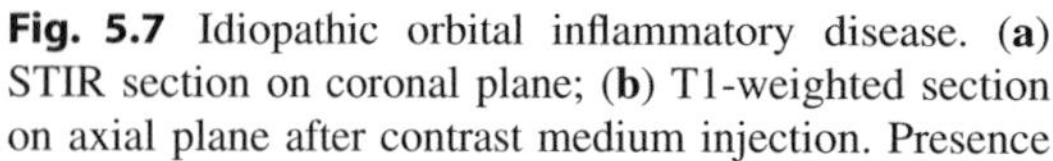

Fig. 5.7 Idiopathic orbital inflammatory disease. (**a**) STIR section on coronal plane; (**b**) T1-weighted section on axial plane after contrast medium injection. Presence of an infiltrating lesion involving the retrobulbar space and the muscular cone, enhancing after contrast medium injection. (**Original to the authors**)

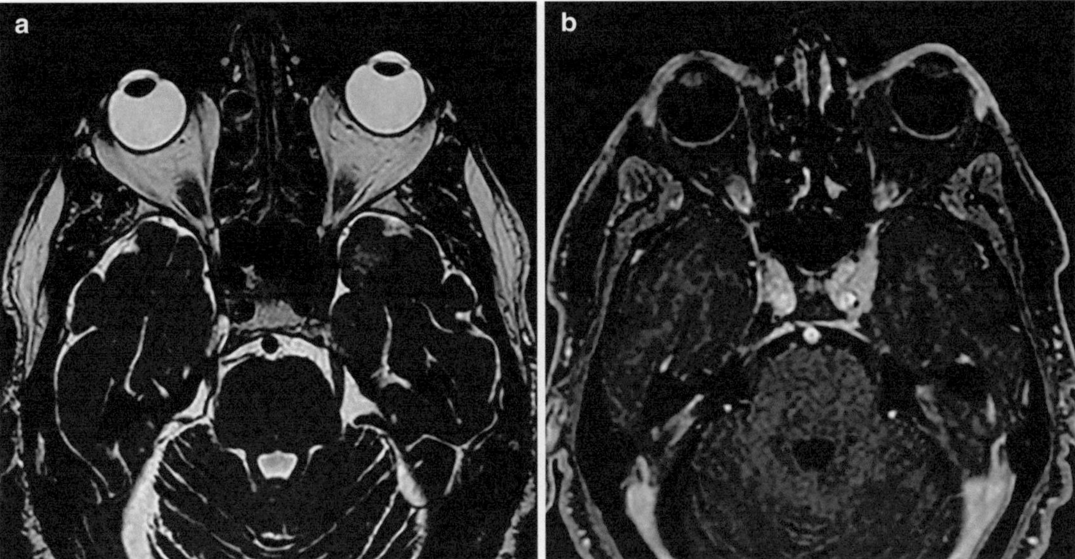

Fig. 5.8 Cavernous sinus meningioma. Presence of a left hypointense cavernous sinus wall lesion, enhancing after contrast medium injection. (**Original to the authors**)

5.5 Extraconal Compartment

The extraconal lesions may be located at the osteodural complex, the extraconal space, and the lacrimal gland.

5.5.1 Mass Lesions of the Osteodural Complex

The osteodural group includes subperiosteal, bony, and paraorbital lesions.

5.5.1.1 Orbital Dermoid and Epidermoid

Orbital dermoids and epidermoids are choristomatous cystic lesions resulting from congenital epithelial inclusions during development; they contain epidermal and dermal structures (hair follicles, sweat, and sebaceous glands) [5].

They are commonly located in the anterior extraconal compartment often adjacent to suture lines, usually in the superolateral or superonasal quadrants [3]; dermoid cysts are more often located at lateral frontozygomatic suture [8]. These cysts are usually encapsulated, may cause bony remodeling, and may extend through a bony canal in the intracranial compartment (dumbbell lesions) [6].

Dermoid cysts may contain areas of fat signal intensity; they are iso- or hypointense on T1-w images or bright with fat-like signal intensity and are usually hyperintense on T2-w images (Fig. 5.9); diffusion may be variable, depending upon their contents, and sometimes restricted [8]. These cysts may be subperiosteal (20%) with extensive bone remodelling.

Epidermoid cysts do not contain mesodermal derivatives [5]; thus, they show fluid signal intensity similar to cerebrospinal fluid and characteristically demonstrate hyperintense signal on DW images due to the accretion of keratin debris [3] (Fig. 5.10).

Both lesions show faint postcontrast rim enhancement; wall calcification is more commonly seen in dermoids [3, 5]. Irregular margins with perilesional edema and enhancement suggest rupture with inflammation.

Differently from epidermoid and dermoid cysts, post-traumatic hemorrhagic cysts are T1 hyperintense due to the presence of subacute blood products [3].

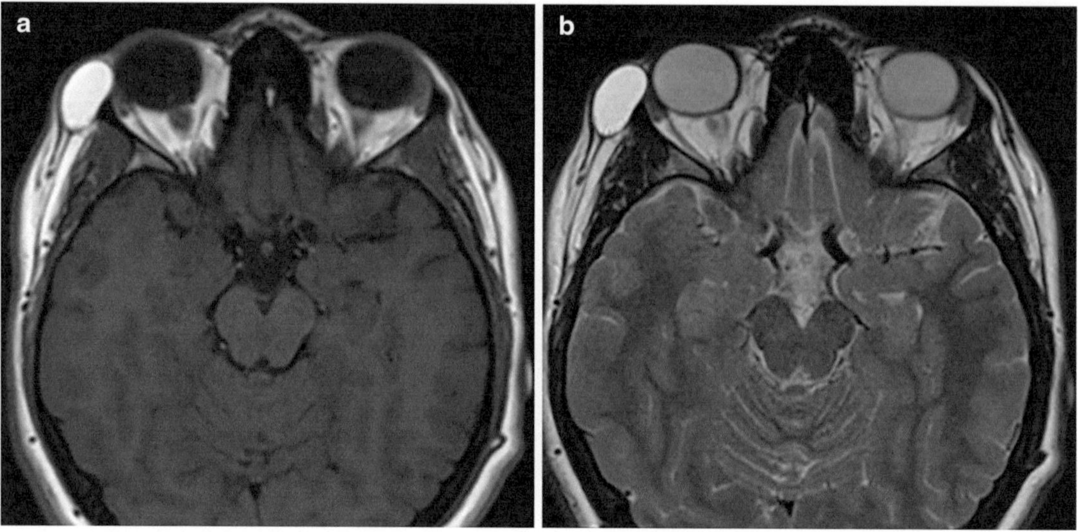

Fig. 5.9 Dermoid cyst. (**a**) T1-weighted section on axial plane; (**b**) T2-weighted section on axial plane. Presence of a fat signal intensity lesion extending through the right fronto-zygomatic suture into the temporal fossa. (**Original to the authors**)

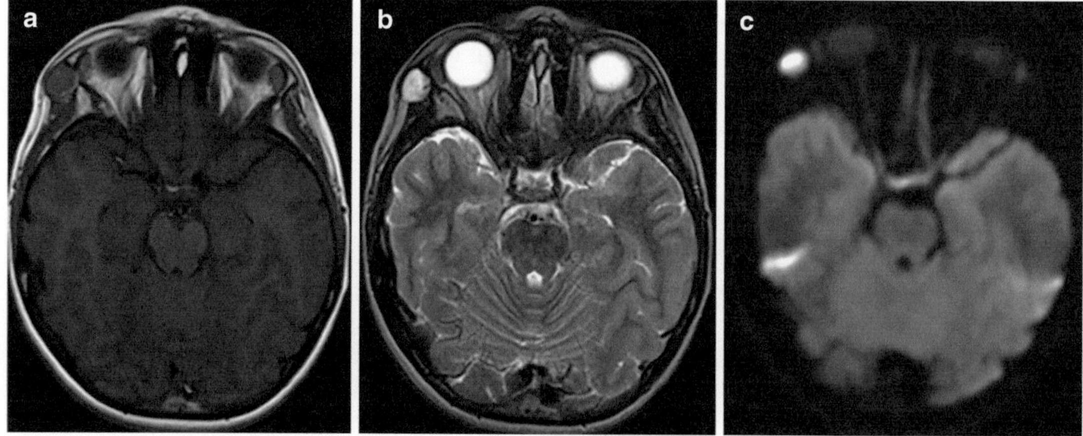

Fig. 5.10 Epidermoid cyst. (**a**) T1-weighted section on axial plane; (**b**) T2-weighted section on axial plane; (**c**) DWI on axial plane. Presence of a fluid signal intensity lesion, with restricted diffusion, extending through the right fronto-zygomatic suture into the temporalis fossa. (**Original to the authors**)

5.5.2 Fibrous Dysplasia

Cranio-facial fibrous dysplasia may involve the frontal, ethmoid, or sphenoid bones; it is frequent in children and adolescents with slight female predilection, mostly monostotic (70–80%) [8]. Orbital bony involvement may lead to hypertelorism, exophthalmos, visual impairment, and blindness [8] due to replacement of normal bone with abnormal metaplastic immature woven bone, forming irregular curvilinear trabeculae, where hemorrhage and cystic changes may be seen [8].

MRI is superior in assessing marrow involvement and neurovascular impingement [6]. Fibrous dysplasia appears as diploic space widening with a variable signal intensity depending on the degree of sclerosis [3]. The involved bone

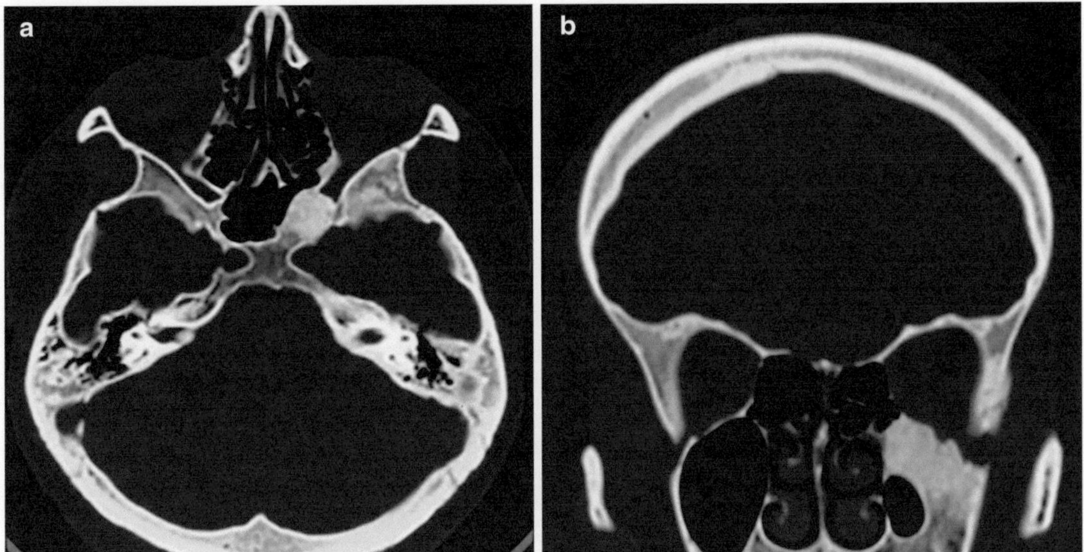

Fig. 5.11 Fibrous dysplasia. (**a**) CT axial section; (**b**) CT coronal reconstruction. Dysplastic marrow involvement of the left maxillary bone with "ground-glass" appearance. (**Original to the authors**)

appears heterogeneous, usually T1 hypo-isointense and T2 hypointense (sometimes with foci of T2 hyperintensity and fluid-fluid levels) and with heterogeneous contrast enhancement [3, 8]. Similar to benign lesions elsewhere in the head and neck, the fibrous dysplasia shows significantly higher ADC values compared to malignant bone tumors.

CT is essential in demonstrating the ground-glass appearance of the expanded diploic space (Fig. 5.11) with sparing of the inner table (differently from the Paget's disease) [6, 11]; it is useful in evidencing narrowing of the optic canal and impingement of the optic nerve.

aerated sinuses and resembling the cortical bones in its ivory form or taking on a ground-glass appearance in its spongy form; these two features can coexist in the same lesion (mixed form) [17]. MRI is less effective because small compact osteomas might not be detected and can be confused with intrasinus air; it is more accurate for the study of the adjacent structures such as optic nerve, eyeball, orbit's vascular structures, and muscles [17].

The differential diagnosis includes meningioma of the frontal plate with orbital extension, orbital focal spot of fibrous dysplasia, ossifying fibroma, or Paget disease [17].

5.5.3 Fronto-Orbital Osteoma

Fronto-orbital osteomas account for 0.4–5% of orbital tumors. They can variably extend to the orbit causing signs and symptoms including proptosis, diplopia, and limitation of ocular movements [17].

CT and MRI allow the correct diagnosis. According to its degree of mineralization, osteoma appears at CT as a well-defined dense, polycyclic mass, in contrast to the hypodensity of

5.5.4 Subperiosteal Abscess and Hemorrhage

Subperiosteal abscess is lentiform shaped, usually along the superior or medial orbital wall and is secondary to paranasal sinus inflammation. The phlegmonous stage appears with T1- and T2-w hyperintense signal and homogeneous contrast enhancement; the mature organized abscesses show fluid signal intensity with peripheral rim enhancement. Pus characteristically shows diffusion restriction. Perilesional fat stranding and extraocular muscles edema usually show a hazy hyperintense signal on STIR sequences [3].

Subperiosteal hemorrhage can mimic the appearance of an abscess, particularly when a history of trauma is not evident. Acute hemorrhage appears as hyperdensity on CT, while chronic hematoma shows T1- and T2-w hypointense signal with a fibrous rim [3] (Fig. 5.12).

5.5.4.1 Paranasal Sinus Mucocele

Paranasal sinus mucoceles result in the expansion of the involved sinus and are completely fluid-filled,

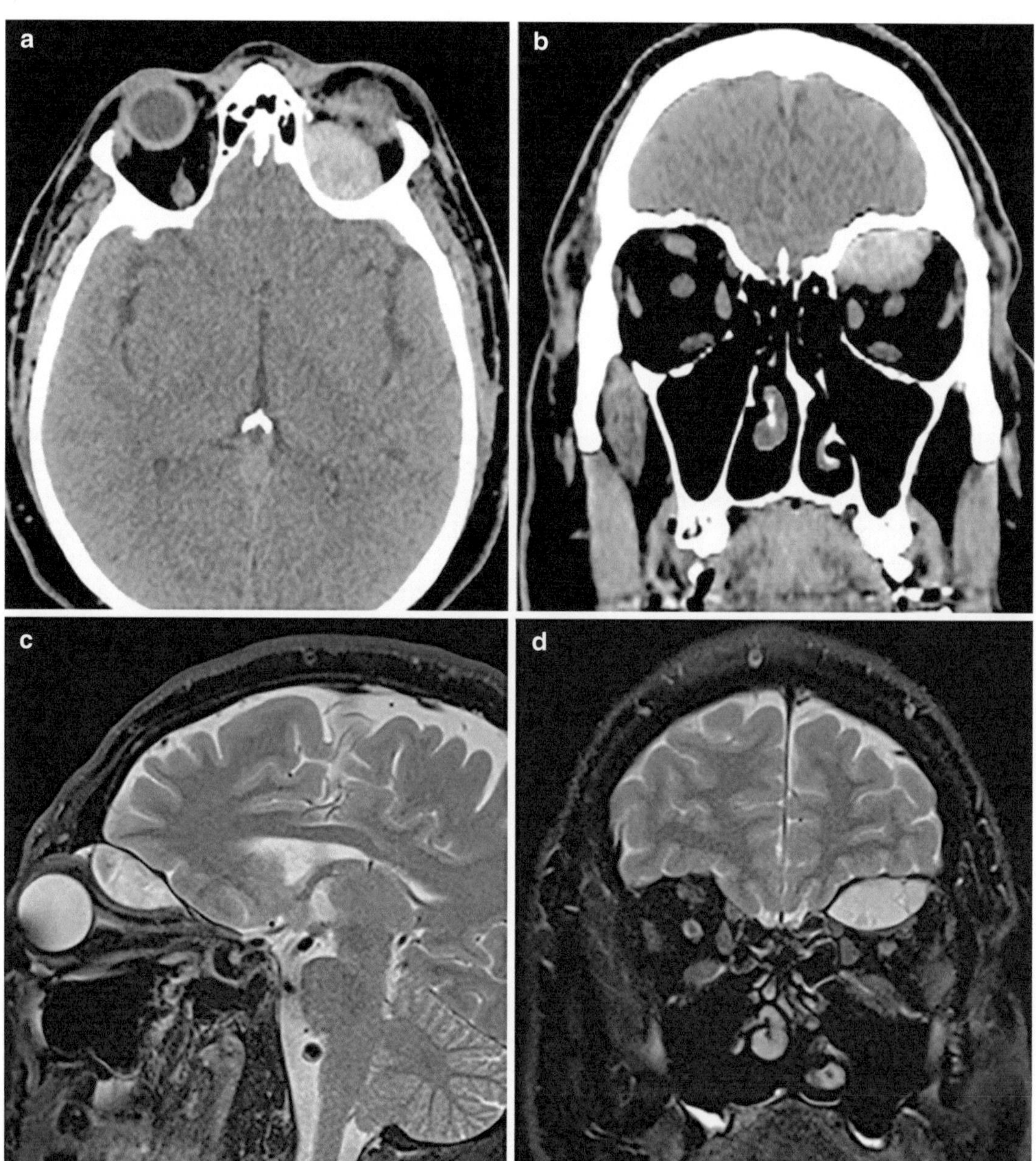

Fig. 5.12 Subperiosteal hemorrhage. (**a**) CT axial section; (**b**) CT coronal reconstruction; (**c**, **d**) T2-weighted section on sagittal and coronal plane. (**e**, **f**) T1-weighted section on axial plane before and after contrast medium injection. Presence of a lentiform hemorrhagic collection along the superior orbital wall, not enhancing after contrast medium injection. (**Original to the authors**)

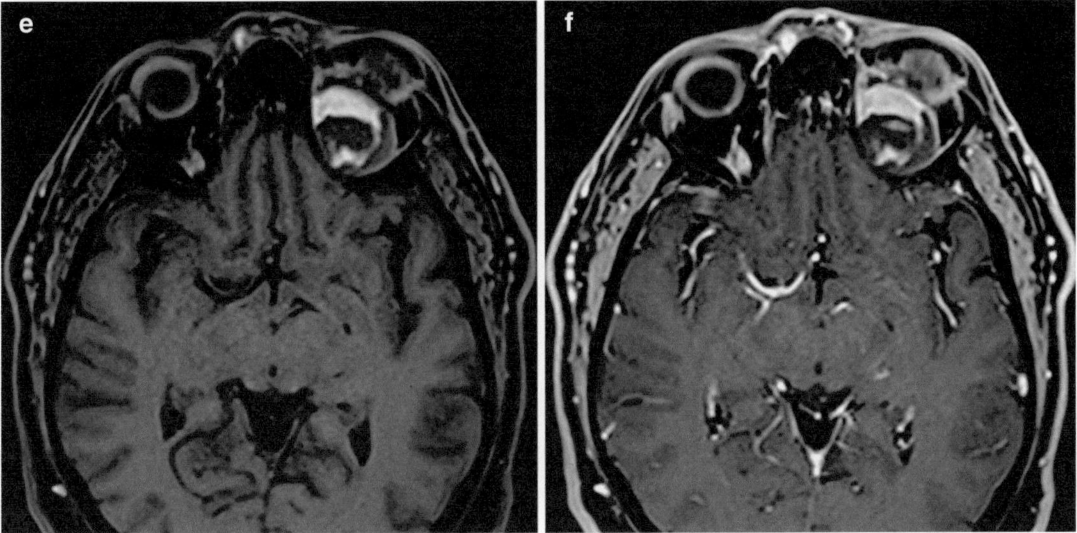

Fig. 5.12 (continued)

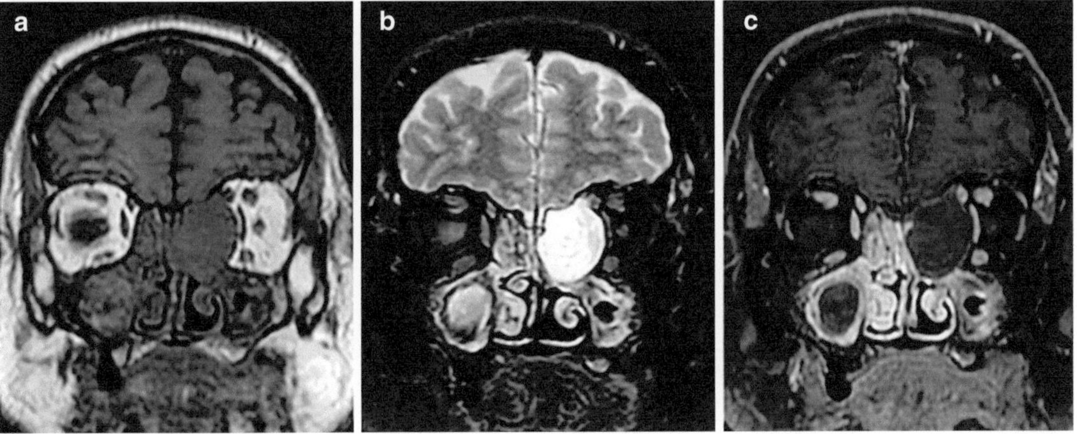

Fig. 5.13 Paranasal sinus mucocele. (**a**) T1-weighted section on coronal plane; (**b**) STIR sequence on coronal plane; (**c**) T1-weighted section on axial plane after contrast medium injection. Left ethmoid fluid, expansile collection remodeling the lamina papyracea and extending toward the medial extraconal space; note the opacified maxillary and right ethmoid sinuses with inspissated secretions. (**Original to the authors**)

showing fluid signal intensity on MRI (T1-hypointense and T2-w hyperintense). With decreased of the water content and the relative increased protein content of the fluid, the lesion appears T1-hyperintense with variable T2-w hypointensity. The presence of air within the cyst rules out the mucocele and should suggest a superimposed infection. Bony involvement is best delineated on CT, while MRI better delineates impingement on the orbital structures [3] (Fig. 5.13).

5.5.5 Mass Lesions of the Extraconal Space

5.5.5.1 Orbital Lymphoproliferative Diseases

Orbital lymphoproliferative lesions, particularly those involving the ocular adnexa [11], are the most common primary orbital malignancy in older adults (≥60 years of age) [6, 10].

These diseases comprise a wide spectrum of lesions from benign to malignant. Benign orbital lymphoproliferative diseases include noninfectious chronic inflammatory diseases (such as atypical and benign reactive lymphoid hyperplasia); malignant lymphomas are usually primary low-grade B cell non-Hodgkin's lymphomas [3]; they can be primary or secondary, the latter occurring in 2–5% of patients with advanced systemic lymphoma [10].

Orbital lymphoma can be unilateral (more frequent) or bilateral [11]; they can occur anywhere in the orbit, mostly in the lacrimal gland (nearly 40% of cases), conjunctiva, and eyelid [9].

Differentiating these lesions has obvious therapeutic implications since the latter requires radiotherapy and the former responds to steroid therapy [3]. Both the benign and malignant orbital lymphoproliferative diseases have similar CT and MRI findings with T1- and T2-w isointensity, restricted diffusion, and homogeneous contrast enhancement [3, 10]. However, orbital lymphomas tend to be more ill-defined (Fig. 5.14) than benign orbital lymphoproliferative diseases, which have more well-defined lobulated margins [3, 10]. Lymphoma can also cause focal or fusiform enlargement of the extraocular muscles (mimicking myositis or thyroid disease-related).

A characteristic feature of these tumors is their tendency to mold and encase surrounding orbital structures, such as the globe, optic nerve, and orbital wall; bone remodeling and osseous erosion are quite rare, although it may occasionally occur with diffuse large B-cell lymphoma [8, 10]. Bony destruction or perineural spread suggests an aggressive histology [8].

Malignant orbital lymphoproliferative diseases tend to be hypoenhancing (assessed by contrast enhancement ratio of signal intensity to the temporal muscle) compared to benign orbital lymphoproliferative diseases, which show increased vascularity and abundant fibrotic component; hypervascularity of benign orbital lymphoproliferative diseases also leads to the "flow-void sign" on T2-w images.

Quantitative MR techniques may aid in the differentiation of benign and malignant orbital

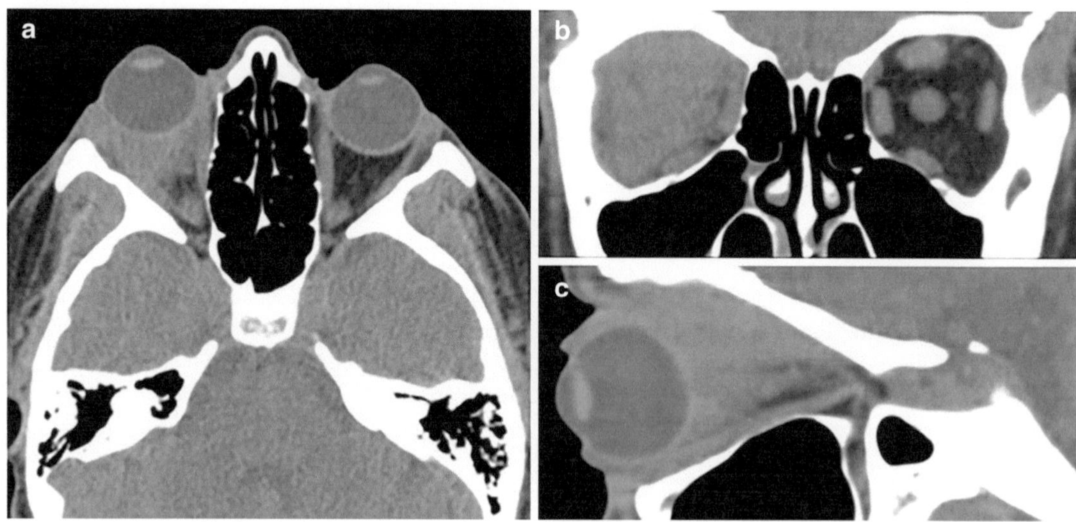

Fig. 5.14 Orbital lymphoma. (**a**) CT axial section; (**b**) CT coronal reconstruction; (**c**) CT sagittal reconstruction. Ill-defined, relatively hyperdense retrobulbar mass. (**Original to the authors**)

lymphoproliferative diseases [3]. Malignant orbital lymphoproliferative diseases show higher diffusion restriction (lower ADC values) reflecting increased cellular density, than benign orbital lymphoproliferative diseases showing increased interstitial fluid content. Advanced imaging techniques such as T1 dynamic contrast enhancement can also allow differentiation between the two types of orbital lymphoproliferative diseases [3].

Whole body staging, most often with FDG PET-CT [11] is necessary when orbital lymphoma is diagnosed.

Differentiation of orbital lymphoma from pseudotumor is often challenging at imaging; the findings of infiltration or thickening of ocular muscles favor a diagnosis of pseudotumor [10]. Patient's clinical history is often useful for the diagnosis, as acute onset of pain suggests an inflammation, while patients with orbital lymphoma typically have no pain [10]. Ultimately, however, biopsy may be required for diagnosis [10].

5.5.5.2 Rhabdomyosarcoma

Rhabdomyosarcoma, a mesenchymal tumor, is the most common extraocular malignancy in childhood. It represents up to 25% of head and neck rhabdomyosarcomas and has a better prognosis due to the early clinical presentation. It occurs most commonly in the extraconal compartment, either in the superonasal or superior quadrants.

The rhabdomyosarcoma may appear well circumscribed if small, but larger lesions are infiltrative and encase (not invade) the adjacent soft tissue structures and the globe (which is distorted but intact). Bone destruction is seen in up to 40% of cases and best demonstrated on CT; the paranasal sinuses may also be invaded.

The tumor usually appears homogeneous, although areas of necrosis or hemorrhage may lead to heterogeneity; calcifications are rare and are usually secondary to adjacent bone destruction. On MRI, the mass appears T1-isointense (hyperintense areas may represent hemorrhage), heterogeneously T2 hyperintense with moderate to intense contrast enhancement; necrotic areas are nonenhancing with the surrounding enhancing viable tissue giving a ring enhancement pattern. MRI is superior to CT in delineating dural involvement and intracranial extension. Paranasal sinus invasion is best differentiated from trapped secretions by comparing pre- and postcontrast T1 images. These findings may be mimicked by a ruptured dermoid cyst with inflammatory changes (look for T1 hyperintense fat components), neuroblastoma metastases, or Langerhans cell histiocytosis (more prominent bony involvement) [3].

5.5.5.3 Langerhans Cell Histiocytosis, Erdheim Chester Disease, Rosai Dorfman Disease

Langerhans cell histiocytosis is a multisystem disorder that most commonly involves the skeleton, particularly the skull and ribs. Single lesion is referred to eosinophilic granuloma and appears as a punched-out lytic lesion with cortical and medullary bone destruction; the soft tissue component demonstrates T1 hypointense, T2 and STIR hyperintense signal with diffuse postcontrast enhancement [6].

Erdheim Chester disease is a non-Langerhans cell histiocytosis entity occurring in a similar age group as orbital lymphoproliferative diseases, but with a male predominance. It is indistinguishable from orbital lymphoproliferative diseases on imaging and often presents as bilateral or unilateral intraconal masses. The presence of bony involvement (sclerosis), intracranial dural mass, or pachymeningitis are clues to the diagnosis [3].

Rosai Dorfman disease is another non-Langerhans cell histiocytosis, more commonly presenting as an extraconal mass associated with massive lymphadenopathy in children and young adults [3].

5.5.5.4 Schwannoma

Orbital schwannomas are rare and more often sporadic, although they may occur in the context of neurofibromatosis type 2 and schwannomatosis [5].

They mostly arise from branches of the ophthalmic division of the trigeminal nerve (commonly the frontal); branches of the oculomotor, trochlear, abducens nerves, parasympathetic and sympathetic fibers, and the ciliary ganglia are more rare sites of origin [3, 10].

Clinical symptoms are nonspecific and include proptosis, pain, and blurred vision [5].

Orbital schwannomas are typically extraconal and located at the superior quadrant [2, 3], owing to their frequent origin from the frontal branch of the ophthalmic nerve [10]. The tumor may extend in the cranial cavity in a dumbbell shape form through the orbital apex and superior orbital fissure [3].

MR imaging reveals the tumor location and extent [10]; defining the nerve of origin is best done on coronal images by following it up to the orbital apex [3].

Orbital schwannomas are well circumscribed, isointense on T1-weighted images, and heterogeneously hyperintense on T2-weighted images relative to the brain cortex; they show avid and heterogeneous enhancement after intravenous gadolinium contrast medium [5, 10].

The MRI signal heterogeneity reflects the solid and cystic components of the tumor. No consistent MR appearance can be attributed to histopathologically delineated areas (Antoni A and B); regardless of cell type, central fibrocollagenous components appear T2 hypointense while the peripheral myxoid components appear T2 hyperintense, often giving these lesions a target appearance [3]. Degenerative changes such as cysts, calcifications, and hemorrhage are described in long-standing tumors [5].

MRI features can help in differentiating schwannoma from cavernous malformation. Schwannomas are usually T2 hyperintense, although heterogeneous, a pattern that differs from the relatively homogeneous pattern of cavernous malformations which show progressive enhancement on delayed venous phase images [10].

5.5.5.5 Neurofibroma

Neurofibromas are benign, slow growing, peripheral nerve tumors composed of fibroblasts, schwann cells, and axons [10]. They are associated with neurofibromatosis in approximately 12% of cases. Orbital neurofibromas may demonstrate localized, diffuse (solitary), or plexiform growth pattern [10], the latter being most common and pathognomonic for NF 1 [3].

Like schwannomas, orbital neurofibromas are more commonly superior extraconal lesions, arising from the sensory trigeminal nerve branches [3, 10] and causing downward displacement of the globe.

The distinction between these two entities is often not possible on imaging. The lack of a capsule makes solitary subtypes relatively less well defined; they appear heterogeneous on both T1- and T2-w images with heterogeneous contrast enhancement [6]. The cystic/mucinous components favor the diagnosis of schwannoma [3].

Patient history may be help to diagnosis, since neurofibroma is specific for NF 1 instead schwannoma is more characteristic of NF 2.

5.5.5.6 Orbital Plexiform Neurofibroma

Plexiform neurofibroma is the most common type of peripheral nerve sheath tumor occurring almost exclusively in children with NF 1 [5, 8, 10]. It accounts for 1–2% of all orbital tumors, mainly in the first decade of life [8].

Plexiform neurofibromas usually presents with nodular periorbital masses, causing loss of vision and proptosis. Progressive glaucoma, optic nerve atrophy, and blindness are reported complications [8].

These trans-spatial complex tumors that involve cranial or peripheral nerve branches can be seen within the orbit, periorbital region, scalp, temporal fossa, and skull base [5]. The infiltrative serpentine masses extend in both the intraconal and extraconal compartments [8].

Unlike schwannoma, it is not possible to distinguish the nerve fibers separately from the tumor that shows nerve fascicles irregularly expanded by myxoid accumulation, tumoral schwann cells, fibroblasts, and collagen fibers [8]. The tumor may cross the tissue planes and may involve large portions of the face.

Imaging studies show a typical orbital and periorbital infiltrative soft tissue, often appearing as a conglomerate of wormlike masses ("bag of worms") with more extensive interspatial spread, such as lymphangioma [3, 5, 10]. Plexiform neurofibroma shows heterogeneous signal, typically hypointense on T1-w, hyperintense on T2-w images, with variable contrast enhancement [8]; the nodular masses appear hyperintense with central low signal on T2-w images ("target sign"), considered a distinctive finding [3, 5, 8]; mixed or increased diffusion is also evident. Alternatively, the tumor may also appear amorphous with ill-defined margins [8].

Orbital plexiform neurofibromas are associated with ipsilateral sphenoid wing dysplasia, osseous thinning, and expansion of the middle cranial fossa [5]; this bone defect is called "Harlequin eye" appearance [8]. The bony dysplasia may cause optic nerve compression with proptosis and buphthalmos.

DTI with tractography reconstruction is increasingly used for the pre-operative mapping of neurogenic tumors originating in the head and neck, such as schwannomas and neurofibromas; it can accurately detect alterations of involved nerve fascicles, such as displacement, stretching, bowing, or rupture [8].

Other orbital tumors may mimic plexiform neurofibroma including infantile/capillary hemangioma and rhabdomyosarcoma; however, they are not associated features of NF 1 [8].

The risk of malignant transformation for orbital plexiform neurofibroma in NF 1 is about 10% [8]; suspected features of malignancy are occurrence of pain, rapid tumor growth compared to prior imaging, and presence of soft tissue or bony destruction [3]. FDG-PET CT and MRI PET are sensitive and specific tools to detect the sarcomatous transformation [8].

5.5.5.7 Capillary Hemangioma

Capillary hemangioma is the most common orbit lesion in infancy [3]. It presents a proliferative phase with enlargement in the first year, followed by an involutional phase that may last 7–10 years.

Capillary hemangioma is commonly seen in the orbital preseptal region, although it may occasionally extend into the extraconal compartment. When large, the lesion may cause bony remodeling with orbital expansion [3]. It usually demonstrates T1-hypointense and T2-hyperintense signal with intervening fibrous septa, appearing as interspersed T2 hypointense bands and multiple serpiginous flow voids reflecting increased vascularity, with intense postcontrast enhancement. In the involutional phase, fatty replacement occurs with increase of T1 hyperintense signal and nonenhancing components of the lesion.

Screening of the brain is also useful since the orbital capillary hemangioma may be a part of the posterior fossa brain malformations, hemangioma, arterial lesions, cardiac and eye abnormalities [3].

5.5.5.8 Venolymphatic Malformations

Venolymphatic malformation may be superficial or deep. Deep and small orbital lesions are commonly extraconal, but can become multispatial when larger. They are characterized by cystic (lymphangiomatous) spaces and variable, more solid appearing (venous) components. The cystic spaces may contain hemorrhages of varying ages causing fluid-fluid levels. They appear T2 hyperintense with acute blood showing T2 hypointense and subacute blood products demonstrating characteristic T1 hyperintense signal. Solid components rarely show the presence of phleboliths. The cystic components may present rim enhancement, while the venous components show more homogeneous enhancement. Perilesional fat stranding may be present in case of acute presentation [3].

5.5.5.9 Orbital Metastases

Orbital metastases are relatively uncommon, but their detection has increased in recent decades, due to the improved treatments with increasing of the median survival of the neoplastic patients [13, 14]. Breast cancer is the most common type of neoplasm metastasizing to the orbit [3], followed by prostate carcinoma, melanoma, and lung cancer [6, 13].

Metastatic disease may infiltrate orbital muscles, fat, and bone. Some malignancies show distinct tissue selectivity in metastatic disease, with specific localizations to orbital and periorbital tissues; for instance, prostate cancer tends toward bone, breast to orbital fat, melanoma and carcinoid tumor to muscle [10, 14].

Lateral (40%), superior (30%), medial (20%), and inferior (10%) quadrants are affected by metastatic tumors with decreasing frequency; the anterior orbit, adjacent to the lymphatic rich conjunctiva and eyelids, is mostly involved [14]. Besides, secondary involvement may also occur by direct invasion of the orbit by cancers of the nasopharynx, paranasal sinuses, or cranium [3].

Clinical manifestation consists in rapid onset of proptosis and motility disturbances, also with frequent pain and decreased vision [10]. A paradoxical enophthalmos is observed in 10% of metastatic orbital lesions, most often from scirrhous breast and gastrointestinal tract tumors, with infiltrative and fibrotic contraction of orbital fat, leading to posterior globe retraction [10].

The morphology and appearance of orbital metastases depend on the primary tumor and may range from solid homogeneous lesions to mixed solid-cystic lesions or almost completely cystic, with variable enhancement patterns [3] (Fig. 5.15). They may result in a well-defined round or fusiform mass involving the extraocular muscles with variable signal intensity and contrast enhancement [3]. The retrobulbar fat demonstrates diffuse enhancement with abnormally heterogeneous T1 and T2 hypointensity, due to fibrotic infiltration; this pattern may also be observed with metastatic scirrhous carcinomas [10].

Differentiating orbital metastasis from nonneoplastic infiltrative processes may pose a diagnostic challenge. A solitary lesion may be difficult to differentiate from other masses, while multiplicity is an indicator of metastasis [3].

Differential diagnostic considerations include thyroid disease-related, which is often bilateral and spares tendinous insertions, as well as orbital pseudotumor, which is typically painful and involves the tendinous insertion [10]; granulomatous disease, such as sarcoidosis, can involve the extraocular muscles, optic nerve, optic chiasm, or lacrimal gland, and may also mimic metastatic disease.

5.5.6 Mass Lesions of the Lacrimal Gland

Lacrimal gland lesions represent 5–14% of biopsied orbital masses; approximately half are benign and half are malignant [3, 10]. Most tumors occur in the deeper orbital lobe rather than the anterior palpebral lobe [6]. Mass lesions of the lacrimal gland may be classified as epithelial and nonepithelial [8, 10].

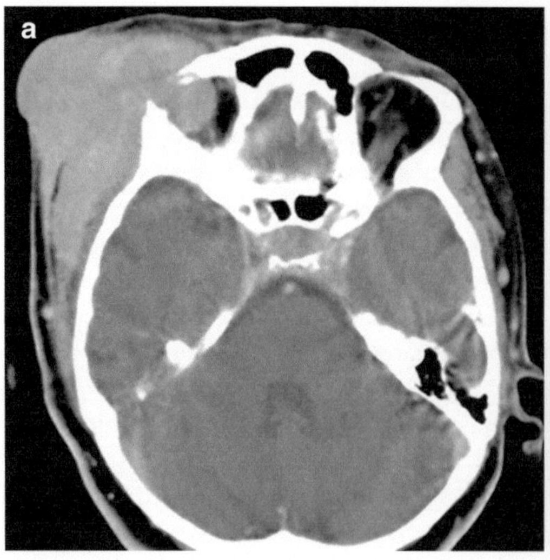
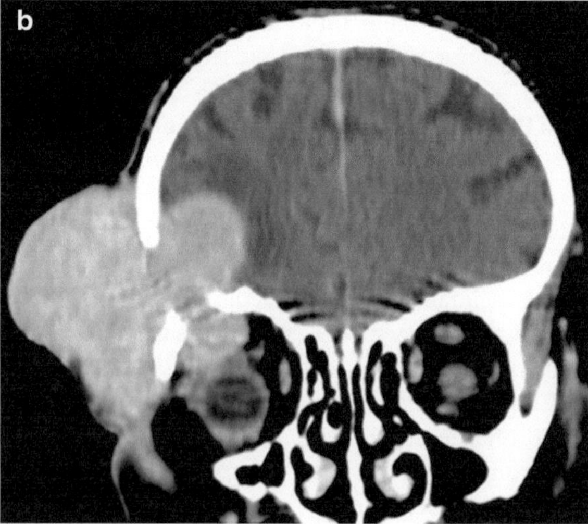

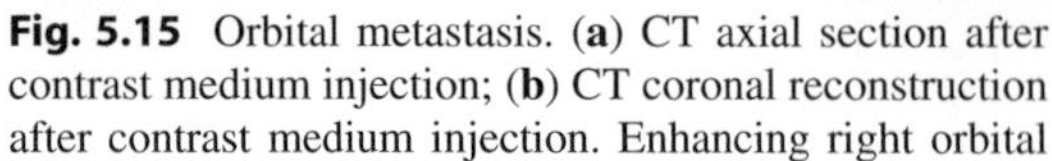

Fig. 5.15 Orbital metastasis. (**a**) CT axial section after contrast medium injection; (**b**) CT coronal reconstruction after contrast medium injection. Enhancing right orbital soft tissue mass leading to bone erosion with intracranial and infratemporal invasion. (**Original to the authors**)

5.5.6.1 Pleomorphic Adenoma

Pleomorphic adenoma, also called benign mixed tumor, originates mainly from the orbital lobe of the ductal system [8] and is the most common benign neoplasm of the lacrimal gland, accounting for up to 57% of epithelial lesions [13].

This tumor occurs in the fourth or fifth decade of life, without gender predilection. Clinical signs include a painless, slow-growing mass in the lateral orbit, causing downward displacement of the globe and proptosis usually persisting for more than 12 months [8].

Pleomorphic adenoma is an encapsulated round tumor, consisting of interspersed epithelial and stromal components; necrosis, hyalinization, myxoid, and mucinous degeneration may be seen. Larger lesions may be heterogeneous due to cystic degeneration, hemorrhage, serous or mucous collections, or necrosis. This results in moderate and heterogeneous or homogenous contrast enhancement [8].

Bone remodeling, typically with a smooth concavity at the lacrimal fossa and calcifications may be seen on bone window CT. Bone erosion, infiltration of the adjacent orbital tissue, and poorly defined margins and nodularity are rare and suggestive of malignancy [8, 10]. ADC values are sensitive in differentiating pleomorphic adenoma from malignant tumors of the lacrimal gland (Fig. 5.16).

5.5.6.2 Adenoid Cystic Carcinoma

Approximately, 50% of epithelial lacrimal gland tumors are malignant, including adenoid cystic carcinoma, mucoepidermoid carcinoma, adenocarcinoma, squamous cell carcinoma, and undifferentiated carcinoma types, such as the similar secretory carcinoma of salivary origin [5].

Adenoid cystic carcinoma is the most common malignancy of the lacrimal gland. Most patients present with a hard mass in the upper lateral orbit, often with pain, due to perineural spread or bony invasion [8].

Adenoid cystic carcinoma appears hypointense on T1-weighted images, hypo- or hyperintense on T2-weighted images with prominent contrast enhancement [8]. T1-weighted FS contrast enhancement MRI is ideal for tumor staging and for evaluating perineural spread. In general, most adenoid cystic carcinomas show perineural spread at microscopic examination; however, radiologically, perineural spread may remain undetected on the radiological studies unless involvement of major nerve trunks occurs, such as the supraorbital nerve [11].

Early lesions may be indistinguishable from pleomorphic adenoma (well-circumscribed margin without bony destruction) but intratumoral calcifications are more common in undifferentiated epithelial tumors [11].

Irregular tumor borders with distortion of the globe and orbital contents may be seen in patients with more advanced disease [10]. Some authors report mean ADC value of significantly lower than other lesions like pleomorphic adenoma, but significantly higher than lymphomas; thus, ADC values can help in differential diagnosis [8].

Adenoid cystic carcinoma is hypermetabolic on PET CT, which is useful in detecting both the primary lesion and distant metastases [8].

5.5.6.3 Lymphoproliferative Disorders

Lymphoproliferative disorders account for up to 50% of nonepithelial lacrimal lesions; they are more frequently malignant lymphoma of non-Hodgkin B-cell type, although they are only 1% of biopsied orbital masses [10].

Lacrimal gland lymphoma occurs mainly in the seventh decade of life as a painless mass in the superotemporal orbit.

The imaging features are a nonspecific, homogeneously enhancing mass at the lacrimal fossa usually without bone erosion, and displacing the eye globe. The older patient age, the presence of lymphadenopathy elsewhere, and lack of osseous remodeling are all suggestive of lymphoma. Lower ADC values may also be indicative of lymphoma, respect to other lacrimal gland diseases [10].

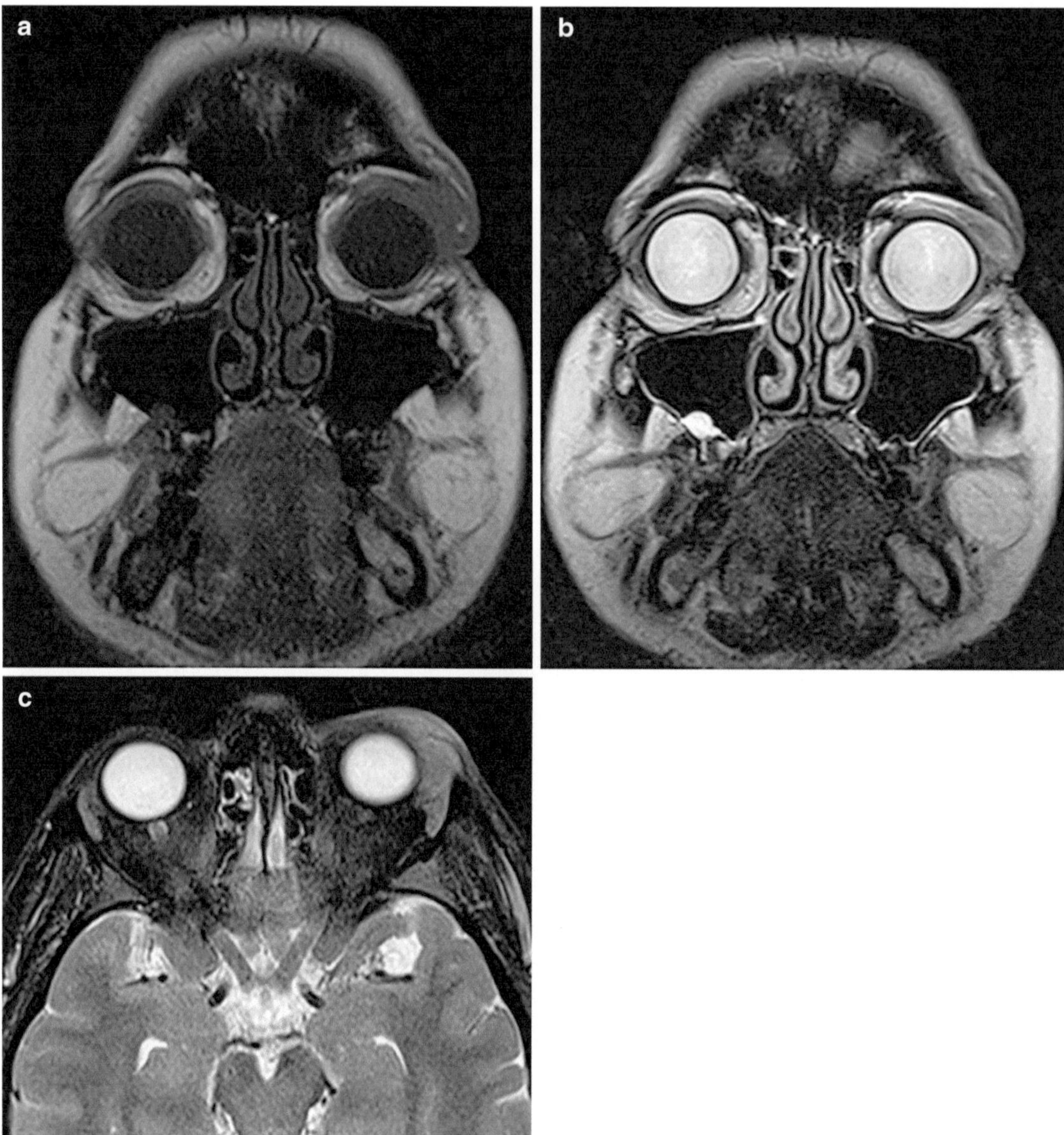

Fig. 5.16 Pleomorphic adenoma. (**a**) T1-weighted section on coronal plane; (**b**) T2-weighted section on coronal plane; (**c**) STIR section on axial plane. Well-circumscribed, oval lesion in the left superotemporal orbit that did not extend beyond the equator. (**Original to the authors**)

5.6 Conclusion

A wide variety of tumoral and non-tumoral mass lesions may be encountered in the cranio-orbital region; thus, imaging is essential to their correct definition.

MRI is especially valuable for assessing extent, characterization, and precise location of the lesions, the involved orbital compartments (intraconal, extraconal, orbital apex, perineural spread), and the intraconal extension. CT better shows calcifications and bony erosion especially in malignant tumors.

Knowledge of the most common orbit-cranial lesions, their clinical presentation, imaging appearance, and key features may help to the correct diagnosis and to the correct management.

References

1. Nagesh CP, Rao R, Hiremath SB, Honavar SG. Magnetic resonance imaging of the orbit, part 1: basic principles and radiological approach. Indian J Ophthalmol. 2021;69:2574–84. https://doi.org/10.4103/ijo.IJO_3141_20.
2. Gala F. Magnetic resonance imaging of optic nerve. Indian J Radiol Imaging. 2015;25:421–38. https://doi.org/10.4103/0971-3026.169462.
3. Nagesh CP, Rao R, Hiremath SB, Honavar SG. Magnetic resonance imaging of the orbit, part 2: characterization of orbital pathologies. Indian J Ophthalmol. 2021;69:2585–616. https://doi.org/10.4103/ijo.IJO_904_21.
4. Mombaerts I, Ramberg I, Coupland SE, Heegaard S. Diagnosis of orbital mass lesions: clinical, radiological, and pathological recommendations. Surv Ophthalmol. 2019;64(6):741–56. https://doi.org/10.1016/j.survophthal.2019.06.006.
5. Joseph AK, Guerin JB, Eckel LJ, et al. Imaging findings of pediatric orbital masses and tumor mimics. Radiographics. 2022;42:880–97. https://doi.org/10.1148/rg.210116.
6. Kılıç M, Özöner B, Aydın L, Özdemir B, Yılmaz İ, Müslüman AM, Yılmaz A, Çavuşoğlu H, Aydın Y. Cranio-orbital tumors: clinical results and a surgical approach. Sisli Etfal Hastan Tip Bul. 2019;53(3):240–6. https://doi.org/10.14744/SEMB.2018.82698.
7. Khan SN, Sepahdari AR. Orbital masses: CT and MRI of common vascular lesions, benign tumors, and malignancies. Saudi J Ophthalmol. 2012;26(4):373–83. https://doi.org/10.1016/j.sjopt.2012.08.001.
8. Purohit BS, Vargas MI, Angeliki A, et al. Orbital tumours and tumour-like lesions: exploring the armamentarium of multiparametric imaging. Insights Imaging. 2016;7(1):43–68. https://doi.org/10.1007/s13244-015-0443-8.
9. Ferreira TA, Saraiva P, Genders SW, Buchem MV, Luyten GPM, Beenakker J-W. CT and MR imaging of orbital inflammation. Neuroradiology. 2018;60:1253–66. https://doi.org/10.1007/s00234-018-2103-4.
10. Tailor TD, Gupta D, Dalley RW, Keene CD, Anzai Y. Orbital neoplasms in adults: clinical, radiologic, and pathologic review. Radiographics. 2013;33(6):1739–58. https://doi.org/10.1148/rg.336135502.
11. Karcioglu ZA. Overview and imaging of orbital tumors. In: Chaugule S, Honavar S, Finger P, editors. Surgical ophthalmic oncology. Cham: Springer; 2019. https://doi.org/10.1007/978-3-030-18757-6_10.
12. Sheng J, Li Q, Liu T, Wang X. Cerebrospinal fluid dynamics along the optic nerve. Front Neurol. 2022;13:931523. https://doi.org/10.3389/fneur.2022.931523.
13. Conforti R, Cirillo M, Sardaro A, Caiazzo G, et al. Dilated perivascular spaces and fatigue: is there a link? Magnetic resonance retrospective 3Tesla study. Neuroradiology. 2016;58(9):859–66. https://doi.org/10.1007/s00234-016-1711-0. Epub 2016 Jul 16. PMID: 27423658.
14. Conforti R, Marrone V, Sardaro A, Di Maio N, et al. The cerebral perivascular spaces: review of the literature on diffuse or focal expansion. Recenti Prog Med. 2013;104(7–8):291–4. https://doi.org/10.1701/1315.14562. PMID: 24042394.
15. Menon S, Sandesh O, Anand D, Menon G. Spheno-orbital meningiomas: optimizing visual outcome. J Neurosci Rural Pract. 2020;11(3):385–94. https://doi.org/10.1055/s-0040-1709270.
16. Badakere A, Patil-Chhablani P. Orbital apex syndrome: a review. Eye Brain. 2019;11:63–72. https://doi.org/10.2147/EB.S180190. PMID: 31849556; PMCID: PMC6913296.
17. Haddar S, Nèji H, Dabbèche C, et al. Fronto-orbital osteoma. Answer to the e-quid "unilateral exophthalmos in a 30-year-old man" diagnostic and interventional. Imaging. 2013;94:119–22. https://doi.org/10.1016/j.diii.2012.05.005.

Part III

Surgical Approaches to the Cranio-Orbital Region

The Supraorbital Pterional Approach

Francesco Maiuri ⓘ, Giuseppe Mariniello ⓘ, and Sergio Corvino

6.1 Introduction

The approach to the cranio-orbital lesions is evolved over the years with the aims to obtain better control of the intraorbital structures and lesser brain retraction.

In the first years of the past century, some neurosurgeons [1, 2] proposed resecting the supraorbital arch in the frontal approach. In 1982, Jane et al. [3] reviewed this approach and considered it the best supraorbital route for orbital tumors. Al-Mefty and Fox [4] suggested a supero-lateral approach and reconstruction to improve the orbital exposure. The pterional approach, first described by Heuer [5], was refined by Yasargil [6], who suggested drilling of the sphenoid ridge and occasional removal of part of the orbital ridge and roof.

All the above cited approaches are not adequate for large tumors extending in both intracranial and intraorbital compartments. To this aim, Al-Mefty [7] proposed the supraorbital pterional approach, which conjugates the pterional approach with removal of the lateral orbital wall and roof.

6.2 Surgical Technique

6.2.1 Patient Positioning and Skin Flap

The patient is positioned in the operating table with the head fixed at the Mayfield head holder and rotated 30° toward the contralateral side. The neck is slightly extended, allowing spontaneous retraction of the frontal lobe.

The scalp incision (Fig. 6.1) begins at level of the zygomatic arch, 1 cm anterior to the tragus, then it proceeds up to the superior temporal line and curves anterior and medially, up to the midline, about 2 cm posterior to the hairline. The temporal muscle flap is detached from the temporal fossa and the lateral orbital wall is exposed; a small muscle margin is left attached to the bone to be used for the muscle closure. During the scalp dissection, the periosteum and galea must be preserved with the aim of being used over an eventual defect of the frontal sinus. The frontal and supraorbital nerves must be preserved to avoid paralysis of the frontal muscle and anesthesia in the forehead.

F. Maiuri (✉) · G. Mariniello · S. Corvino
Division of Neurosurgery, Department of
Neurosciences, Reproductive and
Odontostomatological Sciences, University of Naples
"Federico II", Naples, Italy
e-mail: frmaiuri@unina.it; giumarin@unina.it

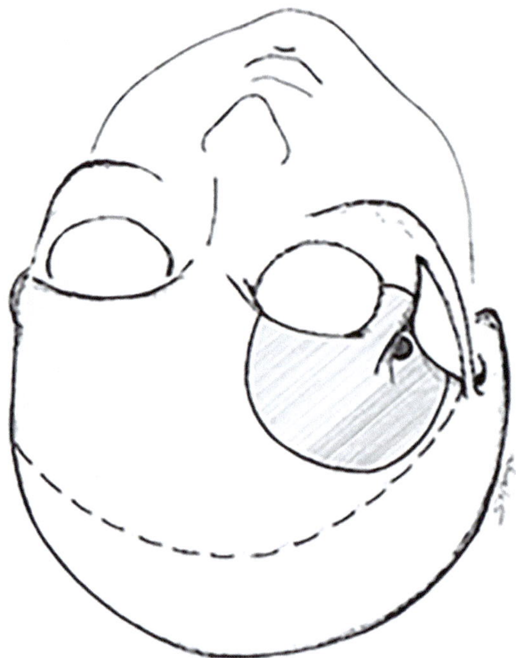

Fig. 6.1 Schematic draw of the scalp incision and craniotomy of the right supraorbital pterional approach. (Courtesy of Simona Buonamassa, MD)

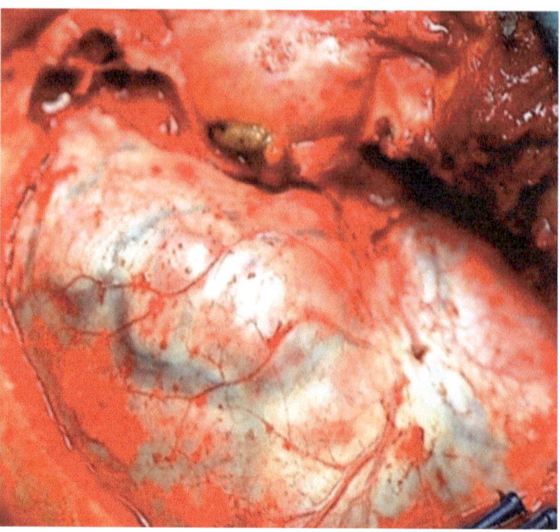

Fig. 6.2 Intraoperative image after the craniotomy: the superior and lateral orbital walls and the frontotemporal region are well exposed

6.2.2 Craniotomy

The craniotomy (Figs. 6.1 and 6.2) is performed by using 2 or 3 burr holes. A craniotome is used to create a fronto-temporal bone flap centered on the sphenoid wing that exposes the anterior and middle cranial fossa floors and temporal tip. Through a burr hole over the frontal sinus an osteotomy is made posterior to the orbital rime to detach the orbital roof. In this way, when the bone flap is elevated, the orbital roof remains attached to the flap itself. During the flap elevation, careful dissection of the dura mater and periorbita is necessary to avoid interruption. The superior orbital rime remains intact. When tumor invasion of the orbital roof and rime is evidenced, these structures may be resected using a rongeur. If the frontal sinus has been opened, the mucosa must be exenterated and the sinus must be filled with antibiotics and occluded by cottonoids.

6.2.3 Management of the Skull Base Structures

The skull base structures, including orbital apex, optic canal, optic strut, anterior clinoid and superior orbital fissure, must be managed by microsurgical technique and the use of a high-speed diamond drill, and by extradural route. The orbital apex may be exposed by extending posteriorly the resection of the orbital roof. The optic canal must be opened by drilling its wall with a diamond drill during continuous washing, to avoid excessive heating. No attempt must be made to use rongeurs in the optic canal, because this maneuver may result in optic nerve damage.

The supraorbital pterional approach allows good exposure and opening of the superior and lateral walls of the optic canal and the optic strut; on the other hand, the inferomedial wall is less controlled [8, 9]. Thus, the circumferential decompression of the optic canal may be accomplished with an anterior clinoidectomy and removal of the optic strut.

The resection of the skull base structures depends on the direction of tumor growth and orbital location. If the tumor is in the apex or in the optic canal, the entire orbital roof must be removed, and the optic canal must adequately be opened. If the tumor enters to the orbit through its lateral wall without involvement of the optic canal, it may not be opened [8–11].

6.2.4 Incision of the Dura Mater and Periorbita

The incision of the dura mater and periorbita must follow rigorous criteria to obtain good exposure and to allow watertight closure. The dura mater is opened in a semicircular fashion, then the dural flap is bisected by a second dural incision that points toward the optic canal. The dural incision along the optic canal must be made by leaving a cuff of the dura around the optic nerve for an adequate closure [12]. The incision of the anulus of Zinn and the periorbita must be made medial to the levator and superior rectus muscles to avoid injury to the oculomotor nerve.

6.2.5 Reconstruction

The closure of the dura mater must be watertight also over the optic canal, when preserved. The frontal sinus must be obliterated by muscle tissue and covered by a galeal flap mobilized and sutured to the dura mater and reinforced by fibrin glue.

We do not reconstruct the orbital roof in our cases. This usually does not result in cosmetic problems. The bone flap is replaced and fixed by wires and the temporal muscle is sutured to the small muscle margin left attached to the bone. Then, the skin is closed in layers.

Postoperatively, moderate periorbital ecchymosis and slight-to-moderate swelling occur for several days.

6.3 Complications

Complications of the supraorbital pterional approach may be observed during both intraoperative and post-operative periods.

Intraoperative complications may occur in all phases of the approach. During the turning of the skin flap, the frontal and supraorbital nerves may be injured, resulting in frontal nerve palsy or decreased sensation of the forehead, respectively; it may be avoided by carefully dissecting the nerves from the subcutaneous tissues and supraorbital notch.

At the elevation of the bone flap, the frontal sinus may accidentally be opened; this often results in post-operative cerebrospinal fluid (CSF) rhinorrhea. In such event, the careful closure of the defect by periosteum and galea flaps must be achieved.

Injuries to the cranial nerves may occur during the bone resection at the skull base and/or at the entry into the orbit. The injury to the optic nerve may be due to excessive retraction, particularly in presence of adherent tumors, to the occlusion of the central retinal artery, and particularly to heat transmission during drilling of the optic nerve canal. This complication is serious and not an exception (5% in the series of Maroon et al. [13]). It may be avoided by careful microsurgical drilling using a high-speed drill and a diamond bur with continuous irrigation. The injury to the oculomotor nerves may occur at the superior orbital fissure, when opened, or within the orbit. This complication may be prevented by avoiding undue retraction of levator and superior rectus muscles and by approaching the intraorbital tumor component medially, between the superior rectus and levator and medial rectus muscles.

Intraoperative bleeding from the internal carotid and ophthalmic arteries, although very rare, may occur mainly at the reoperations for tumor recurrence.

Postoperative complications include pulsating proptosis, enophthalmos, hematoma, CSF rhinorrhea, and meningitis.

Pulsating proptosis is rare and may be due to cerebral edema and CSF; remission usually occurs within 1–2 months. Enophthalmos may occur after resection of large tumors with significant residual cavity, but it is not significant. In exceptional cases, where the cosmetic problem is severe, the reoperation for orbital repair may be evaluated.

Postoperative intraorbital hematoma is rare and results from insufficient hemostasis of the surgical field. As already discussed, moderate periorbital ecchymosis lacks pathological significance, while severe chemosis should suggest a hematoma. The evacuation of the blood collection is often required to prevent eye damage.

The CSF rhinorrhea may occur because of accidental opening of the frontal and/or ethmoidal sinus or not correct repair of the sinus wall after resection of an invading tumor. Its incidence is about 3%. Most CSF fistulas undergo remission by lumbar puncture and antibiotic therapy, as done for other surgical approaches and sites. Cases where the CSF leak persists with the risk of meningitis must undergo reoperation with careful closure of the communication.

6.4 Supraorbital Pterional Versus Other Approaches: Advantages and Limits

The choice of the best surgical approach to the cranio-orbital mass lesions depends on several factors, including route of the orbital spread, intraorbital location, and mass size [14–16] (Table 6.1).

Table 6.1 The supraorbital pterional approach versus other approaches: advantages and limits

Approach	Exposure	Advantages	Limits
Supraorbital pterional	– Supero-lateral orbital compartment – Medial orbital compartment above the optic nerve – Orbital apex – Anterior and middle fossae	– No damage to the orbital structures – Less risk of enophthalmos	– Need of craniotomy – Bad exposure of the infratemporal fossa and infero-medial orbital region
Mini-pterional	– Lateral compartment – Optic canal – Orbital apex – Middle fossa	– Smaller incision – Smaller craniotomy	– Smaller working corridor – Poor orbital medial exposure
Supraorbital	– Anterior cranial fossa – Superior orbital compartment	– Minimal disruption of the temporalis muscle	– Large frontotemporal skin incision – Risk of injury to the frontal branch of the facial nerve
Supraorbital "Keyhole"	– Anterior cranial fossa – Superior orbital compartment	– Minimally invasive approach through eyebrow incision	– Limited maneuverability of instruments – Cosmetic damage of the eyebrow
Lateral orbito-cranial	– Superolateral orbital compartment – Lateral wall of the optic canal – Orbital apex – Temporal fossa	– Limited orbitotomy – Wide exposure of the superolateral orbital compartment	– Poor control of the inferomedial orbital compartment
Fronto-temporal-orbito-zygomatic (FTOZ)	– Orbital cavity – Orbital apex – Middle fossa – Infratemporal fossa	– Enhanced exposure – Less brain retraction	– More invasive – Periorbital hematoma
Endoscopic endonasal	– Medial orbital compartment – Medial aspect of the orbital apex	– Minimally invasive – No orbitotomy – No craniotomy – No scar	– Limited exposure of the orbital apex – Risk of CSF leak and infection
Endoscopic transorbital	– Inferomedial and lateral orbital compartments – Good exposure of the optic canal and superior orbital fissure	– Less invasive – No orbitotomy – No craniotomy – No scar – Less distance to the orbital target	– Poor sphenoid wing, middle fossa and orbital apex exposure

The **supraorbital pterional approach** provides good exposure of the lateral, superior, and partly medial orbital compartments, anterior and middle cranial fossa, orbital apex, optic canal, and superior orbital fissure [4, 8–10, 17, 18]. Its limits include the need for a large craniotomy, the bad exposure of the infratemporal fossa, and the infero-medial orbital region below the medial side of the optic foramen. Thus, mass lesions with significant infratemporal extension require a frontotemporal-orbitozygomatic approach; on the other hand, mass lesions of the medial intra-orbital compartment with significant extension in the ethmoidal sinus may require a medial transorbital approach [15, 19].

Several other approaches may be used for cranio-orbital mass lesions. These include the mini-pterional craniotomy, the frontotemporal-orbitozygomatic approach, the lateral supraorbital, supraorbital key-hole and lateral orbital-cranial approaches, the endoscopic endonasal and transorbital approaches.

The **mini-pterional craniotomy** [20] is a less invasive modification of the standard pterional craniotomy [18, 21, 22]. However, the smaller craniotomy size may limit the space for frontal and temporal lobe mobilization in larger lesions. Moreover, the exposure at the medial orbital roof and inferolateral orbital wall is significantly more limited. Thus, the mini-pterional approach may be used only for small cranio-orbital lesions with no or limited extension in the medial orbital compartment.

The **frontotemporal-orbitozygomatic** approach is a frontotemporal approach with orbital roof opening associated to the resection of the zygomatic process [23, 24]. It allows good exposure of the orbital cavity, orbital apex, and middle fossa; the downward extension of the bone resection allows to expose the infratemporal fossa [25].

This approach enhances the surgical exposure and allows less brain retraction. However, it is more invasive and carries the risk of periorbital hematoma and enophthalmos. Thus, in the cranio-orbital surgery, this approach should be limited to more extensive tumors, mainly to those with significant extension into the infratemporal fossa [10].

The **supraorbital approach** is a variant of the pterional approach with no removal of the temporal bone [3]. It includes a standard pterional skin incision to provide supraorbital frontal bone exposure with minimal disruption of the temporalis muscle [15, 26]. Removal of the orbital roof and superior orbital rime allows to expose the orbital cavity.

The supraorbital approach provides good access to the anterior cranial fossa and superior orbital compartment; on the other hand, the access to the lateral intraorbital compartment is less easy. This approach may be used for cranio-orbital lesions extending in the superior compartment of the orbital region. It also carries the risk of injury to the frontal branch of the facial nerve.

The **supraorbital keyhole approach**, first introduced in 1998 by Perneczsky [27], is realized through an incision within the eyebrow and a supraorbital enlarged keyhole. The minimal soft-tissue dissection and the small craniotomy size reduce postoperative orbital and frontotemporal swelling [28]. The limited exposure and the risk of frontal sinus contamination are the main disadvantages.

This approach, more limited than the previously cited, may be used for treating orbital intraconal and extraconal lesions superior to the optic nerve.

The **lateral orbito-cranial approach** [29] includes a lateral orbitotomy and a small craniotomy at the level of the temporal fossa. It allows good exposure of the superolateral intraorbital compartments, the lateral wall of the optic canal, and the anterior temporal region [30, 31].

This approach is useful for cranio-orbital mass lesions located at the lateral compartment of the orbital cavity also when involving the wall of the optic canal [29]. On the other hand, the mass lesions extending medially to the axis of the optic nerve are not sufficiently controlled.

The **endoscopic approaches** to the orbit include the transorbital, the transsphenoidal endonasal, and the combined endonasal-transorbital approaches. The transorbital approaches [32–34] are realized by palpebral incision through medial and/or lateral surgical corridors; they allow to expose the sphenoid wing, the roof of the optic canal, and the superior orbital fissure. The endoscopic endonasal approach provides exposure to the inferomedial orbital region and the inferomedial wall of the optic canal [35–37].

Although these approaches are less invasive than the cranio-orbital microsurgical ones, they are often too limited for large cranio-orbital mass lesions.

6.5 Conclusion

The supraorbital pterional approach is, in our experience, the most useful approach to the cranio-orbital mass lesions of middle and large size. Those located in the lateral orbital compartment may be approached through a less invasive lateral orbito-cranial approach. On the other hand, the indication to the fronto-temporal-orbito-zygomatic approach may be limited to more extensive mass lesions with significant infratemporal extension. The significant tumor extension in the ethmoidal sinus and below the medial wall of the optic canal, although often exposed by the supraorbital pterional approach, may require a medial transorbital approach. The less invasive endoscopic endonasal and transorbital approaches may be used for treating not large mass lesions.

References

1. McArthur L. An aseptic surgical access to the pituitary body and its neighborhood. JAMA. 1912;58:2009–11.
2. Frazier CHI. An approach to the hypophysis through the anterior cranial fossa. Ann Surg. 1913;57(2):145–50. https://doi.org/10.1097/00000658-191302000-00001.
3. Jane JA, Park TS, Pobereskin LH, Winn HR, Butler AB. The supraorbital approach: technical note. Neurosurgery. 1982;11(4):537–42.
4. Al-Mefty O, Fox JL. Superolateral orbital exposure and reconstruction. Surg Neurol. 1985;23(6):609–13. https://doi.org/10.1016/0090-3019(85)90012-6.
5. Heuer G. Surgical experience with an intracranial approach to chasmal lesions. Arch Surg. 1920;1:368–81.
6. Yasargil M, Fox J, Ray M. The operative approach to aneurysms of the anterior communicating artery. In: Advances and technical standards in neurosurgery. Berlin: Springer-Verlag; 1975.
7. Al-Mefty O. Supraorbital-pterional approach to skull base lesions. Neurosurgery. 1987;21(4):474–7. https://doi.org/10.1227/00006123-198710000-00006.
8. Mariniello G, de Divitiis O, Bonavolontà G, Maiuri F. Surgical unroofing of the optic canal and visual outcome in basal meningiomas. Acta Neurochir. 2013;155(1):77–84. https://doi.org/10.1007/s00701-012-1485-z.
9. Mariniello G, Bonavolontà G, Tranfa F, Maiuri F. Management of the optic canal invasion and visual outcome in spheno-orbital meningiomas. Clin Neurol Neurosurg. 2013;115(9):1615–20. https://doi.org/10.1016/j.clineuro.2013.02.012.
10. Mariniello G, Maiuri F, Strianese D, Donzelli R, Iuliano A, Tranfa F, et al. Spheno-orbital meningiomas: surgical approaches and outcome according to the intraorbital tumor extent. Zentralbl Neurochir. 2008;69(4):175–81. https://doi.org/10.1055/s-2008-1077077.
11. Mariniello G, de Divitiis O, Corvino S, Strianese D, Iuliano A, Bonavolontà G, et al. Recurrences of spheno-orbital meningiomas: risk factors and management. World Neurosurg. 2022;161:e514. https://doi.org/10.1016/j.wneu.2022.02.048.
12. Mariniello G, Maiuri F. Letter: mini-pterional craniotomy and extradural clinoidectomy for clinoid meningioma: optimization of exposure using augmented reality template: 2-dimensional operative video. Oper Neurosurg (Hagerstown). 2020;20(1):E75. https://doi.org/10.1093/ons/opaa353.
13. Maroon JC, Kazim M, Kennerdell JS. Orbital meningiomas and other tumors. In: Brain surgery: complications avoidance and management, vol. 1. London: Churchill Livingstone; 1992.
14. Paluzzi A, Gardner PA, Fernandez-Miranda JC, Tormenti MJ, Stefko ST, Snyderman CH, et al. "Round-the-clock" surgical access to the orbit. J Neurol Surg B Skull Base. 2015;76(1):12–24. https://doi.org/10.1055/s-0033-1360580.
15. Abou-Al-Shaar H, Krisht KM, Cohen MA, Abunimer AM, Neil JA, Karsy M, et al. Cranio-orbital and orbitocranial approaches to orbital and intracranial disease: eye-opening approaches for neurosurgeons. Front Surg. 2020;7:1. https://doi.org/10.3389/fsurg.2020.00001.
16. Abussuud Z, Ahmed S, Paluzzi A. Surgical approaches to the orbit: a neurosurgical perspective. J Neurol Surg B Skull Base. 2020;81(4):385–408. https://doi.org/10.1055/s-0040-1713941.
17. Andrade-Barazarte H, Jägersberg M, Belkhair S, Tymianski R, Turel MK, Schaller K, et al. The extended lateral supraorbital approach and extradural anterior clinoidectomy through a frontopterio-orbital window: technical note and pilot surgical series. World Neurosurg. 2017;100:159–66. https://doi.org/10.1016/j.wneu.2016.12.087.
18. Martínez-Pérez R, Albonette-Felicio T, Hardesty DA, Prevedello DM. Comparative anatomical analysis between the minipterional and supraorbital

approaches. J Neurosurg. 2020;134(3):1276–84. https://doi.org/10.3171/2019.12.JNS193196.

19. Galbraith JE, Sullivan JH. Decompression of the perioptic meninges for relief of papilledema. Am J Ophthalmol. 1973;76(5):687–92. https://doi.org/10.1016/0002-9394(73)90564-3.

20. Figueiredo EG, Deshmukh P, Nakaji P, Crusius MU, Crawford N, Spetzler RF, et al. The minipterional craniotomy: technical description and anatomic assessment. Neurosurgery. 2007;61(5 Suppl 2):256–64; discussion 64–5. https://doi.org/10.1227/01.neu.0000303978.11752.45.

21. Jägersberg M, Brodard J, Qiu J, Mansouri A, Doglietto F, Gentili F, et al. Quantification of working volumes, exposure, and target-specific maneuverability of the pterional craniotomy and its minimally invasive variants. World Neurosurg. 2017;101:710–717.e2. https://doi.org/10.1016/j.wneu.2017.02.011.

22. Rychen J, Croci D, Roethlisberger M, Nossek E, Potts M, Radovanovic I, et al. Minimally invasive alternative approaches to pterional craniotomy: a systematic review of the literature. World Neurosurg. 2018;113:163–79. https://doi.org/10.1016/j.wneu.2018.02.016.

23. Pellerin P, Lesoin F, Dhellemmes P, Donazzan M, Jomin M. Usefulness of the orbitofrontomalar approach associated with bone reconstruction for frontotemporosphenoid meningiomas. Neurosurgery. 1984;15(5):715–8. https://doi.org/10.1227/00006123-198411000-00016.

24. Hakuba A, Liu S, Nishimura S. The orbitozygomatic infratemporal approach: a new surgical technique. Surg Neurol. 1986;26(3):271–6. https://doi.org/10.1016/0090-3019(86)90161-8.

25. Dunklebarger M. Multimodal approaches in the management of malignancies involving the orbit. Oper Tech Otolaryngol-Head Neck Surg. 2018;29:232–42.

26. Park HH, Sung KS, Moon JH, Kim EH, Kim SH, Lee KS, et al. Lateral supraorbital versus pterional approach for parachiasmal meningiomas: surgical indications and esthetic benefits. Neurosurg Rev. 2020;43(1):313–22. https://doi.org/10.1007/s10143-019-01147-8.

27. Perneczky A. The keyhole concept in neurosurgery: with endoscope-assisted microsurgery and case studies. New York: Thieme; 1999.

28. Eroglu U, Shah K, Bozkurt M, Kahilogullari G, Yakar F, Dogan İ, et al. Supraorbital keyhole approach: lessons learned from 106 operative cases. World Neurosurg. 2019;124:e667. https://doi.org/10.1016/j.wneu.2018.12.188.

29. Mariniello G, Maiuri F, de Divitiis E, Bonavolontà G, Tranfa F, Iuliano A, et al. Lateral orbitotomy for removal of sphenoid wing meningiomas invading the orbit. Neurosurgery. 2010;66(6 Suppl Operative):287–92; discussion 92. https://doi.org/10.1227/01.NEU.0000369924.87437.0B.

30. Chabot JD, Gardner PA, Stefko ST, Zwagerman NT, Fernandez-Miranda JC. Lateral orbitotomy approach for lesions involving the middle fossa: a retrospective review of thirteen patients. Neurosurgery. 2017;80(2):309–22. https://doi.org/10.1093/neuros/nyw045.

31. Zhou G, Ju X, Yu B, Tu Y, Shi J, Wu E, et al. Navigation-guided endoscopy combined with deep lateral orbitotomy for removal of small tumors at the lateral orbital apex. J Ophthalmol. 2018;2018:2827491. https://doi.org/10.1155/2018/2827491.

32. Dallan I, Sellari-Franceschini S, Turri-Zanoni M, de Notaris M, Fiacchini G, Fiorini FR, et al. Endoscopic transorbital superior eyelid approach for the management of selected spheno-orbital meningiomas: preliminary experience. Oper Neurosurg (Hagerstown). 2018;14(3):243–51. https://doi.org/10.1093/ons/opx100.

33. Zoia C, Bongetta D, Gaetani P. Endoscopic transorbital surgery for spheno-orbital lesions: how I do it. Acta Neurochir. 2018;160(6):1231–3. https://doi.org/10.1007/s00701-018-3529-5.

34. De Rosa A, Pineda J, Cavallo LM, Di Somma A, Romano A, Topczewski TE, et al. Endoscopic endo- and extra-orbital corridors for spheno-orbital region: anatomic study with illustrative case. Acta Neurochir. 2019;161(8):1633–46. https://doi.org/10.1007/s00701-019-03939-9.

35. Abhinav K, Acosta Y, Wang WH, Bonilla LR, Koutourousiou M, Wang E, et al. Endoscopic endonasal approach to the optic canal: anatomic considerations and surgical relevance. Neurosurgery. 2015;11(Suppl 3):431–45; discussion 45–6. https://doi.org/10.1227/NEU.0000000000000900.

36. Cabrilo I, Dorward NL. Endoscopic endonasal intracanalicular optic nerve decompression: how I do it. Acta Neurochir. 2020;162(9):2129–34. https://doi.org/10.1007/s00701-020-04476-6.

37. Jeon C, Hong SD, Woo KI, Seol HJ, Nam DH, Lee JI, et al. Use of endoscopic transorbital and endonasal approaches for 360° circumferential access to orbital tumors. J Neurosurg. 2020;135:103. https://doi.org/10.3171/2020.6.JNS20890.

Ramón Medel, Juan Carlos Sánchez España,
and Francisco Zamorano Martín

7.1 Superomedial Approach

The superomedial orbit can be accessed via Lynch incision, sub-brow incision, or an eyelid crease incision [1]. These incisions allow access to the superior-nasal compartment, to the medial intraconal space and the medial apex between the optic nerve and the medial and superior recti [1–4].

Transcutaneous frontoethmoidal anterior orbitotomy or Lynch incision is used for access to the superomedial extraconal and subperiosteal spaces to reach lesions and tumors of the frontal and ethmoid sinuses [1, 2]. This has been replaced by transcaruncular and superior-nasal lid approaches. For this procedure, an arched incision is placed midway from the medial canthal angle to the bridge of the nose, extending from the inferior to the superior orbital rim in the concavity of the medial canthus. Once the rim is exposed, dissection is carried either subperiosteally or through the orbital septum into the medial orbit, depending on the purpose of the surgery

[3–5]. If additional exposure is needed inferiorly, the anterior crus of the medial canthal tendon can be disinserted from the anterior lacrimal crest and the lacrimal sac dissected from the lacrimal sac fossa to the level of the nasolacrimal duct [1–3]. The main anatomic structures limiting exposure through this incision are the nasolacrimal duct inferiorly and the trochlea superiorly [1, 2]. Although this approach provides excellent exposure, the main disadvantage is the resultant scar, which is not well-camouflaged and can sometimes lead to medial canthal webbing. Thus, this approach is used only when other routes do not give adequate exposure such as for resection of large ethmoid and frontal sinus carcinomas that extend toward the orbit [2, 5, 6].

The cutaneous route in the brow has also been abandoned because of the unaesthetic scar and for not providing a better access than through the upper lid crease, which hides the scar in a few weeks [4, 6]. The latter approach begins through the skin, followed by dissection in the suborbicularis plane, identification of the preaponeurotic fat pad, and incision of the orbital septum [1, 4, 6]. To access the subperiosteal space a dissection superiorly to the periosteum of the orbital rim should be performed, followed by incision into periosteum anterior to the arcus marginalis [4]. On entering the superomedial quadrant, it is important not to injure the tendon of the superior oblique muscle and the supraorbital bundle.

R. Medel (✉)
Instituto de Microcirugía Ocular, Barcelona, Spain
e-mail: medel@imo.es

J. C. S. España
Clínica de la Mirada, Barcelona, Spain

F. Z. Martín
Instituto de Oftalmología, Conde de Valenciana,
Valencia, Spain

The main advantage of this approach is to obtain an adequate exposure of the superomedial quadrant with a better aesthetic result [1, 2, 6, 7].

7.2 Transcaruncular Approach

The transcaruncular anterior orbitotomy provides access to the extraconal and subperiosteal space of the medial orbit [2, 8, 9]. The main uses of this orbitotomy approach are to repair a medial wall fracture and perform and ethmoidectomy as part of orbital decompression [2, 4, 10, 11] (Fig. 7.1).

In this technique, an incision is made in the caruncle and extended superiorly and inferiorly with adequate length to not struggle with exposure later on in the case [4]. The incision can be extended into the superior and inferior fornix to the level of the lacrimal puncta, so that the total length is at least 2 cm [4, 8]. Careful attention is paid to avoid injury to the canalicular system [2, 12]. Curved tenotomy scissors are then inserted and gentle blunt dissection is performed over the posterior lacrimal crest, thereby exposing the periosteum of the medial orbital wall, which can be incised using sharp dissection or fine tip cutting cautery to reach the subperiosteal space (Fig. 7.2a, b) [2, 8, 9]. The anterior and posterior ethmoidal vessels serve as useful landmarks. The assistant can pull the skin of the upper and lower eyelid adjacent to the lacrimal puncta to provide exposure [11]. This can be combined with a lateral orbitotomy for greater exposure. An absorbable suture can be used to close the incision in the caruncle [8]. Through this relatively small incision, access can be obtained to the anterior medial orbital wall, the inferomedial strut, the medial orbital floor, and even the superomedial orbital wall [2, 4, 8, 13, 14].

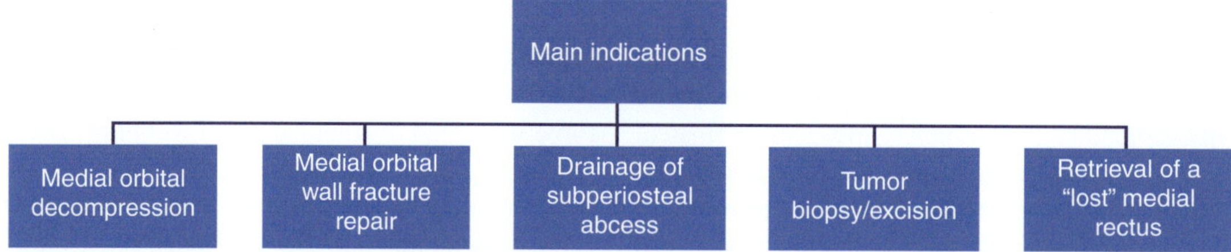

Fig. 7.1 Main indications of medial orbitotomy

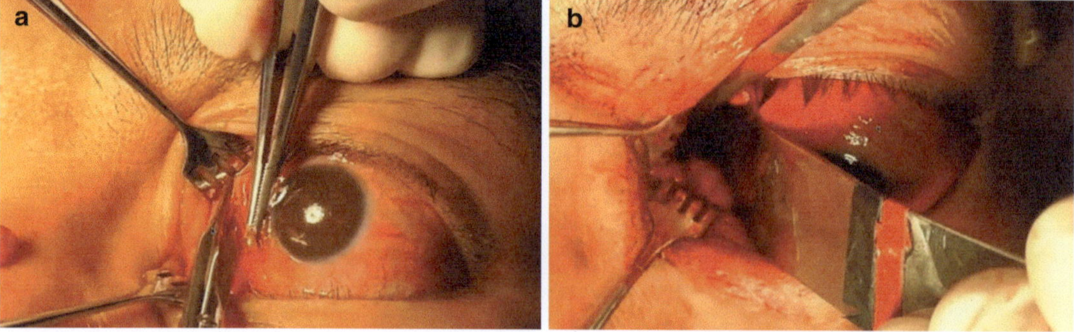

Fig. 7.2 Transcaruncular approach to the medial orbital wall. (**a**) Conjunctival incision between the plica and caruncle. (**b**) Extraconal space exposition with malleable retractors

7.3   Transconjunctival Approach

The transconjunctival medial orbitotomy is used for access to Tenon's capsule, the medial intraconal space, and the anterior one-third of the optic nerve on the medial side [2, 4]. A 180° conjunctival peritomy is performed at the medial limbus, and radial relaxing incisions of the bulbar conjunctiva can be made to improve exposure [4, 8]. Tenon's capsule is then bluntly separated from the sclera with Stevens scissors. If a deep intraconal dissection is anticipated, the medial rectus should be disinserted from the eye to improve exposure and if the exposure is limited, a lateral orbitotomy can be combined to provide more room medially as in the transcaruncular approach (Fig. 7.3a, b) [2, 4]. Once the procedure is complete, the medial rectus is sewn back on the globe and the conjunctiva is closed with absorbable sutures. This approach provides good exposure of medial orbital tumors in the anterior half of the intraconal space [2, 4, 8].

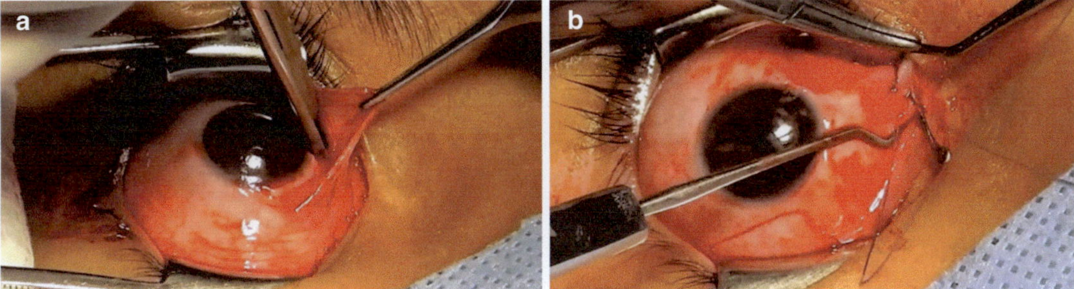

Fig. 7.3 Transconjunctival medial orbitotomy. (**a**) Conjunctival peritomy is performed at the medial limbus. (**b**) Medial rectus isolation

7.4 Inferomedial Approach

The transcaruncular incision allows visualization of the medial half of the orbital floor [8]. For wider exposure of the floor or to create an incision that allows placement of large implant for an inferomedial fracture, it could be necessary to extend the incision toward the inferior conjunctiva [2, 8, 9]. This is considered a complex area for surgery because of the difficulty that manipulation of the inferior oblique muscle presents where it inserts in the inferior-nasal bone wall [2, 4].

References

1. Bosniak SL. Principles and practice of ophthalmic plastic and reconstructive surgery. Philadelphia: Saunders; 1996.
2. Nerad JA. Techniques in ophthalmic plastic surgery: a personal tutorial. Philadelphia: Saunders. p. 696.
3. Lynch RC. The technique of a radical frontal sinus operation which has given me the best results. (Original communications are received with the understanding) that they are contributed exclusively to the laryngoscope. Laryngoscope. 1921;31(1):1–5. https://doi.org/10.1288/00005537-192101000-00001.
4. Karcioglu ZA. Surgical treatment. In: Orbital tumors. New York: Springer; 2005. p. 359–90. https://doi.org/10.1007/0-387-27086-8_31.
5. Pelton RW. The anterior eyelid crease approach to the orbit. Curr Opin Ophthalmol. 2009;20(5):401–5. https://doi.org/10.1097/ICU.0B013E32832EC3F7.
6. Nerad JA. Diagnostic approach to the patient with proptosis. In: Techniques in ophthalmic plastic surgery; 2021. p. 545–610. https://doi.org/10.1016/B978-0-323-39316-4.00014-4.
7. Pelton RW, Patel BCK. Superomedial lid crease approach to the medial intraconal space: a new technique for access to the optic nerve and central space. Ophthal Plast Reconstr Surg. 2001;17(4):241–53. https://doi.org/10.1097/00002341-200107000-00003.
8. Shorr N, Baylis H. Transcaruncular–transconjunctival approach to the medial orbit and orbital apex. In: Oral presentation at the American Society of Ophthalmic Plastic and Reconstructive Surgeons, 24th annual scientific symposium, Chicago, November 13; 1993.
9. Shorr N, Baylis HI, Goldberg RA, Perry JD. Transcaruncular approach to the medial orbit and orbital apex. Ophthalmology. 2000;107(8):1459–63. https://doi.org/10.1016/S0161-6420(00)00241-4.
10. Graham SM, Thomas RD, Carter KD, Nerad JA. The transcaruncular approach to the medial orbital wall. Laryngoscope. 2002;112(6):986–9. https://doi.org/10.1097/00005537-200206000-00009.
11. Lai PC, Liao SL, Jou JR, Hou PK. Transcaruncular approach for the management of frontoethmoid mucoceles. Br J Ophthalmol. 2003;87(6):699–703. https://doi.org/10.1136/BJO.87.6.699.
12. Fante RG, Elner VM. Transcaruncular approach to medial canthal tendon plication for lower eyelid laxity. Ophthal Plast Reconstr Surg. 2001;17(1):16–27. https://doi.org/10.1097/00002341-200101000-00004.
13. Leone CR, Lloyd WC, Rylander G. Surgical repair of medial wall fractures. Am J Ophthalmol. 1984;97(3):349–56. https://doi.org/10.1016/0002-9394(84)90635-4.
14. Goldberg RA. Is there a "lost" rectus muscle in strabismus surgery? Am J Ophthalmol. 2001;132(1):101–3. https://doi.org/10.1016/S0002-9394(01)01019-4.

The Fronto-Temporo-Orbito-Zygomatic Approach

8

Roberto Delfini, Andrea Gennaro Ruggeri, and Sara Iavarone

8.1 Introduction

Evolution toward the current concept of the frontal-temporo-orbit-zygomatic approach has been progressive. In 1982, Jane et al. described the "supraorbital approach" which allowed access to the floor of the anterior cranial fossa and the superior portion of the orbit with minimal retraction through a craniotomic operculum incorporating the superior orbital rim and part of the roof of the orbit [1]. Al-Mefty [2, 3] modified this approach by incorporating the superior and lateral margins of the orbit with a pterional craniotomy and then removing them in one piece. In 1984, Pellerin et al. [4] described an orbitofrontal craniotomy with removal of the lateral wall of the orbit, malar eminence, and zygomatic arch in surgical treatment of meningiomas of the sphenoid wing. Hakuba et al. [5] described the infratemporal orbitozygomatic approach as a useful technique for lesions located in the parasellar region and interpeduncular fossa, including meningiomas of the medial third of the sphenoid wing, petroclival meningiomas, trigeminal neuromas, and aneurysms of the basilar top. Their method involved preserving a large part of the skull base with three separate bone fragments. Alaywan and Sindou [6], and McDermott et al. [7] described a two-piece orbitozygomatic approach with fronto-temporal and orbitozygomatic bone opercula removal. In 1998, J. Zabramski et al. reported a variant of the orbitozygomatic approach in two pieces according to a technique that is currently the most widely used [8].

8.2 Surgical Technique

8.2.1 Patient Position and Skin Incision

The patient is positioned supine on the operating table with the head locked in the Mayfield head holder and rotated 30° (to a maximum of 60°) toward the side contralateral to the surgical incision. Rotation is greater for tumors and vascular lesions of the anterior and middle cranial fossae and less for those involving the clivus and posterior cranial fossa. The neck is slightly extended so that the malar eminence is positioned at the highest point of the operating field, thus allowing a spontaneous retraction of the frontal lobe with respect to the roof of the orbit [8].

The skin incision begins 1 cm anterior to the tragus, at the level of the lower edge of the zygomatic arch. It then proceeds upward and forward in a slightly curved arc to reach just behind the point where the hairline intersects the contralateral midpupillary line (Fig. 8.1). The inferior portion of the incision must be limited to avoid

R. Delfini (✉) · A. G. Ruggeri · S. Iavarone
Division of Neurosurgery, Department of
Neurological Sciences, University of Rome Sapienza,
Rome, Italy

G. Bonavolontà et al. (eds.), *Cranio-Orbital Mass Lesions*,
https://doi.org/10.1007/978-3-031-35771-8_8

"

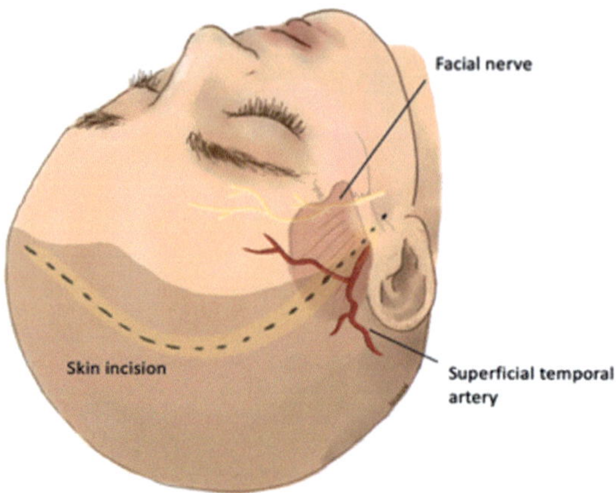

Fig. 8.1 The skin incision extends from the lower edge of the zygomatic arch to the contralateral midpupillary line. (Illustration by Sara Iavarone)

injury to the frontotemporal branch of the facial nerve. The division of the frontotemporal branch into the zygomatic and temporal branches occurs within the parotid gland and the point where the anterior and middle branches diverge from the frontotemporal branch of the facial nerve is approximately 1.1 cm below the tragus [9].

8.2.2 Elevation and Preservation of the Skin Flap and Frontal Branch of the Facial Nerve

The skin flap is mobilized anteriorly to expose the underlying superficial temporal fascia. The frontal periosteum is preserved. The frontotemporal branch of the facial nerve is located in the subgaleal fat pad. To avoid injuring this branch, the subgaleal dissection must be interrupted 2.5–3 cm posterior to the superior margin of the orbit in its lateral portion. Subfascial dissection is then performed via an incision of the superficial temporal fascia. The subfascial dissection begins posteriorly and extends forward along the margin of the superior temporal line. This technique offers the possibility of protecting the branches of the facial nerve located in the superficial portion of this fascial plane (Fig. 8.2). The fronto-temporal branch of the facial nerve emerges from the parotid gland in multiple branches located in the subgaleal space, in the same plane as the

superficial fat pad. In the study described by Ammirati et al. [10], it was found that in 30% of the cases examined, some branches of the middle division of the frontotemporal branch of the facial nerve run within the interfascial space and enter the temporal muscle. This finding may explain why interfascial dissection, conventionally used for pterional craniotomy, carries a 30% risk of injury to these branches.

In order to obtain a better approximation of the temporal muscle in the reconstructive phase, it is useful to leave a myofascial cuff along the superior temporal line.

Dissection proceeds by raising the temporal fascia in the plane between the deep layer and the muscle to anteriorly expose the cheekbone and superior orbital margin. The deep layer of the temporal fascia (fused with the periosteum of the zygomatic process of the frontal bone and the cheekbone) is separated subperiosteally to obtain full exposure of the upper margin of the orbit, the zygomatic process, and the malar eminence as far as the zygomatic-facial foramen and zygomatic arch.

The temporal muscle is incised near the posterior portion of the skin incision and elevated subperiosteally using the retrograde technique described by Oikawa et al. [11], i.e., proceeding from the bottom upward with a dissector, maintaining the integrity of the periosteum and thus protecting the deep vessels as well as nerve and muscle fibers (Fig. 8.3). The prevention of temporal muscle atrophy is an important aspect in the orbitozygomatic approach.

Kadri and Al-Mefty [12] recommended six steps useful for temporal muscle preservation: (1) preservation of the superficial temporal artery; (2) preservation of facial nerve branches by subfascial dissection; (3) zygomatic osteotomy to increase exposure and avoid compression or retraction injuries of the temporal muscle; (4) dissection of the muscle via the retrograde subperiosteal route to preserve the deep vessels and nerves; (5) disengagement of the muscle along the superior temporal line without cutting the fascia; (6) reattachment of the muscle directly to the bone. Alternatively, the muscular cuff can be used to bring the fascia and the temporal muscle

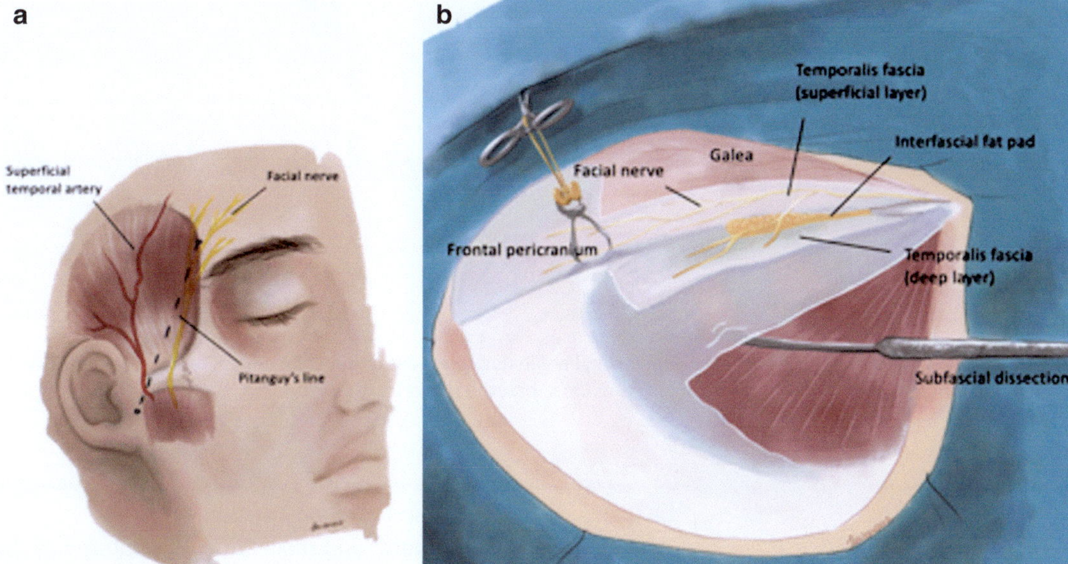

Fig. 8.2 (**a**) The frontal branch of the facial nerve runs posterior to the Pitanguy line: a line passing 0.5 cm below the tragus and 1.5 cm above the lateral end of the eyebrow. (**b**) Illustration of the subfascial dissection of the temporal muscle and the distribution of the fibers of the facial nerve with respect to the anatomical planes. (Illustration by Sara Iavarone)

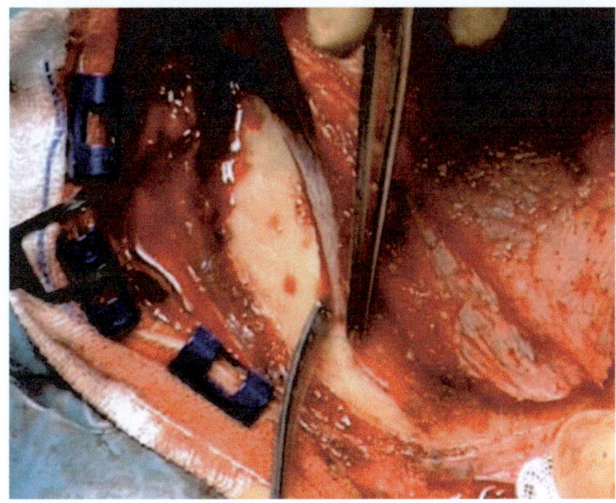

Fig. 8.3 Dissection of the temporal muscle according to the retrograde technique described by Oikawa while preserving the integrity of the periosteum

together according to the technique originally described by Spetzler and Lee [13].

At this point, we proceed medially by blunt dissection to separate the periorbit from the upper and lateral margins of the orbit up to the supraorbital notch (Fig. 8.4). If further medial exposure is required, the supraorbital nerve can be freed from the notch or supraorbital foramen using a small chisel or a burr [9].

8.2.3 Single Piece Orbito-Zygomatic (OZ) Craniotomy

In the single-piece OZ approach, the frontotemporal craniotomy is combined with a series of osteotomies through the orbit and the cheekbone to remove a single craniotomic operculum that includes the roof and lateral wall of the orbit, the lateral surface of the cheekbone, and the zygomatic process of the temporal bone.

Positioning of the keyhole at the MacCarty point (Fig. 8.5) is a fundamental step in order to proceed with the one-piece OZ craniotomy. The keyhole, as described by MacCarty [14, 15], should expose in its upper half the dura mater that lines the frontal lobe and in its lower half the periorbit: the roof of the orbit constitutes the bony bridge that divides the two halves. The drill hole in the MacCarty point is made over the frontosphenoid suture, approximately 1 cm behind

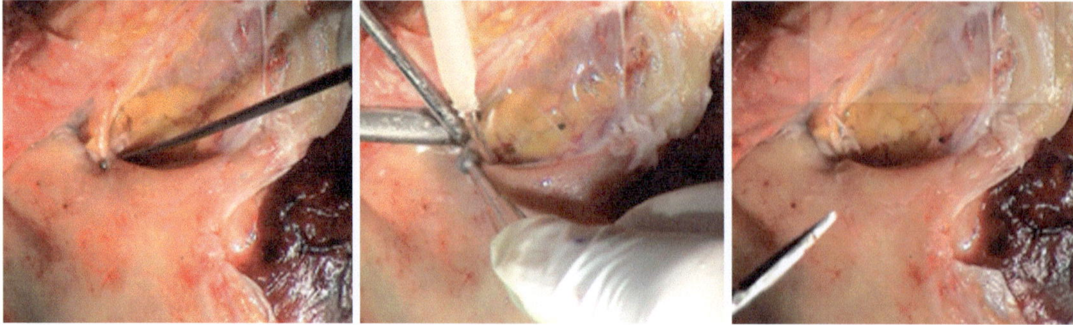

Fig. 8.4 Intraoperative photo showing the supraorbital notch that represents the medial margin of the craniotomy. With the aid of a burr, the supraorbital nerve is freed from the supraorbital notch

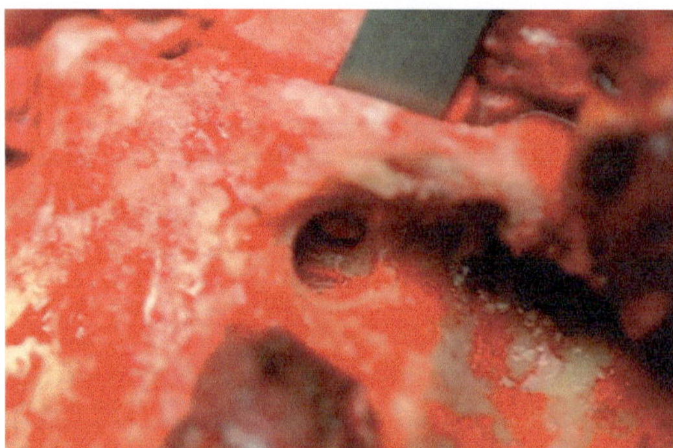

Fig. 8.5 MacCarty point: a bony bridge consisting of the roof of the orbit divides the periorbit from the dura mater that covers the frontal lobe

the frontozygomatic junction. Its diameter is about twice the size of a normal drill hole in order to allow access to the anterior cranial fossa and the orbital cavity.

The six osteotomies are then performed using the craniotome. The first osteotomy extends from the orbital portion of the MacCarty keyhole to the inferior orbital fissure. The second osteotomy crosses the zygomatic body and extends to the inferior orbital fissure: this section is made 1 cm below the angle of junction of the frontal and temporal processes of the zygomatic bone (Fig. 8.6). The osteotomy through the cheekbone meets the cut along the lateral wall of the orbit at the anterolateral edge of the inferior orbital fissure.

The third osteotomy is performed through the anterior root of the zygomatic process of the temporal bone, just in front of the articular tubercle of the zygomatic bone. The zygomatic process is

dissected in an oblique direction, providing a stable base for reconstruction.

The fourth and most critical osteotomy of the one-piece OZ craniotomy involves a cut through the upper edge of the orbit and an intraorbital cut along the roof of the orbit (Fig. 8.7).

The fifth osteotomy extends along the frontal and parietal bones and connects the craniotomy holes. The final osteotomy of the single-piece OZ craniotomy connects a temporal craniotomy hole and the frontal compartment of the MacCarty keyhole (Fig. 8.8) [16].

8.2.4 Two-Piece OZ Craniotomy

The two-piece OZ craniotomy combines the pterional craniotomy with a supraorbital osteotomy and removal of a portion of the zygomatic bone (Fig. 8.9).

First, a classic frontotemporal craniotomy is performed. Subsequently, before proceeding with bone cuts, the dura mater must be separated from the frontal bone, from the small wing of the sphenoid and from the middle cranial fossa.

The small wing of the sphenoid is drilled until it reaches the lateral margin of the superior orbital fissure.

During the initial part of the two-piece OZ craniotomy, the osteotomies of the skull base through the anterior root of the zygomatic process of the temporal bone and the zygomatic body are similar to those described in the one-piece OZ craniotomy. The remaining osteotomies

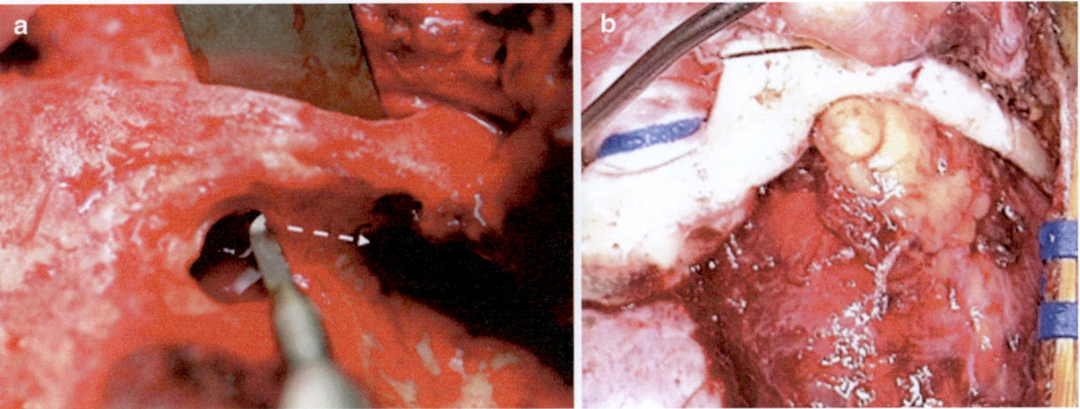

Fig. 8.6 The first cut extends from the orbital portion of the MacCarty keyhole to the inferior orbital fissure (**a**). The second cut crosses the body of the zygomatic bone and reconnects to the first cut at the level of the inferior orbital fissure. The third cut crosses the zygomatic process of the temporal bone just in front of the articular tubercle (**b**)

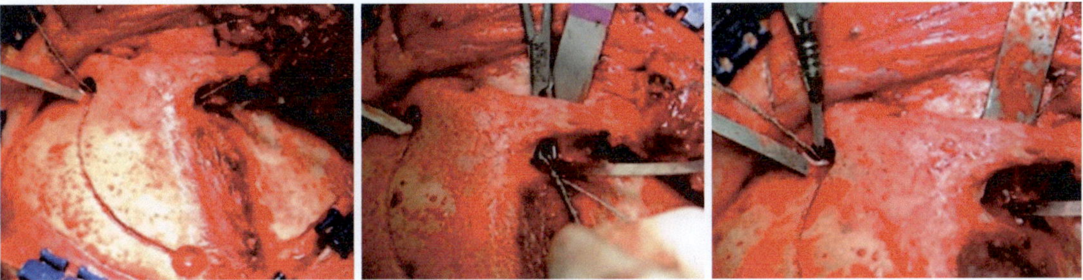

Fig. 8.7 The cut along the roof of the orbit is made using the Gigli saw, connecting the medial margin of the craniotomy at the level of the supraorbital notch to the orbital portion of the MacCarty keyhole

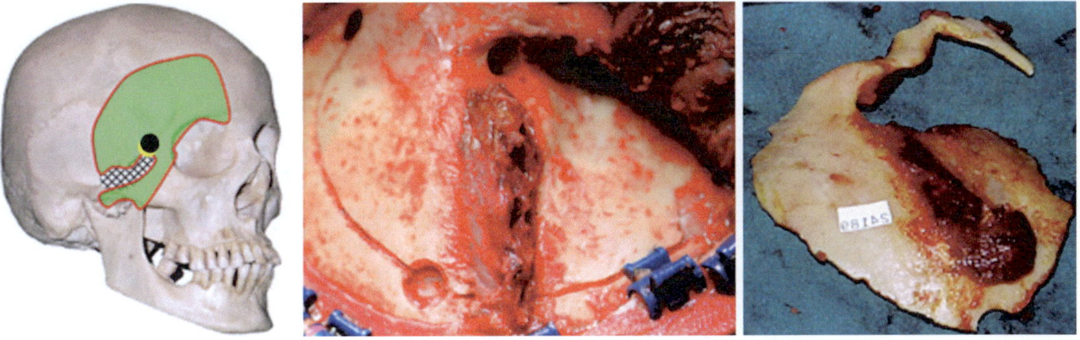

Fig. 8.8 Final craniotomy connecting the individual craniotomy holes and final appearance of the single piece bone operculum

are specific for the two-piece OZ craniotomy. As described by Zabramski et al. [8], a small craniotomy is made using a burr hole along the antero-lateral wall of the temporal fossa, thus creating a space for the craniotome used to perform the osteotomy along the lateral wall of the orbit. The

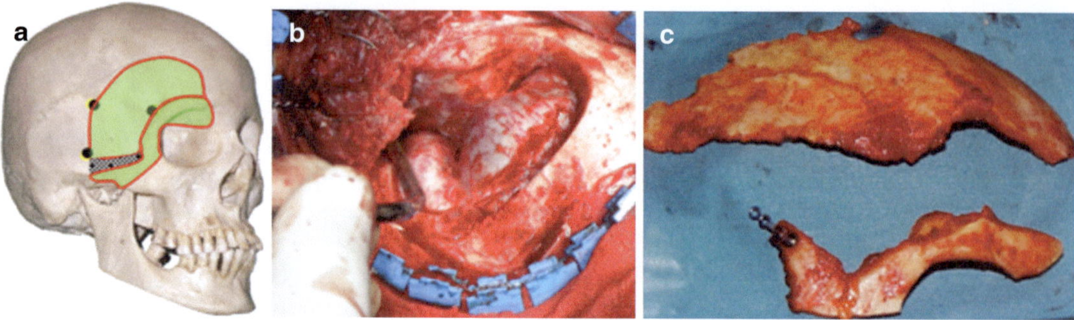

Fig. 8.9 The two-piece orbitozygomatic approach essentially consists of the combination of a pterional craniotomy with an orbitozygomatic osteotomy (**a**). Figure (**b**) shows the intraoperative view after completing the craniotomy with the two removed pieces next to it (**c**)

first osteotomy begins along the roof of the orbit lateral to the supraorbital notch and is directed toward the superolateral margin of the superior orbital fissure. The subsequent osteotomy frees the lateral wall of the orbit by connecting the posterolateral end of the first osteotomy and the anterolateral part of the inferior orbital fissure (Fig. 8.9). The inferior orbital fissure can be visualized in most craniotomies, and this portion of the osteotomy passes through the craniotomy hole previously made on the anterolateral part of the temporal bone [16].

8.2.5 Modified Supraorbital Orbitozygomatic Craniotomy

The periorbit is separated by blunt dissection from the upper and lateral margins of the orbit and medially up to the level of the supraorbital notch. The depth of the dissection rarely exceeds 2–3 cm. If further medial exposure is required, the supraorbital nerve is freed from the supraorbital notch or foramen with a small chisel or diamond burr. Typically, the limits of exposure include the supraorbital notch medially and the frontozygomatic suture laterally (Fig. 8.7). The first osteotomy is performed at the upper edge of the orbit, lateral to the supraorbital nerve (Fig. 8.7a). This cut can be extended medially if more medial frontal exposure is desired. The second osteotomy is made in the lateral wall of the orbit toward the inferior orbital fissure. The third osteotomy is made to connect these two osteotomies in the roof of the orbit. Modified supraorbital orbitozygomatic craniotomy can be performed using a 1- or 2-piece method [9].

8.2.6 Reconstruction

The galea can be used as an autologous patch graft in the event of duroplasty or for a possible cranialization of the frontal sinus. To obtain a better osteosynthesis, it is also possible to perform a pre-plating before proceeding with the zygomatic osteotomy in order to reduce the risk of postoperative facial asymmetry. Care must also be taken in the reconstruction of the roof of the orbit to limit the risk of enophthalmos. Titanium plates and 4 or 5 mm self-tapping screws are used for osteosynthesis of the craniotomic operculum. The temporal muscle is brought back to the myofascial cuff at the level of the superior temporal line. An interrupted suture with 3/0 vicryl stitches can be used for the superficial temporal fascia and galea. Subcutaneous drainage is left in place for 2 days to prevent blood collection. The skin suture can be performed using either resorbable sutures or metallic staples [16].

8.3 Clinical Use

The OZ approach makes it possible to follow four different surgical corridors: (1) subfrontal, (2) trans-Sylvian, (3) pretemporal, and (4) subtemporal. The trans-Sylvian and pretemporal corridors allow access to deep regions, including (1) optic-carotid; (2) carotid-oculomotor; (3) supracarotid; (4) oculomotor-tentorial [16] .

The orbitozygomatic craniotomies in either one and two pieces both have the advantage of providing a wider exposure of the anterior skull base than the frontotemporal approach (Figs. 8.9 and 8.10), thus minimizing the need for retraction of the brain parenchyma. By removing the upper and lateral walls of the orbit and cheekbone, a wide angle of exposure is obtained for lesions involving the apex of the orbit, the paraclinoid and parasellar regions, the apex of the basilar artery, the cavernous sinus, and the floor of the anterior and middle fossa [8].

In the one-piece OZ approach, the zygomatic osteotomy is generally less extensive and mainly involves the frontal process. Therefore, the one-piece OZ approach is theoretically more suitable for tumors of the parasellar and orbital regions (Figs. 8.11 and 8.12), in which greater mobiliza-tion of the zygomatic arch does not really improve lesion exposure.

In contrast, the one-piece OZ approach is less indicated for ruptured aneurysms [17], hyperostotic spheno-orbital and sphenoid meningiomas, and for large intraorbital tumors with increased intraocular pressure. In ruptured aneurysms, coexisting cerebral edema increases the risk of damage to the parenchyma during extracranial osteotomy of the roof of the orbit. In tumors characterized by severe hyperostosis of the roof and lateral wall of the orbit, accidental fracture of the single block bone flap may give rise to force vectors involving the optic canal and the sphenoid sinus with consequent risk of damaging the optic nerve and the CSF fistula. In the case of intraocular hypertension, the greater manipulation of the eyeball necessary to dissect the roof of the orbit from the extracranial intraorbital side increases the risk of blindness as well as the risk of dangerous bradyarrhythmias resulting from the elicitation of the Aschner-Dagnini oculocardiac reflex [18].

Supraorbital craniotomy is usually used for injuries of the anterior, middle, and sella turcica cranial fossae. The major fields of application are aneurysms of the anterior communicating artery and supraclinoid ICA aneurysms. Lemole et al.

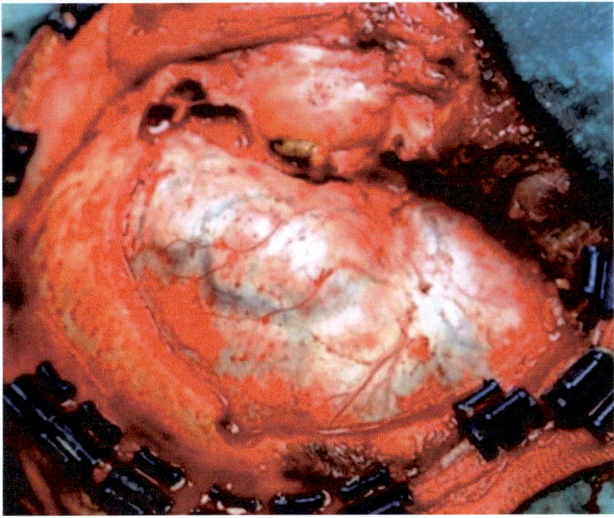
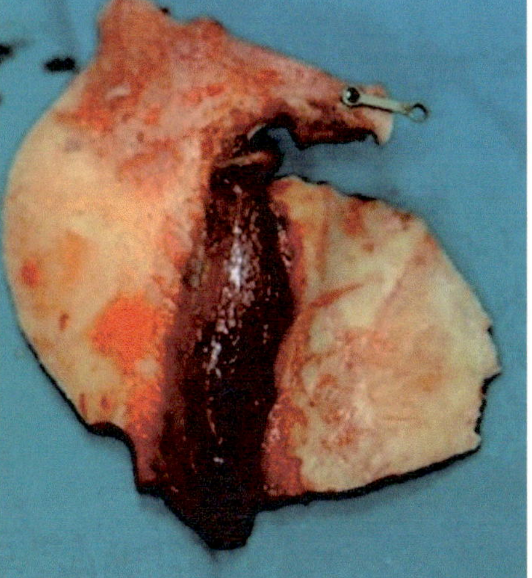

Fig. 8.10 Intraoperative photo of the supraorbital orbitozygomatic craniotomy and the removed craniotomic operculum

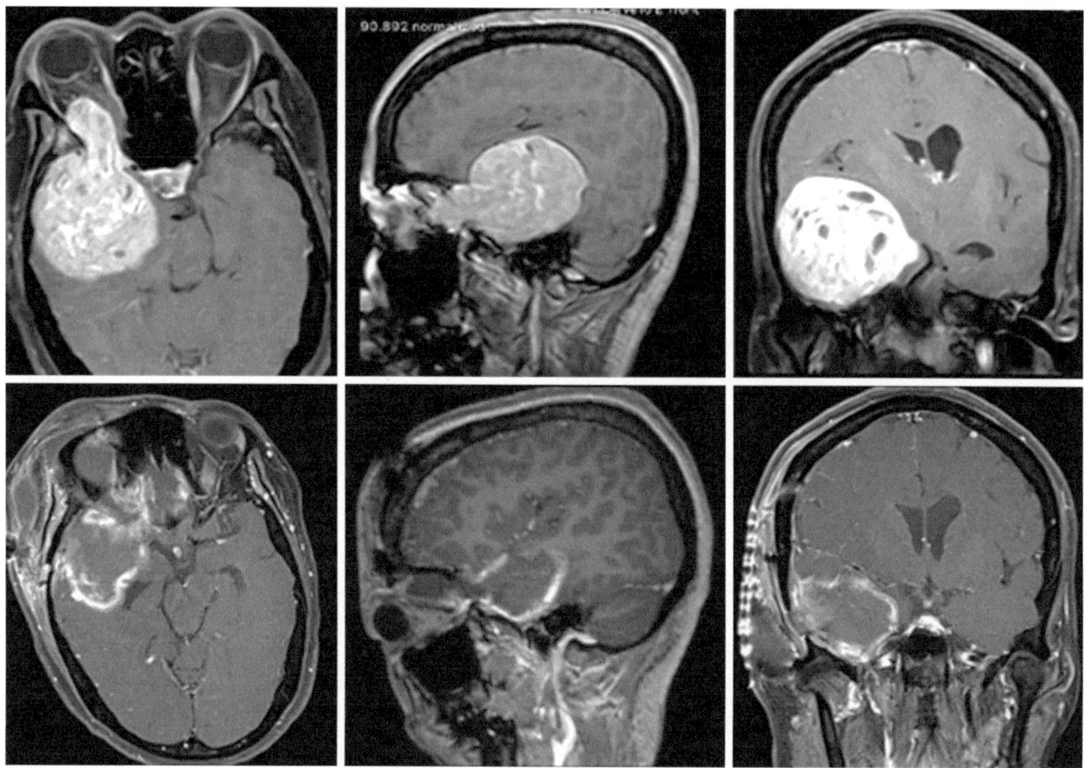

Fig. 8.11 Clinical case of voluminous spheno-orbital wing meningioma removed using a fronto-temporo-orbito-zygomatic approach, obtaining a complete removal

[19] also proposed the use of this approach for the treatment of sellar lesions.

The increased exposure offered by OZ craniotomy comes at the expense of an increased risk of cosmetic deformity, CSF leakage, enophthalmos, pulsating exophthalmos, and blindness [18].

As emerges in the study described by Tanriover et al., the two-piece OZ allows for significantly greater orbital roof removal than the one-piece variety. However, permanent removal of the roof of the orbit carries an inherent risk of inadequate reconstruction and consequent cosmetic defect, meaning that at least 2.5–3 cm of the anterior-posterior length of the roof of the orbit must be preserved with the osteotomy to prevent enophthalmos [17]. In the two-piece OZ, the frontotemporal bone operculum is lifted as the initial step and the orbitozygomatic osteotomy is performed as a second separate step. The roof of the orbit and the side wall are then removed under direct vision, achieving a more precise orbitotomy than in the single-piece OZ.

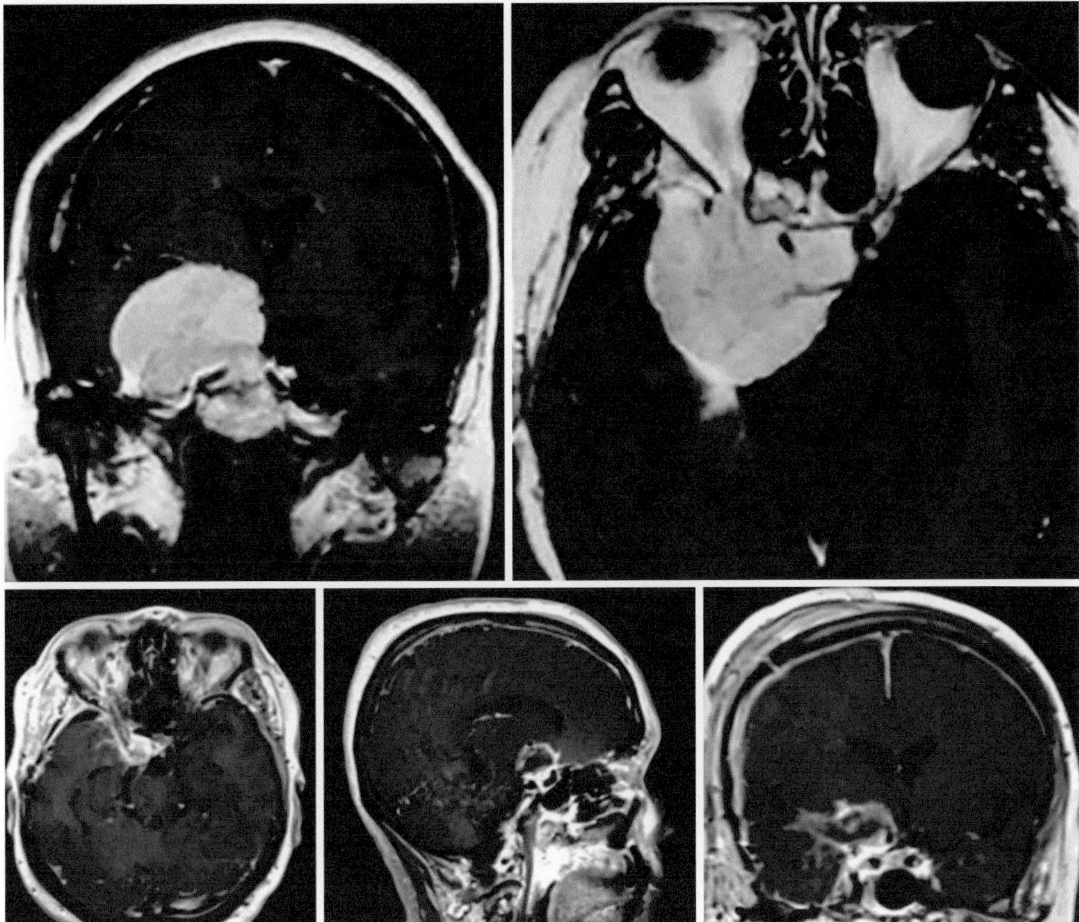

Fig. 8.12 Clinical case of spheno-petro-clival meningioma removed using a fronto-temporo-orbito-zygomatic approach

References

1. Jane JA, Park TS, Pobereskin LH, Winn HR, Butler AB. The supraorbital approach: technical note. Neurosurgery. 1982;11(4):537–42.
2. Al-Mefty O. Supraorbital-pterional approach to skull base lesions. Neurosurgery. 1987;21(4):474–7. https://doi.org/10.1227/00006123-198710000-00006.
3. Al-Mefty O, Anand VK. Zygomatic approach to skull-base lesions. J Neurosurg. 1990;73(5):668–73. https://doi.org/10.3171/jns.1990.73.5.0668.
4. Pellerin P, Lesoin F, Dhellemmes P, Donazzan M, Jomin M. Usefulness of the orbitofrontomalar approach associated with bone reconstruction for frontotemporosphenoid meningiomas. Neurosurgery. 1984;15(5):715–8. https://doi.org/10.1227/00006123-198411000-00016.
5. Hakuba A, Liu SS, Nishimura S. The orbitozygomatic infratemporal approach: technique a new surgical technique. Surg Neurol. 1986;26(3):271–6. https://doi.org/10.1016/0090-3019(86)90161-8.
6. Alaywan M, Sindou M. Fronto-temporal approach with orbito-zygomatic removal surgical anatomy. Acta Neurochir. 1990;104:79–83. https://doi.org/10.1007/BF01842824.
7. McDermott MW, Durity FA, Rootman J, Woodhurst WB. Combined frontotemporal-orbitozygomatic approach for tumors of the sphenoid wing and orbit. Neurosurgery. 1990;26:107. https://doi.org/10.1097/00006123-199001000-00015.
8. Zabramski JM, Sankhla SK, Cabiol J, Spetzler RF. Orbitozygomatic craniotomy technical note. J Neurosurg. 1998;89(2):336–41. https://doi.org/10.3171/jns.1998.89.2.0336.
9. Seçkin H, Avci E, Uluç K, Niemann D, Başkaya MK. The work horse of skull base surgery: orbitozygomatic approach. Technique, modifications, and applications. Neurosurg Focus. 2008;25(6):E4. https://doi.org/10.3171/FOC.2008.25.12.E4.

10. Ammirati M, Spallone A, Ma J, Cheatham M, Becker D. An anatomicosurgical study of the temporal branch of the facial nerve. Neurosurgery. 1993;33(6):1038–44. https://doi.org/10.1227/00006123-199312000-00012.

11. Oikawa S, Kobayashi S. Retrograde dissection of the temporalis muscle preventing muscle atrophy for pterional craniotomy technical note. J Neurosurg. 1996;84(2):297–9. https://doi.org/10.3171/jns.1996.84.2.0297.

12. Kadri PAS, Al-Mefty O. The anatomical basis for surgical preservation of temporal muscle. J Neurosurg. 2004;100(3):517–22. https://doi.org/10.3171/jns.2004.100.3.0517.

13. Spetzler RF, Lee KS. Reconstruction of the temporalis muscle for the pterional craniotomy technical note. J Neurosurg. 1990;73(4):636–7. https://doi.org/10.3171/jns.1990.73.4.0636.

14. Maccarty CS. Surgical techniques for removal of intracranial meningiomas. Clin Neurosurg. 1959;7:100–11. https://doi.org/10.1093/neurosurgery/7.cn_suppl_1.100.

15. MacCarty CS. Meningiomas of the sphenoidal ridge. J Neurosurg. 1972;36(1):114–20. https://doi.org/10.3171/jns.1972.36.1.0114.

16. Tanriover N, Ulm AJ, Rhoton AL, Kawashima M, Yoshioka N, Lewis SB. One-piece versus two-piece orbitozygomatic craniotomy: quantitative and qualitative considerations. Neurosurgery. 2006;58(SUPPL 2):ONS-229. https://doi.org/10.1227/01.NEU.0000210010.46680.B4.

17. Sekhar LN, Kalia KK, Yonas H, Wright DC, Ching H. Cranial base approaches to intracranial aneurysms in the subarachnoid space. Neurosurgery. 1994;35(3):472–83. https://doi.org/10.1227/00006123-199409000-00016.

18. Luzzi S, Lucifero AG, Spina A, et al. Cranio-orbito-zygomatic approach: core techniques for tailoring target exposure and surgical freedom. Brain Sci. 2022;12(3):405. https://doi.org/10.3390/brainsci12030405.

19. Lemole GM, Henn JS, Zabramski JM, Spetzler RF. Modifications to the orbitozygomatic approach. J Neurosurg. 2003;99(5):924–30. https://doi.org/10.3171/jns.2003.99.5.0924.

The Lateral Orbito-Cranial Approach

9

Diego Strianese, Giuseppe Mariniello [ID],
Marco Lorenzetti, and Francesco Maiuri [ID]

9.1 Introduction

The lateral approach to the orbit was first proposed in 1889 by Kronlein [1] who suggested a curved skin incision and removing the lateral orbital wall to improve the access to the retrobulbar lesions. Berke [2] modified the Kronlein skin incision into a transverse incision extending 30–35 mm from the lateral canthus. Later Maroon and Kennerdel [3] suggested to add to the lateral microsurgical orbitotomy the removal of a portion of the greater sphenoid wing with the aim to expose the temporal dura and the deep orbit.

Since the early 1990s, several technical modifications of the classical lateral orbitotomy have been proposed to improve the surgical exposure of the orbital apex and superior orbital compart-

ment [4–7]. In the surgical practice, both classical lateral orbitotomy and modified lateral orbital approaches are mainly used for removing bone lesions of the lateral orbital wall and intraorbital lesions of the lateral and superolateral compartments of the orbit and orbital apex.

This chapter discusses the indications, advantages, and limits of the lateral orbitotomy coupled with resection of the sphenoid wing for removing mass lesions with both intraorbital and intracranial extension. This approach may better be defined "orbito-cranial" because it includes an orbitotomy and a small craniotomy [8].

9.2 Surgical Technique

A curvilinear skin incision is made along the upper eyelid crease extending to 2 cm lateral to the canthal angle along a natural skin crease (Fig. 9.1). The orbital and temporal portions of the greater sphenoid wing are exposed by dissecting the temporal muscle from the superior temporal line, the anterior third of the zygomatic arch, and the lateral orbital rim (Fig. 9.2). The frontal process of the zygomatic bone is isolated from the surrounding tissue (Fig. 9.3) and removed by using the oscillating saw. The bone is drilled from the sphenozygomatic junction through the temporal portion of the greater sphenoid wing to the lateral edge of the superior orbital fissure. This bone resection allows to expose the anterior pars of the

D. Strianese
Division of Ophthalmology, Department of
Neurosciences, Reproductive and
Odontostomatological Sciences, School of Medicine,
University "Federico II", Naples, Italy

G. Mariniello · M. Lorenzetti · F. Maiuri (✉)
Division of Neurosurgery, Department of
Neurosciences, Reproductive and
Odontostomatological Sciences, School of Medicine,
University "Federico II", Naples, Italy
e-mail: giumarin@unina.it

F. Maiuri (✉)
Division of Neurosurgery, Department of
Neurosciences, Reproductive and
Odontostomatological Sciences, University of Naples
"Federico II", Naples, Italy
e-mail: frmaiuri@unina.it

© The Author(s), under exclusive license to Springer Nature Switzerland AG 2023
G. Bonavolontà et al. (eds.), *Cranio-Orbital Mass Lesions*,
https://doi.org/10.1007/978-3-031-35771-8_9

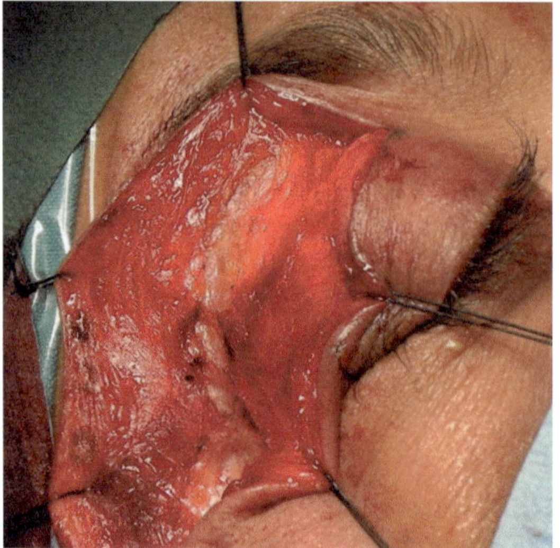

Fig. 9.1 Curvilinear skin incision along the right upper eyelid crease extending 2 cm lateral to the canthal angle

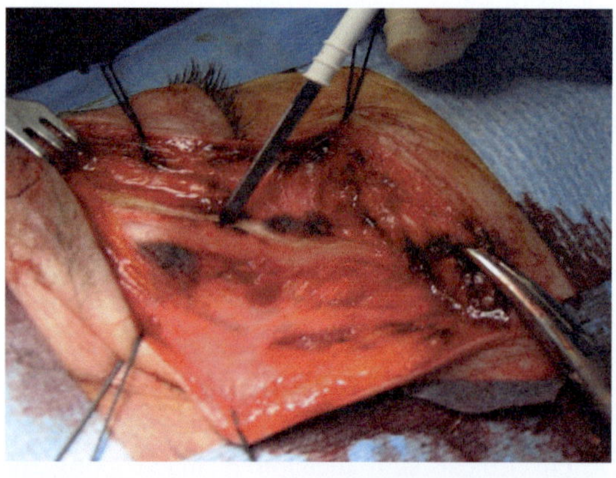

Fig. 9.2 Dissection of the temporal muscle from the superior temporal line and the lateral orbital rim

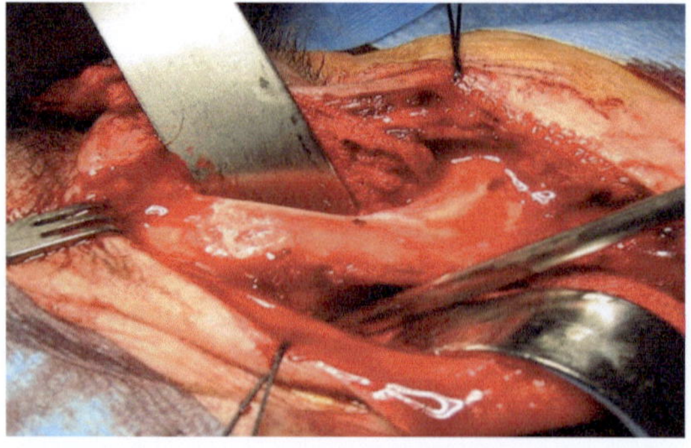

Fig. 9.3 The frontal process of the zygomatic bone is isolated and well exposed

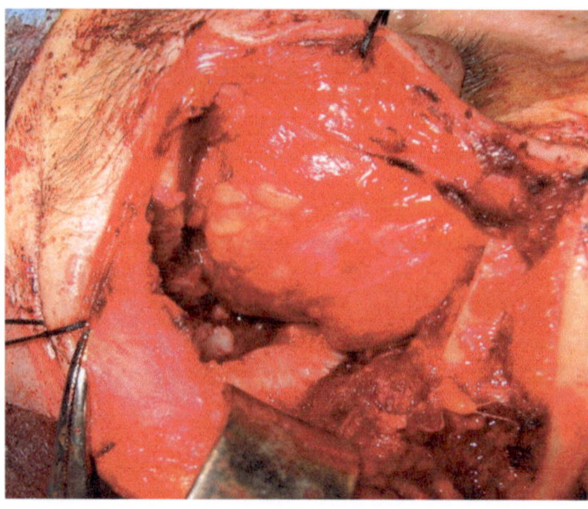

Fig. 9.4 The lateral periorbita is widely exposed after removal of the frontal process of the zygomatic bone

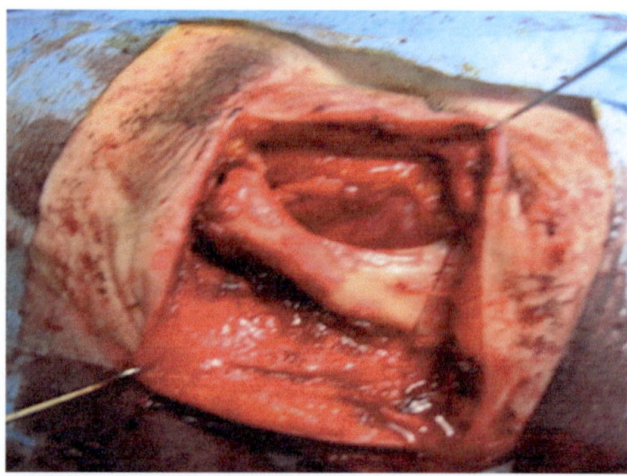

Fig. 9.5 The frontal process of the zygomatic bone is replaced and fixed by wires

temporal fossa and the lateral periorbita (Fig. 9.4). Thus, the dura is opened and the intracranial tumor component is exposed and removed by microsurgical technique.

Then, a horizontal incision of the periorbita allows to expose and remove the intraorbital component of the mass lesion. The lateral wall of the optic canal may also be resected, if necessary.

The reconstruction must involve both the periorbita and dura. If they are infiltrated, as for spheno-orbital meningiomas, they must be resected and the residual defect must be repaired using a flap of dural substitute. Then, the frontal process of the zygomatic bone is replaced and fixed by wires or miniplats (Fig. 9.5).

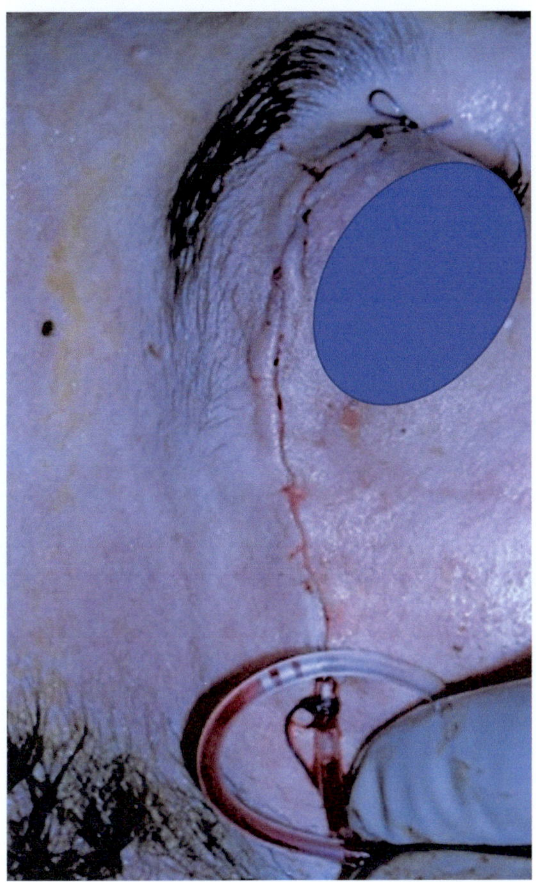

Fig. 9.6 The skin is closed with aesthetic suture

Reconstruction of the orbital roof and wall is not performed. The skin is closed with 3-0 uninterrupted suture (Fig. 9.6).

This approach allows good exposure of the lateral and superolateral orbital compartment and temporal fossa.

The subfascial dissection of the temporal muscle permits to expose a large bone field with no risk of injuring the frontal branch of the facial nerve. The resection of the frontal branch of the zygomatic process and whole lateral orbital wall allows a wide exposure of the orbital cavity; the resection may be extended, if necessary, to the external two-third of the orbital roof. The resection of the greater sphenoid wing may be extended to the anterior temporal bone (up to 3 cm), according to the size and extension of the mass lesion. The medial limits of the bone removal are the superior orbital fissure and the anterior cli-

noid process, which are not sufficiently controlled. The lateral wall of the optic canal may be opened to decompress the optic nerve; however, the circumferential invasion of the optic canal is a contraindication to this approach.

The lateral orbital rim must be resected and reimplanted to increase the size of the surgical field, mainly in cases with large intraorbital tumor component.

Although the reconstruction of the orbital wall and orbital roof is advised in several studies [9–11], we do not believe it is necessary.

9.3 Indication and Patient Selection

The selection criteria for patient/candidate to surgery by lateral orbito-cranial approach include:

- Tumor location at the lateral or superolateral orbital compartment and eventually to the anterior portion of the temporal fossa;
- No evidence of involvement of the anterior clinoid process and superior orbital fissure; and
- No evidence of tumor extension around or beyond the optic canal.

Patients with cranio-orbital mass lesions who do not agree with these criteria must be operated on through sovraorbital-pterional or fronto-temporo-orbito-zygomatic approach.

The lateral orbito-cranial approach may be used for lateral extradural mass lesions, such as bone tumors of the sphenoid wing and lateral orbital wall, as well as for lateral intradural mass lesions, such as spheno-orbital meningiomas [8].

9.4 Advantages and Limits

The main advantage of the lateral orbitocranial approach is its lesser invasiveness of both skin and bone steps. The skin incision along the upper eyelid crease and up to 2 cm lateral to the canth angle results in good cosmetic outcome, when the skin closure is made in a cosmetic manner.

Thus, large skin flaps, such as bicoronal and fronto-temporal, are avoided.

The resection of the greater wing of the sphenoid bone allows to expose the anterior temporal fossa through a small craniotomy. In this way, this approach is significantly, less invasive than the supraorbital-pterional and fronto-temporal-orbito-zygomatic approaches, which require large craniotomies.

Because of the limited skin incision and small craniotomy, this approach is significantly more rapid. However, this lateral orbito-cranial approach is only reserved to a selected group of patients with mass lesions located in the supero-lateral orbital compartment and anterior part of the temporal fossa. The skin scar, although usually cosmetic, is visible. Finally, the postoperative enophthalmos, although not observed in our surgical material of cranio-orbital tumors and our series of spheno-orbital meningiomas [8], is sometimes reported.

9.5 Modified Lateral Orbitocranial Approaches

Several modifications of the above described lateral orbitocranial approach have been proposed [12–14].

The *total lateral orbitotomy* [15, 16] is similar to the lateral orbitocranial approach, but the bone flap is extended to encompass the superior orbital rim up to the superior orbital notch and inferiorly the body of the zygoma extending medially to the midpoint of the inferior orbital rim. This more extensive approach, by removing the superior and inferior orbital rims, improves the surgical exposure and allows access to anterior cranial fossa and infraorbital region. It may be used for more extensive tumors involving the orbital apex and superior and inferior orbital fissures. The surgical risks mainly include injury to the lateral rectus muscle and optic nerve.

The *modified lateral orbitotomy*, proposed by Couldwell [13, 17, 18], includes a lateral canthotomy incision forked along the superior eyelid and opening of the lateral orbital rim to allow direct access to the sphenoid wing with partial sparing of the lateral orbital wall. The drilling of the sphenoid wing exposes the periorbita and the temporal dura, the superior orbital fissure, which can be unroofed, the cavernous sinus, the anterior clinoid, and the middle fossa structures. The lateral orbital rim is replaced and fixed at the end of the procedure.

This less invasive lateral approach provides exposure of the primary working corridor of the pterional craniotomy: it may be used for cranio-orbital mass lesions mainly located at the superior orbital fissure and cavernous sinus with no large intraorbital component.

9.6 Conclusion

The lateral orbito-cranial approach is a less invasive procedure which allows good exposure of the supero-lateral orbital compartment and anterior temporal fossa through a lateral orbitotomy and resection of the external sphenoid wing without a classic craniotomy. It may be used in a selected group of patients with cranio-orbital mass lesions located in the lateral orbital compartment, lateral to the axis of the optic nerve.

References

1. Krönlein RU. Zur pathologie and operative Behandlung der dermoidcysten der orbita. Beitr Klin Chir. 1889;4:149–63.
2. Berke RN. A modified Krönlein operation. Trans Am Ophthalmol Soc. 1953;51:193–231. https://pubmed.ncbi.nlm.nih.gov/13216779/. Accessed 14 Dec 2022.
3. Maroon JC, Kennerdell JS. Lateral microsurgical approach to intraorbital tumors. J Neurosurg. 1976;44(5):556–61. https://doi.org/10.3171/JNS.1976.44.5.0556.
4. Mourier KL, Cophignon J, D'Hermies F, Clay C, Lot G, George B. Superolateral approach to orbital tumors. Minim Invasive Neurosurg. 1994;37(1):9–11. https://doi.org/10.1055/S-2008-1053441.
5. Cossu M, Pau A, Viale GL. Postero-lateral microsurgical approach to orbital tumors. Minim Invasive Neurosurg. 1995;38(3):129–31. https://doi.org/10.1055/S-2008-1053472.
6. Paolini S, Santoro A, Missori P, Pichierri A, Esposito V, Ciappetta P. Surgical exposure of lateral orbital lesions using a coronal scalp flap and lateral orbitozygomatic approach: clinical experience.

Acta Neurochir. 2006;148(9):959–63. https://doi.org/10.1007/S00701-006-0859-5.

7. Nemet A, Martin P. The lateral triangle flap—a new approach for lateral orbitotomy. Orbit. 2007;26(2):89–95. https://doi.org/10.1080/01676830600974571.

8. Mariniello G, Maiuri F, de Divitiis E, et al. Lateral orbitotomy for removal of sphenoid wing meningiomas invading the orbit. Neurosurgery. 2010;66(6 Suppl Operative):ons287. https://doi.org/10.1227/01.NEU.0000369924.87437.0B.

9. Bikmaz K, Mrak R, Al-Mefty O. Management of bone-invasive, hyperostotic sphenoid wing meningiomas. J Neurosurg. 2007;107(5):905–12. https://doi.org/10.3171/JNS-07/11/0905.

10. de Jesús O, Toledo MM. Surgical management of meningioma en plaque of the sphenoid ridge. Surg Neurol. 2001;55(5):265–9. https://doi.org/10.1016/S0090-3019(01)00440-2.

11. Evans BT, Neil-Dwyer G, Lang D. Reconstruction following extensive removal of meningioma from around the orbit. Br J Neurosurg. 1994;8(2):147–55. https://doi.org/10.3109/02688699409027961.

12. Paluzzi A, Gardner PA, Fernandez-Miranda JC, et al. "Round-the-clock" surgical access to the orbit. J Neurol Surg B Skull Base. 2015;76(1):12–24. https://doi.org/10.1055/S-0033-1360580.

13. Abou-Al-Shaar H, Krisht KM, Cohen MA, et al. Cranio-orbital and orbitocranial approaches to orbital and intracranial disease: eye-opening approaches for neurosurgeons. Front Surg. 2020;7:1. https://doi.org/10.3389/FSURG.2020.00001.

14. Abussuud Z, Ahmed S, Paluzzi A. Surgical approaches to the orbit: a neurosurgical perspective. J Neurol Surg B Skull Base. 2020;81(4):385. https://doi.org/10.1055/S-0040-1713941.

15. Lihua Xiao XLHTHW. The clinical study of lateral orbitotomy. Zhonghua Yan Ke Za Zhi. Published online July; 2002.

16. Kim JW, Yates BS, Goldberg RA. Total lateral orbitotomy. Orbit. 2009;28(6):320–7. https://doi.org/10.3109/01676830903334028.

17. Altay T, Patel BCK, Couldwell WT. Lateral orbital wall approach to the cavernous sinus. J Neurosurg. 2012;116(4):755–63. https://doi.org/10.3171/2011.12.JNS111251.

18. Alzhrani GA, Gozal YM, Sherrod BA, Couldwell WT. A modified lateral Orbitotomy approach to the superior orbital fissure: a video case report and review of anatomy. Oper Neurosurg (Hagerstown). 2019;16(6):685–91. https://doi.org/10.1093/ONS/OPY199.

The Trans-Sphenoidal Trans-Ethmoidal Endoscopic Approach to the Orbit

Domenico Solari, Ciro Mastantuoni, Teresa Somma, Paolo Cappabianca, and Luigi M. Cavallo

10.1 Introduction

The orbit can be considered as a gateway pooled by neurocranium and facial skeleton as per its inner features, location, and connections; over years many specialties, i.e., skull base neurosurgeons, ENT surgeons, and ophthalmologists have claimed access to it and the sovereign over its disease management. These controversies are mirrored in a historical background dotted with manifold surgical corridors and approaches proposed toward and through the orbit that over the years hogged the debate of the stakeholders.

The orbit can be engaged by several traumatic, medical, and oncologic diseases leading to four basics anatomical modifications, namely, inflammatory signs, mass effect, infiltration, and vascular changes, as firstly described by Rootman and Durity [1]. The most common pathologies affecting the orbit and requiring surgical management, either via direct approach or indirect decompression, are traumas causing fractures [2, 3], foreign bodies, vascular lesions, as hemangiomas and cavernomas [4], idiopathic inflammations, thy-

roid orbitopathy [5–8], and tumors, such as meningiomas, and metastasis, hematomas, and abscess [9–12].

10.2 Surgical Approach to the Orbit

The available surgical techniques are defined upon the location of the pathology and can be divided into anterior or soft-tissue approaches, orbital marginotomies or osseous approaches, and craniofacial approaches. Among the marginotomies, the topographical division of the orbit allows to medial, lateral, inferior and superior orbitotomies, which can be further combined to fulfill the surgical goal [13–20]. In the neurosurgical scenario, approaches to the orbit are the unilateral subfrontal, frontotemporal, orbitozygomatic—along with its variants—and the transbasal approach: they were meant as skull base approaches for tumor extending into the orbital compartment, and then further borrowed for the management of purely orbital pathologies [13, 18, 21]. A fortiori, esthetic issues must be addressed when considering a proper corridor to and through the orbit, thus opening the door to the minimally invasive surgery; therefore, the introduction of the endoscopic endonasal approach represented a breakthrough in the management of orbital pathology.

D. Solari (✉) · C. Mastantuoni · T. Somma
P. Cappabianca · L. M. Cavallo
Division of Neurosurgery, Department of
Neurosciences, Reproductive and
Odontostomatological Sciences, Università degli
Studi di Napoli "Federico II", Naples, Italy
e-mail: domenico.solari@unina.it

The first description of the ventro-basal route to the orbit dates back to the 1950s when Walsh and Ogura described an anterior transantal approach for orbital decompression [22]; later on, with the ongoing expertise gained in endoscopic sino-nasal surgery, the first portrayals of the endoscopic orbital decompression by Kennedy et al. [23] and Michel et al. [24] appeared.

The endonasal corridor allows a direct access to both medial and inferior orbital walls and the orbital apex enabling either osseous decompression of the orbit and optic nerve or direct access to lesions located in the medial intra and extraconal space. Moreover, as compared with classic anterior, anterolateral, transorbital, or craniofacial routes, EEA grants an excellent magnification and visualization of the surgical field, entails no skin incisions, obviates the need of brain and globe retraction, thus reducing the risk for brain and orbital trauma, and, through a proper technique, limits fat herniation into the field of visualization [18].

The possibilities unveiled by the deployment of this route allowed skull base surgeons to push further beyond their paraphernalia by proposing four endoscopic endonasal orbital approaches for addressing an ongoing growing number of pathologies, namely, orbital decompression, optic canal decompression, endonasal orbitotomy for endo-orbital lesion removal, and the combined anterior/endoscopic approaches [14, 18, 25]. However, the EEA approach toward the orbit should rely on a rigorous knowledge of the sino-nasal anatomy whose most surgeons are unaware.

The aim of this chapter is to disclose the technique and possibility of EEA for orbit and optic nerve decompression, focusing on the orbital anatomy and its challenge via the endonasal perspective, the most common pathologies suitable for the endonasal corridor, the surgical technique, and pros and cons as compared with the classic transcranial approaches.

10.3 Relevant Endoscopic Endonasal Anatomy

The medial orbital wall is perceived as the lateral nasal wall in an endoscopic endonasal perspective. The middle and posterior portions of the medial orbit wall and the orbital apex are separated from the nose by the lamina papyracea of the ethmoid whilst the intracanalicular portion of the optic nerve is accessible through the superolateral wall of the sphenoid sinus. The lateral nasal wall is made up of six bones, namely, maxillary, lacrimal, ethmoid, sphenoid, vertical portion of palatine, and inferior nasal turbinate. Its surface is extremely irregular due to the presence of the three conchae, also known as turbinates, and respective meatus whose deepest part presents orifices and canals placing the nasal cavity in communication with the other paranasal sinuses.

The superior and middle turbinate are parts of the ethmoid bone, contrariwise the inferior turbinate is an independent bone.

The anterior portion of the lateral nasal wall contains the lacrimal system, namely, the inferior part of the lacrimal gland and the naso-lacrimnal duct (Fig. 10.1a), hosted into the lacrimal fossa, that is featured by the frontal process of the maxilla (anterior crest), and lacrimal bone (posterior crest). The naso-lacrimal duct origins from the homonymous sac in the eye socket, between the maxilla and lacrimal bone, running downward and backward to open into the inferior meatus of the nasal cavity (Fig. 10.1b). Its orifice is partially covered by a mucosal fold called Hasner valve or plica lacrimalis. Within the inferior meatus is present also the opening and Woodruff's vascular plexus.

Posteriorly, the middle turbinate may be affected by different types of abnormal pneumatization. The "concha bullosa" is defined by a pneumatization of the inferior portion of the middle turbinate, whereas if the pneumatization regards the vertical lamella above the osteomeatal com-

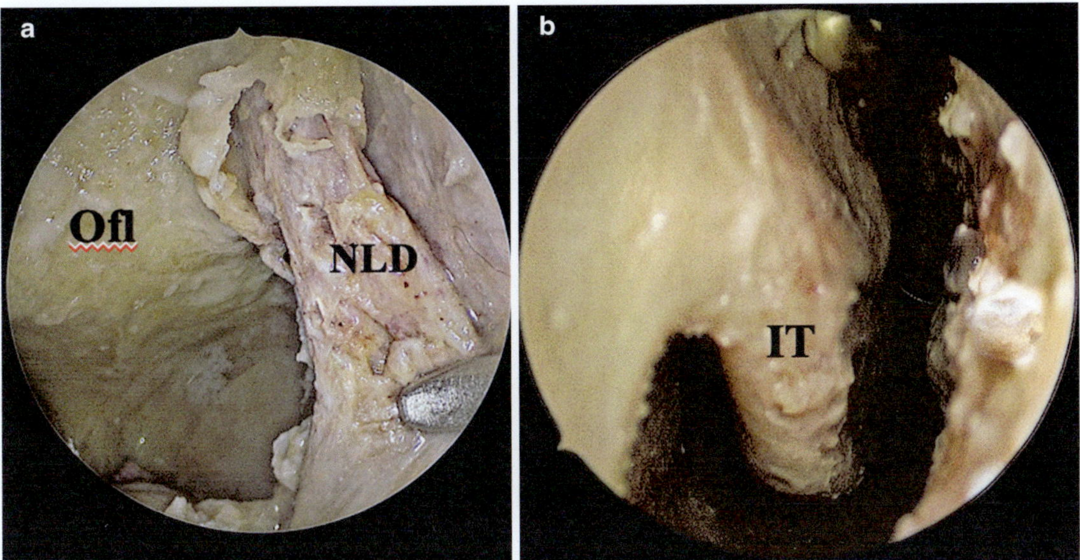

Fig. 10.1 Close-up view of the nasolacrimal duct (NDL) (**a**) and the inferior turbinate (IT) (**b**). *NLD* nasolacrimal duct, *IT* inferior turbinate, *Ofl* orbital floor)

partment is described as "Grunwald's cells," "lamellar bulla," or "conchal air neck" [26].

The middle meatus contains the uncinate process, the ethmoid bulla, the frontal recess, and the ostium of the maxillary sinus. The uncinate process is the first lamella that is identified, and it is a projection of the ethmoid bone and is attached to the lacrimal bone anteriorly and to the inferior turbinate inferiorly, whilst superiorly, it may be attached to the lamina papyracea, to the middle turbinate, or to the ethmoid sinus roof [27]. It is lined by mucosa on both its medial and lateral aspects, and its posterior edge is free within the middle meatus defining along with the ethmoid bulla a two-dimensional cleft, called hiatus semilunaris [28]. Thus, the hiatus semilunaris may be described as a crescent-shaped virtual space between the ethmoid bulla postero-superiorly and the uncinate process antero-inferiorly, where the maxillary and ethmoid sinuses drain into the nasal cavity. Antero-superiorly it extends into the ethmoidal infundibulum, a three-dimensional curved channel, bounded by the uncinate process medially, the lamina papyracea laterally, and the ethmoidal bulla posteriorly whose extreme medial opening is hiatus semilunaris [29] (Fig. 10.2). The hiatus semilunaris has been characterized by Dahlstrom et al. in five types, namely: type I, gen-

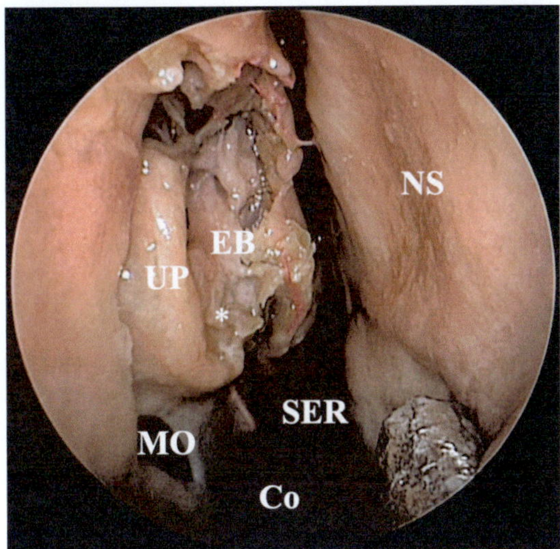

Fig. 10.2 The middle meatus after removal of the middle turbinate. The uncinate process (UP) is the first lamella that is identified. Its posterior edge is free within the middle meatus defining along with the ethmoid bulla (EB) a crescent-shaped virtual cleft, called the hiatus semilunaris (∗) extending antero-superiorly into the ethmoidal infundibulum. *UP* uncinate process, *EB* ethmoid bulla, *MO* maxillary ostium, *Co* choana, *NS* nasal septum, *SER* sphenoethmoidal recess

tle curve; type II, "J" shaped; type III, "L" shaped; type IV, "U" shaped; type Va, straight vertical; type Vb, straight oblique [30].

In this context, the maxillary line is a curvilinear eminence which projects from the anterior attachment of the middle turbinate superiorly to the root of the inferior turbinate inferiorly [31], corresponding, extranasally, to the suture between the lacrimal bone and the maxilla within the lacrimal fossa and intranasally to the attachment of the uncinate process. In an axial plane, the midpoint of the maxillary line approximates the superior aspect of the maxillary sinus ostium, laying approximately 11 mm posteriorly, and the inferior aspect of the junction of the lacrimal sac and the nasolacrimal duct anteriorly [32].

According to a modern vision of the functional anatomy of the nose, the structures lying laterally to the middle turbinate feature the osteomeatal complex draining the anterior ethmoid cells, the maxillary and frontal sinuses, being not a discrete structure but a series of components working synergistically, including anterior ethmoid air cells, maxillary sinus ostium, ethmoid infundibulum, frontal recess, the middle meatus, the hiatus semilunaris, the bulla ethmoidalis, and the uncinate process [33]. The posterior ethmoidal cells are larger and less numerous than the anterior cells. They drain either into the superior or the supreme meatus [34].

Lateral to the sphenoetmoidal recess, there is the sphenoethmoidal air cell, also known as Onodi cell, the posteriormost ethmoidal air cell. It lies superolaterally to the sphenoid sinus being close to the optic nerve and internal carotid artery. It may extend into the anterior clinoid process. The optic nerve can often course through the lateral aspect of the Onodi cell instead of through the sphenoid sinus. When a four-quadrant sphenoid sinus is observed on coronal computed tomographic (CT), the presence of an Onodi cell should be suspected [23].

The sphenoethmoidal recess extends between the choana and the natural ostium of the sphenoid sinus: this latter can be found following the tail of the superior and supreme turbinate, which can also hide it (Fig. 10.3).

The sphenoid sinus itself can vary in size, pneumatization, and for the presence of septa whose behavior and anatomical location is often inconstant. In most cases, a large septum divides

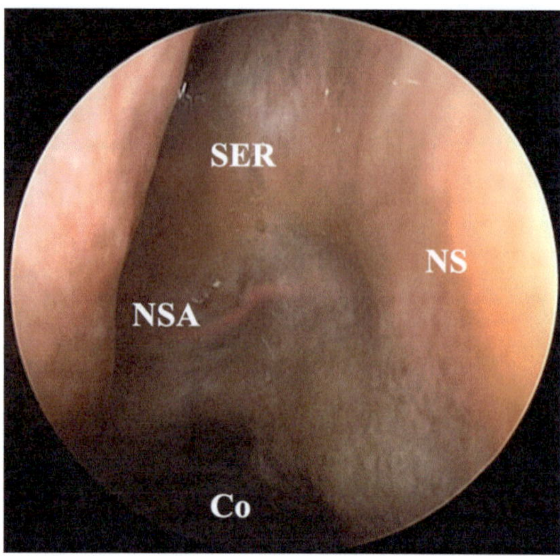

Fig. 10.3 Close-up view of the naso-septal artery (NSA) crossing the spheno-ethmoidal recess (SER) toward the nasal septum (NS). *NSA* naso-septal artery, *SER* spheno-ethmoidal recess, *NS* nasal septum, *Co* Choana

the sphenoid sinus into two sides, which is further crossed by other septa dividing it into multiple smaller cavities.

After removing the septa, some crucial bony landmarks on the posterior wall of the sphenoid sinus should be identified. The sellar floor is the center of the posterior sinus wall and the planum sphenoidale lies above it, with the suprasellar notch, corresponding to the tuberculum sellae seen from a ventral perspective [35] and the clival indentation below. The bony prominences of the internal carotid arteries can be divided into a paraclival segment and the "C-shaped parasellar segment" [36]. The optic nerves can be identified supero-laterally to the sellar floor and carotid prominences on both sides: in between, there are the lateral optocarotid recesses, molded by the pneumatization of the optic strut of the anterior clinoid process, and the medial optocarotid recesses representing the joint between the optic canal and the medial aspect of paraclinoid carotid canal [37].

The optic canal's endocranial opening is situated superiorly to the medial border of the lateral optocarotid recess. The optic nerve travels into the optic canal for 10 mm surrounded by an arachnoid space in communication with the

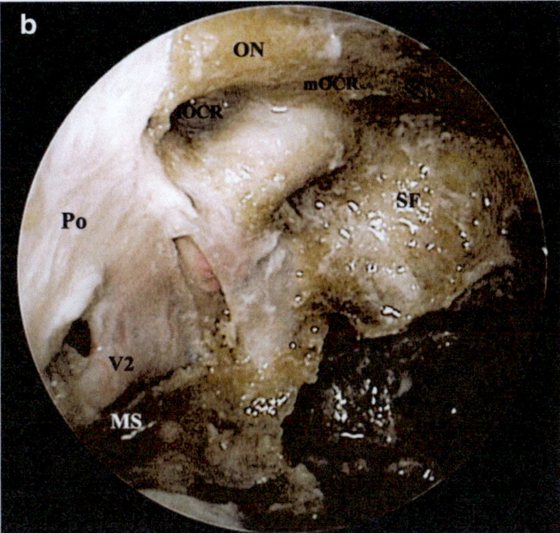

Fig. 10.4 (**a**) The medial periorbita is exposed after medial wall removal and optic canal opening. (**b**) Close-up view of the lateral recess of the sphenoid sinus. The parasellar area presents four bony protrusions: the optic nerves (ON); the superior orbital fissure (red circle); and V1 and V2. Among those, three bony depressions can be found: the lateral optocarotid recess (lOCR), the ventral projection of the maxillary strut (MS), and the depression between the maxillary and mandibular nerves. *SF* sellar floor, *PS* planum sphenoidale, *C* clivus, *SSN* suprasellar notch, *ICAc* cavernous segment of the internal carotid artery, *ON* optic nerves, *lOCR* lateral optocarotid recesses, *mOCR* medial optocarotid recesses, *Po* periorbita, *MS* maxillary strut, *V2* maxillary division of the trigeminal nerve

chiasmatic cistern while its dural sleeve is continuous with the periorbita at the level of orbital apex [38, 39].

Lateral to the internal carotid artery, the parasellar area presents four bony protrusions and three bony depressions. From rostrally to caudally, the optic canal, the superior orbital fissure, the maxillary nerve protuberance, and mandibular nerve bulge can be identified. The three bony depressions are the lateral optocarotid recess, the depression between the cavernous sinus apex, and the trigeminal maxillary division, that is, the ventral projection of the maxillary strut and the depression between the maxillary and mandibular nerves [36, 40, 41]. The maxillary strut is the inferior border of the SOF, and it is useful for inferring SOF location and thus the "front door" of the cavernous sinus [42] (Fig. 10.4).

The periorbital layers are continuous with the parasellar dura, the periosteum covering both the inferior orbital fissure, and the pterygopalatine fossa. Muller's muscle occupies the inferior orbital fissure: it crosses the ventral surface of the maxillary strut and enters the superior orbital fis-

sure, presenting a close relationship with the cavernous sinus. The medial orbital vein is a constant landmark located between SOF, optic nerve, and Muller muscle, immediately beneath the periosteum that runs toward the medial aspect of the cavernous sinus.

10.4 Surgical Indications

The endonasal route toward the orbit recognizes four main surgical indications: orbital decompression, optic canal decompression, endoscopic orbitotomy, and the combined transcranial endonasal approaches. We will focus on the endoscopic endonasal medial orbital wall and optic canal decompression.

The endoscopic endonasal medial orbital wall decompression is mostly used for the treatment of moderate to severe symptoms of Graves orbitopathy, also known as thyroid-eye disease; it is also indicated for any other congestive orbital process causing proptosis and/or vision compromise, namely tumors arising from the medial orbital wall, as meningiomas, hemangiomas, or metastasis [43] fibrous dysplasia, inverted papilloma, pseudotumor, or for sinonasal pathologies extending into the orbit. Likewise, it can be deployed for the decompression of orbital abscesses and hematomas, biopsy of indeterminate lesions, palliative therapy for malignant tumors causing visual symptoms [16], and ligation of the anterior ethmoid artery [44, 45].

The endoscopic endonasal optic nerve decompression can be performed in cases of primary or secondary tumors developing from the lesser sphenoid wing or the sinonasal cavity, such as nasopharyngeal carcinoma, triggering optic nerve compression. It is also useful for tumors of the intracanalicular segment of the optic nerve, in selected cases of traumatic optic neuropathy [46–48], although several controversies still stand, for intracerebral idiopathic hypertension [49] and in the thyroid-related compressive optic neuropathy [18, 50]. In this scenario, it stands clear that it represent a valid minimally invasive surgical option for meningiomas of the optic sheaths [51], type III clinoidal meningiomas according to the Al-Mefty classification [52] and cavernous sinus meningiomas [14, 53–55]. In these cases, the optic decompression is part of a multimodal strategy encompassing adjuvant radiotherapy [53, 56, 57].

10.5 Surgical Procedure

The operating room set up may vary widely according to the technique and surgeon preferences. Depending on the stage of the surgery, we use 0°, 30° and 45°, rigid endoscopes, 18 cm in length and 4 mm of diameter. The endoscope is held freehand during the whole procedure, by the first surgeon during the nasal step and by the second surgeon over the sellar step. This shrewdness allows a dynamic visualization of the surgical field, and the endoscope dynamic movements aid to achieve 3D orientation and depth perception of the surgical field, representing de facto the key for the tridimensionality, even without 3D scopes. Moreover, the two-surgeons four-hands technique afford the first surgeon to work bimanually

with two instruments, according to the "microsurgical technique" and thus, depending on the circumstances, two or three instruments can be inserted into the surgical field.

The patient is placed supine, with the head in neutral position and the trunk raised 10°. The head is properly accommodated in a horse-shoe headrest. Rigid three-pin fixation is reserved to the cases requiring the neuronavigation, namely, in presence of a conchal-type sphenoid configuration or in cases of recurrent lesions.

Two cottonoids soaked in 50% povidone-iodine are placed in the nasal cavity, along the nasal floor and between the nasal septum and middle turbinate. They are left in place for 5 min. Afterward, disinfection of nasal skin is performed. Using a small KILLIAN-type nasal speculum, eight cottonoids (four per nostril) soaked in decongestant solution (2 mg adrenaline, 5 mg of 20% diluted lidocaine, 4 mL of saline solution) are placed between the nasal septum and the middle turbinate. Such procedure is enacted for achieving an effective vasoconstriction on the high vascularized structures involved in the subsequent procedures.

The sterile draping is made in a pyramid-fashion around the nose, completely covering both the eyes and the forehead [58].

10.5.1 Endoscopic Endonasal Medial Orbital Wall Decompression

For the medial orbital wall decompression, a mono-nostril approach may be adequate. The 0° endoscope is inserted along the floor of the nasal cavity in the nostril ipsilateral to the decompression side; the ipsilateral middle turbinate is removed for gaining an adequate access to the medial orbital wall, so the uncinate process is removed with the aid of Kerrison rongeurs. A wide maxillary antrostomy in the posterior direction is then performed to get access to the orbital floor. Care must be taken to prevent the clogging of the osteomeatal complex by the orbital fat and to preserve the nasolacrimal duct. The infraorbital nerve can be identified running along the floor of the orbit (Fig. 10.5).

A comprehensive ethmoidectomy and wide sphenoidotomy should be carried out (Fig. 10.6a). The lamina papyracea is then unveiled from the frontal sinus anteriorly to the orbital apex posteriorly (Fig. 10.6b).

Once the lamina papyracea is exposed, the medial orbital wall should be penetrated and the

periorbita elevated with a spoon curette or a dissector. A dissector or a periosteal elevator is deployed for fracturing and removing it without disrupting the periorbita. Otherwise, a 4- or 5-mm diamond drill can be used to eggshell the bone before breaking it. The dissection should be carried from the lacrimal sac, whose nasal landmark is the maxillary line, anteriorly, to the orbital apex, posteriorly, and from the ethmoid roof, superiorly, to the orbital floor, inferiorly. The bone of the lamina papyracea will get progressively thicker moving from anterior to posterior, thus the drill should be used for the posterior portion removal. The classical medial orbital decompression encompasses the removal of the medial orbital wall alone (Fig. 10.7). Nevertheless, some lesions require orbital floor removal. In those cases, floor removal should be started from the ethmoid-maxillary suture, also known as inferonasal strut, orbital strut or orbitoethmoid strut, with the aid of a diamond drill or Kerrison rongeurs up to the infraorbital canal. A 30° endoscope may facilitate the maneuvers into the maxillary sinus. The anterior third of the floor should be spared, in order to avoid diplopia and enophthalmos.

If the periorbita is disrupted during the maneuvers on the bone, the orbital fat can herniate into

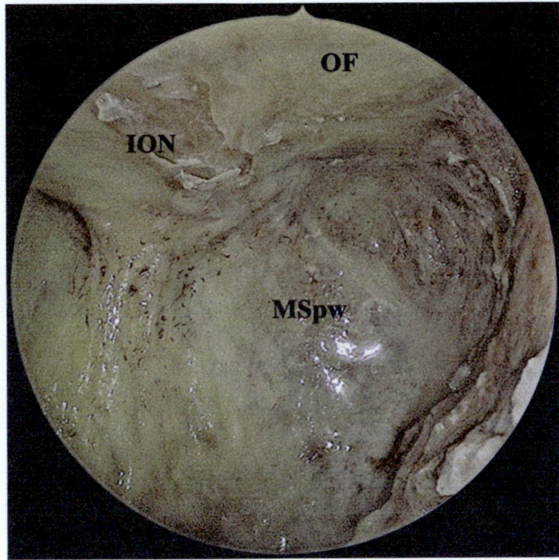

Fig. 10.5 The infraorbital nerve (ION) coursing through the orbital floor (OF). *ION* infraorbital nerve, *MSpw* poster wall of maxillary sinus, *OF* orbital floor

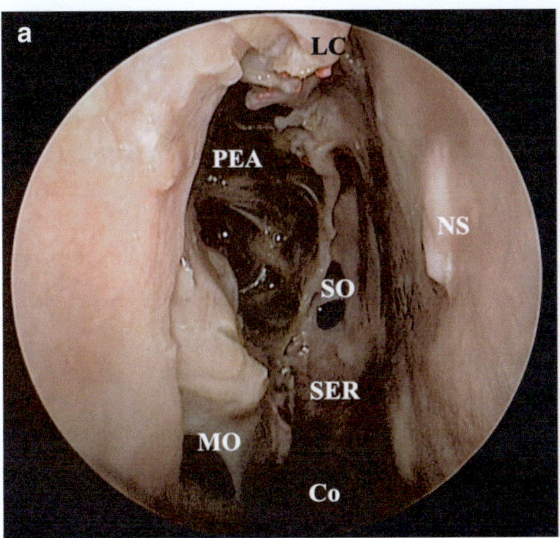

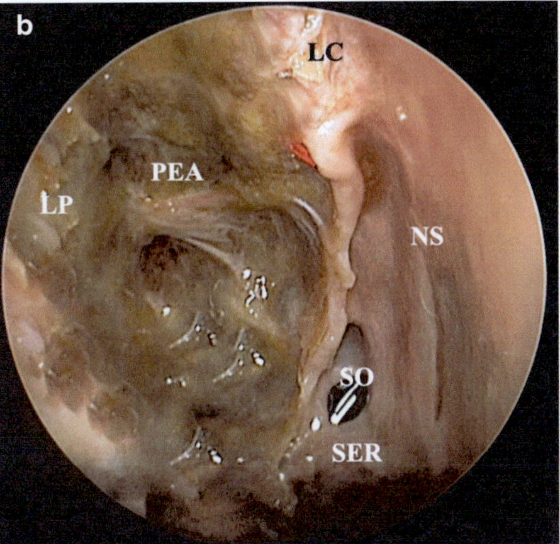

Fig. 10.6 (**a**) Anterior and middle ethmoidectomy. (**b**) Close-up view of the medial orbital wall and lamina papyracea. *LC* lamina cribrosa, *PEA* posterior ethmoidal

artery, *SO* sphenoid ostium, *SER* spheno-ethmoidal recess, *Co* choana, *MO* maxillary ostium, *NS* nasal septum, *LP* lamina papyracea

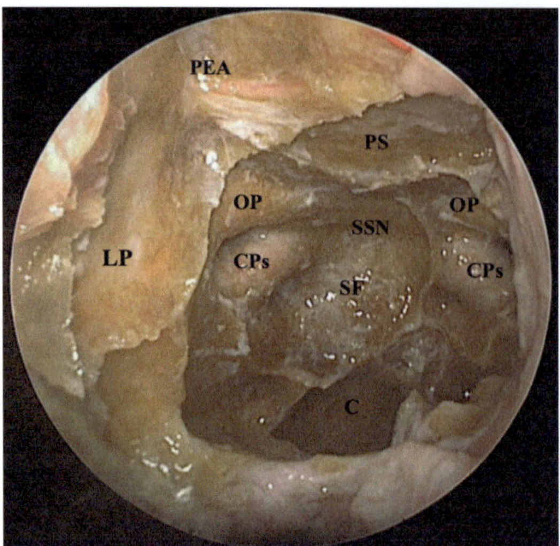

Fig. 10.7 Exposure of the lamina papyracea and medial orbital decompression. The posterior ethmoidal artery (PEA) is placed approximately 7 mm in front of the orbital end of the optic foramen. *SF* sellar floor, *PS* planum sphenoidale, *C* clivus, *SSN* suprasellar notch, *C* clivus, *CPs* carotid protuberances, *OP* optic protuberance, *LP* lamina papyracea, *PEA* posterior ethmoidal artery

the surgical field obstructing the view. Thus, it should be gently cauterized with the bipolar, taking care to not damage the medial rectus muscle [18].

Finally, the periorbita can be opened in a dorso-ventral direction with a sickle knife, and care should be taken in avoiding the medial rectus muscle that lies just deep to the periorbita. Upon the completion of the procedure, the fat prolapses into the ethmoid and maxillary cavities. Nevertheless, the osteomeatal complex should be left unsealed.

10.5.2 Endoscopic Endonasal Optic Nerve Decompression

For the endoscopic endonasal optic nerve decompression, our set up at the department of neurosurgery of University of Naples, Federico II, is based upon the bi-nostril corridor with "two surgeons four-hands technique."

To perform an optic nerve decompression, an extensive ethmoidectomy is performed and the lamina papyracea is exposed up to the anterior

wall of the sphenoid sinus and then removed, as described above. The mucosa of spheno-ethmoidal recess is then coagulated and detached subperiosteally from the anterior wall of the sphenoid sinus. The incision should be superior to the naso-palatine artery running in the inferior aspect of the spheno-ethmoidal foramen. The anterior wall of the sphenoid sinus is removed using a microdrill and Kerrison rongeurs. A minimal posterior septostomy is performed. The sphenoid rostrum and the paramedian septa are drilled flush and removed with a Kerrison rongeurs. When multiple septa are present, care must be taken since they may lead to the optic or carotid prominences.

A wide view over the entire posterior wall of the sphenoid sinus is achieved and the key landmarks can be identified, namely sellar floor, optocarotid recesses, planum sphenoidale and tuberculum sellae, clivus and carotid, and optic protuberances. The medial wall of the orbit is decompressed exposing the periorbita until the optic canal is reached (Fig. 10.4). With the aid of a high-speed 3- or 4-mm diamond drill, the medial wall and the floor of the optic canal are thinned down to eggshell thickness, from the orbital apex to the optic canal's endocranial opening. The optic canal should be opened from distal to proximal, consuming the bony surface in a parallel direction to the optic nerve. Attention should be paid particularly at optic prominence's inferior aspect; finally, the bone can be elevated from the medial canal enabling a 180° decompression. At the end, the nerve should be checked for ruling out the presence of an intraneural hematoma. The incision of the optic sheath is rarely required, and it should be placed in the superomedial quadrant in order to prevent eventual injuries to the ophthalmic artery and it should include the annulus of Zinn.

10.6 Complications

Epiphora is a typical complication of medial orbital wall decompression, and it arises when the maxillary antrostomy is extended too far anteriorly with transection of the naso-lacrimal duct. It can be managed with an endoscopic dacryocystorhinostomy.

Post-operative diplopia may occur in up to one-third of the patients undergoing medial orbital decompression as a rearrangement of the vector in the pull of the extraocular muscles. It is mostly temporary resolving spontaneously over the weeks. As reported by Finn et al. [16] and Yao et al. [49] preservation of the inferomedial orbital strut can reduce rates of diplopia.

The most frequent complications of endoscopic endonasal optic nerve decompression include bleeding from the sphenopalatine artery, vision loss or lack of improvement in vision, CSF leak, and meningitis with an overall complication rate of 9.1% [25]. If sphenopalatine artery is injured and when bleeding occurs, it should be properly coagulated with the bipolar for preventing post-operative bleeding from the nose.

Carotid and optic nerve injuries are rare but catastrophic occurrences whose risk is increased by the presence of paramedian septa leading directly to these structures or by the Onodi air cell. Therefore, a comprehensive surgical planning should be carried out for identifying skull base and neurovascular potential paraphysiological or pathological variations. In this context, neuronavigation should be used in cases of recurrent tumors or not-well pneumatized sphenoid sinus when the anatomic landmarks on the posterior wall of the sphenoid sinus are not discernible. Finally, a proper reconstruction [59] should be tailored upon the size of the osteodural defect and the grade of CSF leak [60].

10.7 Post-Operative Considerations

A nasal packing with Merocel is required due to the middle turbinectomy at the side of the decompression. High doses of steroids are usually administrated for reducing the edema caused by the pathology itself and the surgical maneuvers.

Serial ophthalmologic examinations, including visual acuity assessment, optical coherence tomography (OCT), and Hess test or Rumpel-Leede test should be performed to guide steroid tapering.

Patient instructions should include to limit their activity and avoid nose blowing and straining and twice-daily nasal saline irrigations from post-operative day 7. The patient should also be instructed to recognize and report symptoms and signs of complications as hemorrhages and late occurring CSF leak.

In our institution, we use to discharge the patient from post-operative day 2.

For medial orbital decompression, the expected ocular recession is on average 3.5 mm while an additional lateral decompression can provide further 2 mm of global recession [61].

10.8 Endoscopic Endonasal Approach Vs Transcranial

The natural conformation of the nasal and sinonasal cavity and their intimate relationships with the medial wall and the floor of the orbit makes the endoscopic endonasal route perfectly suited for medial orbital decompression. Moreover, the ventral route toward the optic canal and the optic nerve ensures a direct access to those critical structures without brain retraction or the risk of vascular damages. These advantages further bolster the general perks of EEA for the ventral skull base, namely, the close-up view of the ventral skull base, the illumination and magnification of the surgical field, the absence of surgical scar, and the increased versatility. Nowadays, it is considered the gold standard for the medial orbital pathologies encompassing the possibility of the medial orbital decompression, optic canal decompression, medial orbit or orbital apex tumor removal, direct access to primary sinonasal pathologies with intraorbital extension, such as invasive fungal sinusitis, and subperiosteal abscesses [18].

Indeed, the endoscopic endonasal approach allows a customized 160° to 180° inferomedial optic canal decompression that may be further increased in cases of high degree of pneumatization [62]. Kim et al. reported a mean length of optic canal decompression and a mean circumference of decompression of 13 mm and 252.8° for transcranial approaches and 12.4 mm and 252.8° for endoscopic approach. When finding similar outcomes in their study, Gogela et al. proposed to tailor the approach upon the individual anatomy, the pathology, and the clinical scenario [63].

In this context, EEA is suitable either for lesions extending into the medial or inferomedial canal, whose resection will adequately decompress the nerve or in cases of recurrent tumors encroaching the superolateral canal when the endoscopic route represents a naïve corridor [64, 65]. Contrarily, a wider transcranial decompression of the optic nerve is appropriate for superolateral canal compression, for the presence of significant edema or for the need of intraoperative optic nerve manipulation [66].

The transcranial route, namely anterior and anterolateral approaches, with their minimally invasive variants, allows quite extensive optic decompression with a low risk of CSF leak. Besides, the extradural anterior clinoidectomy, along with the removal of the optic strut, obviates the need for transecting the annulus of Zinn for adequate nerve decompression, thus maintaining its anatomical and functional integrity [67].

In those cases, in which a circumferential decompression of the nerve is required, as for tumor invading the whole optic canal, a combination of the endonasal and transcranial approaches should be considered, yielding a 360° bone removal and decompression: higher risk of CSF leak due to the wide communication between the intracranial space and sphenoid sinus is expected [68].

Therefore, the transcranial and endoscopic endonasal approaches should be considered as complementary route into the skull base surgeon paraphernalia, being possible to choose one or both accordingly to tumor location and expected surgical goals.

The new emerging concept of transorbital route in the scenario of the transorbital neuroendoscopic approaches (TONES) deserve a particular mention, among the paradigm shift of the multiportal surgical strategies [69–71]. Our school recently described the use of transorbital approach for optic nerve decompression, underlying its potential in removing the superolateral portion of the optic canal (an average of 192° decompression) [62]. Moreover, as combining it with the endoscopic endonasal route, complete decompression of the optic canal can be achieved per tailored multiportal minimally invasive accesses [62, 72].

10.9 Conclusions

The endoscopic endonasal approaches toward the orbits harness a straightforward route exploiting the anatomy of the ventral skull base. They allow a direct access to the medial orbital wall and orbital apex avoiding brain retraction and vascular injury. Nevertheless, its use should be carefully considered and tailored upon the location of the pathology and the expected surgical results. Indeed, they warrant a circumscribed decompression of the medial orbital wall and optic nerve, limiting their employment to selected cases. Therefore, they can be integrated into the neurosurgical paraphernalia aimed at bolstering surgeon's mastery for a thorough management of skull base pathologies.

References

1. Rootman J, Durity F. Orbital surgery. In: Sekhar LN, Janecka IP, editors. Surgery of cranial base tumors. New York: Raven Press; 1993. p. 769–85.
2. Bonsembiante A, Valente L, Ciorba A, Galiè M, Pelucchi S. Transnasal endoscopic approach for the treatment of medial orbital wall fractures. Ann Maxillofac Surg. 2019;9(2):411–4. https://doi.org/10.4103/ams.ams_173_19.
3. Suzuki M, Nakamura Y, Ozaki S, Yokota M, Murakami S. Repair of orbital floor fracture with modified transnasal endoscopic approach through anterior space to nasolacrimal duct. J Craniofac Surg. 2017;28(4):998–1002. https://doi.org/10.1097/SCS.0000000000003535.
4. Bachelet JT, Berhouma M, Shipkov H, Kodjikian L, Jouanneau E, Gleizal A. Orbital cavernous hemangioma causing spontaneous compressive hemorrhage. J Craniofac Surg. 2018;29(3):706–8. https://doi.org/10.1097/SCS.0000000000004285.

5. Ong AA, DeVictor S, Vincent AG, Namin AW, Wang W, Ducic Y. Bony orbital surgery for Graves' ophthalmopathy. Facial Plast Surg. 2021;37(6):692–7. https://doi.org/10.1055/s-0041-1735638.

6. Kim SH, Kang SM. Changes in eyelid parameters after orbital decompression according to the surgical approach in thyroid eye disease. Korean J Ophthalmol. 2021;35(6):421–8. https://doi.org/10.3341/kjo.2021.0035.

7. Williams JS, Sahu PD. Surgical management of the orbit in thyroid eye disease: lateral orbital decompression. Curr Opin Otolaryngol Head Neck Surg. 2021;29(4):289–93. https://doi.org/10.1097/MOO.0000000000000728.

8. Tagami M, Honda S, Azumi A. Insights into current management strategies for dysthyroid optic neuropathy: a review. Clin Ophthalmol. 2022;16:841–50. https://doi.org/10.2147/OPTH.S284609.

9. Bowers CA, Sorour M, Patel BC, Couldwell WT. Outcomes after surgical treatment of meningioma-associated proptosis. J Neurosurg. 2016;125(3):544–50. https://doi.org/10.3171/2015.9.JNS15761.

10. Gonen L, Nov E, Shimony N, Shofty B, Margalit N. Spheno-orbital meningioma: surgical series and design of an intraoperative management algorithm. Neurosurg Rev. 2018;41(1):291–301. https://doi.org/10.1007/s10143-017-0855-7.

11. Raheja A, Couldwell WT. Cavernous sinus meningioma with orbital involvement: algorithmic decision-making and treatment strategy. J Neurol Surg B Skull Base. 2020;81(4):348–56. https://doi.org/10.1055/s-0040-1715471.

12. Zawadzki T, Komisarek O, Pawłowski J, Wojtera B, Bilska-Stokłosa J, Osmola K. Orbital abscess: two case reports with review. Indian J Otolaryngol Head Neck Surg. 2021;74:1334–43. https://doi.org/10.1007/s12070-021-02486.

13. Parrilla C, Mele DA, Gelli S, Zelano L, Bussu F, Rigante M, et al. Multidisciplinary approach to orbital decompression. A review. Acta Otorhinolaryngol Ital. 2021;41(Suppl. 1):S90–S101. https://doi.org/10.14639/0392-100X-suppl.1-41-2021-09.

14. Jeon C, Hong SD, Woo KI, Seol HJ, Nam DH, Lee JI, et al. Use of endoscopic transorbital and endonasal approaches for 360° circumferential access to orbital tumors. J Neurosurg. 2020;135:103. https://doi.org/10.3171/2020.6.JNS20890.

15. Oyama K, Watanabe K, Hanakita S, Champagne PO, Passeri T, Voormolen EH, et al. The orbitopterygoid corridor as a deep keyhole for endoscopic access to the paranasal sinuses and clivus. J Neurosurg. 2020;134(5):1480–9. https://doi.org/10.3171/2020.3.JNS2022.

16. Turri-Zanoni M, Lambertoni A, Margherini S, Giovannardi M, Ferrari M, Rampinelli V, et al. Multidisciplinary treatment algorithm for the management of sinonasal cancers with orbital invasion: a retrospective study. Head Neck. 2019;41(8):2777–88. https://doi.org/10.1002/hed.25759.

17. da Silva SA, Yamaki VN, Solla DJF, Andrade AF, Teixeira MJ, Spetzler RF, et al. Pterional, pretemporal, and orbitozygomatic approaches: anatomic and comparative study. World Neurosurg. 2019;121:e398–403. https://doi.org/10.1016/j.wneu.2018.09.120.

18. VanKoevering K, Todeschini AB, Prevedello DL, Carrau RL, Cho RI. Endonasal and transcranial surgical approaches to the orbit. In: Cohen A, Burkat C, editors. Oculofacial, orbital, and lacrimal surgery. Berlin: Springer; 2019.

19. Matsuo S, Komune N, Iihara K, Rhoton AL. Translateral orbital wall approach to the orbit and cavernous sinus: anatomic study. Oper Neurosurg (Hagerstown). 2016;12(4):360–73. https://doi.org/10.1227/NEU.0000000000001145.

20. Norris JH, Norris JS, Akinwunmi J, Malhotra R. Optic canal decompression with dural sheath release; a combined orbito-cranial approach to preserving sight from tumours invading the optic canal. Orbit. 2012;31(1):34–43. https://doi.org/10.3109/01676830.2011.605500.

21. Abussuud Z, Ahmed S, Paluzzi A. Surgical approaches to the orbit: a neurosurgical perspective. J Neurol Surg B Skull Base. 2020;81(4):385–408. https://doi.org/10.1055/s-0040-1713941.

22. Walsh TE, Ogura JH. Transantral orbital decompression for malignant exophthalmos. Laryngoscope. 1957;67(6):544–68. https://doi.org/10.1288/00005537-195706000-00002.

23. Kennedy DW, Goodstein ML, Miller NR, Zinreich SJ. Endoscopic transnasal orbital decompression. Arch Otolaryngol Head Neck Surg. 1990;116(3):275–82.

24. Michel O, Bresgen K, Rüssmann W, Thumfart WF, Stennert E. Endoscopically-controlled endonasal orbital decompression in malignant exophthalmos. Laryngorhinootologie. 1991;70(12):656–62. https://doi.org/10.1055/s-2007-998119.

25. Dhaliwal SS, Sowerby LJ, Rotenberg BW. Timing of endoscopic surgical decompression in traumatic optic neuropathy: a systematic review of the literature. Int Forum Allergy Rhinol. 2016;6(6):661–7. https://doi.org/10.1002/alr.21706.

26. Gibelli D, Cellina M, Gibelli S, Cappella A, Oliva AG, Termine G, et al. Anatomical variants of ethmoid bone on multidetector CT. Surg Radiol Anat. 2018;40(11):1301–11. https://doi.org/10.1007/s00276-018-2057-6.

27. Solari D, Magro F, Cappabianca P, Cavallo LM, Samii A, Esposito F, et al. Anatomical study of the pterygopalatine fossa using an endoscopic endonasal approach: spatial relations and distances between surgical landmarks. J Neurosurg. 2007;106(1):157–63.

28. Isobe M, Murakami G, Kataura A. Variations of the uncinate process of the lateral nasal wall with clinical implications. Clin Anat. 1998;11(5):295–303. https://doi.org/10.1002/(SICI)1098-2353(1998)11:5<295::AID-CA1>3.0.CO;2-P.

29. Hechl PS, Setliff RC, Tschabitscher M. The hiatus semilunaris and infundibulum. In: Endoscopic anatomy of the paranasal sinuses. Vienna: Springer; 1997.

30. Dahlstrom K, Olinger A. Anatomic description of the middle meatus and classification of the hiatus semilunaris into five types based upon morphological characteristics. Clin Anat. 2014;27(2):176–81. https://doi.org/10.1002/ca.22255.

31. Chastain JB, Cooper MH, Sindwani R. The maxillary line: anatomic characterization and clinical utility of an important surgical landmark. Laryngoscope. 2005;115(6):990–2. https://doi.org/10.1097/01.MLG.0000163764.01776.10.

32. Chastain JB, Sindwani R. Anatomy of the orbit, lacrimal apparatus, and lateral nasal wall. Otolaryngol Clin North Am. 2006;39(5):855–64, v-vi. https://doi.org/10.1016/j.otc.2006.07.003.

33. Vaid S, Vaid N. Normal anatomy and anatomic variants of the paranasal sinuses on computed tomography. Neuroimaging Clin N Am. 2015;25(4):527–48. https://doi.org/10.1016/j.nic.2015.07.002.

34. Terrier F, Weber W, Ruefenacht D, Porcellini B. Anatomy of the ethmoid: CT, endoscopic, and macroscopic. AJR Am J Roentgenol. 1985;144(3):493–500. https://doi.org/10.2214/ajr.144.3.493.

35. de Notaris M, Esposito I, Cavallo LM, Burgaya AC, Galino AP, Esposito F, et al. Endoscopic endonasal approach to the ethmoidal planum: anatomic study. Neurosurg Rev. 2008;31(3):309–17. https://doi.org/10.1007/s10143-008-0130-z.

36. de Divitiis O, d'Avella E, de Notaris M, Di Somma A, De Rosa A, Solari D, et al. The (R)evolution of anatomy. World Neurosurg. 2019;127:710–35. https://doi.org/10.1016/j.wneu.2019.03.050.

37. Labib MA, Prevedello DM, Fernandez-Miranda JC, Sivakanthan S, Benet A, Morera V, et al. The medial opticocarotid recess: an anatomic study of an endoscopic "key landmark" for the ventral cranial base. Neurosurgery. 2013;72(1 Suppl Operative):66–76. https://doi.org/10.1227/NEU.0b013e318271f614.

38. Liu JK, Christiano LD, Patel SK, Tubbs RS, Eloy JA. Surgical nuances for removal of tuberculum sellae meningiomas with optic canal involvement using the endoscopic endonasal extended transsphenoidal transplanum transtuberculum approach. Neurosurg Focus. 2011;30(5):E2. https://doi.org/10.3171/2011.3.FOCUS115.

39. Cabrilo I, Dorward NL. Endoscopic endonasal intracanalicular optic nerve decompression: how I do it. Acta Neurochir. 2020;162(9):2129–34. https://doi.org/10.1007/s00701-020-04476-6.

40. Di Somma A, Torales J, Cavallo LM, Pineda J, Solari D, Gerardi RM, et al. Defining the lateral limits of the endoscopic endonasal transtuberculum transplanum approach: anatomical study with pertinent quantitative analysis. J Neurosurg. 2018;130(3):848–60. https://doi.org/10.3171/2017.9.JNS171406.

41. Solari D, Chiaramonte C, Di Somma A, Dell'Aversana Orabona G, de Notaris M, Angileri FF, et al. Endoscopic anatomy of the skull base explored through the nose. World Neurosurg. 2014;82(6 Suppl):S164–70. https://doi.org/10.1016/j.wneu.2014.08.005.

42. Dallan I, Castelnuovo P, de Notaris M, Sellari-Franceschini S, Lenzi R, Turri-Zanoni M, et al. Endoscopic endonasal anatomy of superior orbital fissure and orbital apex regions: critical considerations for clinical applications. Eur Arch Otorhinolaryngol. 2013;270(5):1643–9. https://doi.org/10.1007/s00405-012-2281-3.

43. Lenzi R, Bleier BS, Felisati G, Muscatello L. Purely endoscopic trans-nasal management of orbital intraconal cavernous haemangiomas: a systematic review of the literature. Eur Arch Otorhinolaryngol. 2016;273(9):2319–22. https://doi.org/10.1007/s00405-015-3733-3.

44. Kong DS, Young SM, Hong CK, Kim YD, Hong SD, Choi JW, et al. Clinical and ophthalmological outcome of endoscopic transorbital surgery for cranioorbital tumors. J Neurosurg. 2018;131(3):667–75. https://doi.org/10.3171/2018.3.JNS173233.

45. Castelnuovo P, Turri-Zanoni M, Battaglia P, Locatelli D, Dallan I. Endoscopic endonasal management of orbital pathologies. Neurosurg Clin N Am. 2015;26(3):463–72. https://doi.org/10.1016/j.nec.2015.03.001.

46. Chen B, Zhang H, Zhai Q, Li H, Wang C, Wang Y. Traumatic optic neuropathy: a review of current studies. Neurosurg Rev. 2022;45(3):1895–913. https://doi.org/10.1007/s10143-021-01717-9.

47. Zhao X, Jin M, Xie X, Ye P, He S, Duan C, et al. Vision improvement in indirect traumatic optic neuropathy treated by endoscopic transnasal optic canal decompression. Am J Otolaryngol. 2022;43(3):103453. https://doi.org/10.1016/j.amjoto.2022.103453.

48. Liu J, Zhao J, Wang Y, Wang Z, Li R, Chen Z, et al. Simultaneous endoscopic endonasal decompression of the optic canal, superior orbital fissure, and proper orbital apex for traumatic orbital apex syndrome: surgical anatomy and technical note. Front Surg. 2021;8:811706. https://doi.org/10.3389/fsurg.2021.811706.

49. Tarrats L, Hernández G, Busquets JM, Portela JC, Serrano LA, González-Sepúlveda L, et al. Outcomes of endoscopic optic nerve decompression in patients with idiopathic intracranial hypertension. Int Forum Allergy Rhinol. 2017;7(6):615–23. https://doi.org/10.1002/alr.21927.

50. Berhouma M, Jacquesson T, Abouaf L, Vighetto A, Jouanneau E. Endoscopic endonasal optic nerve and orbital apex decompression for nontraumatic optic neuropathy: surgical nuances and review of the literature. Neurosurg Focus. 2014;37(4):E19. https://doi.org/10.3171/2014.7.FOCUS14303.

51. Solari D, Cavallo LM, Cappabianca P. Commentary: endoscopic endonasal removal of primary/recurrent meningiomas in the medial optic canal: surgical technique and long-term visual outcome. Oper Neurosurg (Hagerstown). 2019;17(5):E192–E4. https://doi.org/10.1093/ons/opz080.

52. Al-Mefty O. Clinoidal meningiomas. J Neurosurg. 1990;73(6):840–9. https://doi.org/10.3171/jns.1990.73.6.0840.

53. Matoušek P, Cvek J, Čábalová L, Misiorzová E, Krejčí O, Lipina R, et al. Does endoscopic transnasal optic nerve decompression followed by radiosurgery improve outcomes in the treatment of parasellar meningiomas? Medicina (Kaunas). 2022;58(8):1137. https://doi.org/10.3390/medicina58081137.

54. Rubino F, Eichberg DG, Shah AH, Luther EM, Lu VM, Saad AG, et al. Is endoscopic resection a useful technique for a cavernous sinus sellar cavernoma? A case report and literature review. Br J Neurosurg. 2021:1–8. https://doi.org/10.1080/02688697.2021.1958154.

55. Koutourousiou M, Vaz Guimaraes Filho F, Fernandez-Miranda JC, Wang EW, Stefko ST, Snyderman CH, et al. Endoscopic endonasal surgery for tumors of the cavernous sinus: a series of 234 patients. World Neurosurg. 2017;103:713–32. https://doi.org/10.1016/j.wneu.2017.04.096.

56. Graillon T, Fuentes S, Metellus P, Adetchessi T, Gras R, Dufour H. Limited endoscopic transsphenoidal approach for cavernous sinus biopsy: illustration of 3 cases and discussion. Neurochirurgie. 2014;60(1–2):42–7. https://doi.org/10.1016/j.neuchi.2014.01.004.

57. Akutsu H, Kreutzer J, Fahlbusch R, Buchfelder M. Transsphenoidal decompression of the sellar floor for cavernous sinus meningiomas: experience with 21 patients. Neurosurgery. 2009;65(1):54–62. https://doi.org/10.1227/01.NEU.0000348016.69726.A6.

58. Cappabianca P, Cavallo LM, de Divitiis O, Solari D, Esposito F, Colao A. Endoscopic pituitary surgery. Pituitary. 2008;11(4):385–90. https://doi.org/10.1007/s11102-008-0087-5.

59. Cavallo LM, Solari D, Somma T, Cappabianca P. The 3F (fat, flap, and flash) technique for skull base reconstruction after endoscopic endonasal suprasellar approach. World Neurosurg. 2019;126:439–46. https://doi.org/10.1016/j.wneu.2019.03.125.

60. Esposito F, Dusick JR, Fatemi N, Kelly DF. Graded repair of cranial base defects and cerebrospinal fluid leaks in transsphenoidal surgery. Oper Neurosurg (Hagerstown). 2007;60(4 Suppl 2):295–303; discussion −4. https://doi.org/10.1227/01.NEU.0000255354.64077.66.

61. Metson R, Dallow RL, Shore JW. Endoscopic orbital decompression. Laryngoscope. 1994;104(8 Pt 1):950–7. https://doi.org/10.1288/00005537-199408000-00008.

62. Di Somma A, Cavallo LM, de Notaris M, Solari D, Topczewski TE, Bernal-Sprekelsen M, et al. Endoscopic endonasal medial-to-lateral and transorbital lateral-to-medial optic nerve decompression: an anatomical study with surgical implications. J Neurosurg. 2017;127(1):199–208. https://doi.org/10.3171/2016.8.JNS16566.

63. Gogela SL, Zimmer LA, Keller JT, Andaluz N. Refining operative strategies for optic nerve decompression: a morphometric analysis of tran-

scranial and endoscopic Endonasal techniques using clinical parameters. Oper Neurosurg (Hagerstown). 2018;14(3):295–302. https://doi.org/10.1093/ons/opx093.

64. Abhinav K, Acosta Y, Wang WH, Bonilla LR, Koutourousiou M, Wang E, et al. Endoscopic endonasal approach to the optic canal: anatomic considerations and surgical relevance. Neurosurgery. 2015;11(Suppl 3):431–45; discussion 45–6. https://doi.org/10.1227/NEU.0000000000000900.

65. Dallan I, Di Somma A, Prats-Galino A, Solari D, Alobid I, Turri-Zanoni M, et al. Endoscopic transorbital route to the cavernous sinus through the meningo-orbital band: a descriptive anatomical study. J Neurosurg. 2017;127(3):622–9. https://doi.org/10.3171/2016.8.JNS16465.

66. Beer-Furlan A, Priddy BH, Jamshidi AO, Shaikhouni A, Prevedello LM, Ditzel Filho L, et al. Improving function in cavernous sinus meningiomas: a modern treatment algorithm. Front Neurol. 2020;11:652. https://doi.org/10.3389/fneur.2020.00652.

67. Yang Y, Wang H, Shao Y, Wei Z, Zhu S, Wang J. Extradural anterior clinoidectomy as an alternative approach for optic nerve decompression: anatomic study and clinical experience. Neurosurgery. 2006;59(4 Suppl 2):ONS253–62; discussion ONS62. https://doi.org/10.1227/01.NEU.0000236122.28434.13.

68. Hainăroşie R, Ioniţă I, Pietroşanu C, Piţuru S, Hainăroşie M, Zainea V. Transnasal endoscopic orbital decompression. Rom J Ophthalmol. 2017;61(3):192–5. https://doi.org/10.22336/rjo.2017.35.

69. Dallan I, Sellari-Franceschini S, Turri-Zanoni M, de Notaris M, Fiacchini G, Fiorini FR, et al. Endoscopic transorbital superior eyelid approach for the management of selected spheno-orbital meningiomas: preliminary experience. Oper Neurosurg (Hagerstown). 2018;14(3):243–51. https://doi.org/10.1093/ons/opx100.

70. Di Somma A, Andaluz N, Cavallo LM, de Notaris M, Dallan I, Solari D, et al. Endoscopic transorbital superior eyelid approach: anatomical study from a neurosurgical perspective. J Neurosurg. 2018;129(5):1203–16. https://doi.org/10.3171/2017.4.JNS162749.

71. Locatelli D, Restelli F, Alfiero T, Campione A, Pozzi F, Balbi S, et al. The role of the transorbital superior eyelid approach in the management of selected spheno-orbital meningiomas: in-depth analysis of indications, technique, and outcomes from the study of a cohort of 35 patients. J Neurol Surg B Skull Base. 2022;83(2):145–58. https://doi.org/10.1055/s-0040-1718914.

72. Alqahtani A, Padoan G, Segnini G, Lepera D, Fortunato S, Dallan I, et al. Transorbital transnasal endoscopic combined approach to the anterior and middle skull base: a laboratory investigation. Acta Otorhinolaryngol Ital. 2015;35(3):173–9.

Alberto Daniele Arosio, Pierlorenzo Veiceschi, Elisa Maria Lazzari, Iacopo Dallan, Davide Locatelli, and Paolo Castelnuovo

Abbreviations

ACF	Anterior cranial fossa
AEA	Anterior ethmoidal artery
CSF-L	Cerebrospinal fluid leakage
CT	Computed tomography
DWI	Diffusion-weighted imaging
EEA	Endoscopic endonasal approaches
ETA	Endoscopic transpalpebral approaches
FS	Frontal sinus
IEA	Inferior eyelid approach
IOF	Inferior orbital fissure
LRM	Lateral rectus muscle
MCF	Middle cranial fossa
MRI	Magnetic resonance imaging
ON	Optic nerve
PEA	Posterior ethmoidal artery
RAOS	Robotic-assisted orbital surgery
RMA	Recurrent meningeal artery

Davide Locatelli and Paolo Castelnuovo authors equally share the last authorship.

Daniele Arosio and Pierlorenzo Veiceschi authors equally contributed to the Manuscript and share the first authorship.

A. D. Arosio · E. M. Lazzari
Division of Otorhinolaryngology,
Department of Biotechnology and Life Sciences,
"Ospedale di Circolo e Fondazione Macchi",
University of Insubria, Varese, Italy

P. Veiceschi
Division of Neurosurgery, Department of
Biotechnology and Life Sciences, "Ospedale di
Circolo e Fondazione Macchi", University of
Insubria, Varese, Italy

I. Dallan
ENT Unit, Azienda Ospedaliero-Universitaria Pisana,
Pisa, Italy

Head and Neck and Forensic Dissection Research
Center (HNS and FDRc), Department of
Biotechnology and Life Sciences, University of
Insubria, Varese, Italy

D. Locatelli
Division of Neurosurgery, Department of
Biotechnology and Life Sciences, "Ospedale di
Circolo e Fondazione Macchi", University of
Insubria, Varese, Italy

Head and Neck and Forensic Dissection Research
Center (HNS and FDRc), Department of Biotechnology
and Life Sciences, University of Insubria, Varese, Italy

Research Center for Pituitary Adenomas and Sellar
Pathology, University of Insubria, Varese, Italy

P. Castelnuovo (✉)
Division of Otorhinolaryngology, Department of
Biotechnology and Life Sciences, "Ospedale di
Circolo e Fondazione Macchi", University of
Insubria, Varese, Italy

Head and Neck and Forensic Dissection Research
Center (HNS and FDRc), Department of Biotechnology
and Life Sciences, University of Insubria, Varese, Italy

Research Center for Pituitary Adenomas and Sellar
Pathology, University of Insubria, Varese, Italy
e-mail: paolo.castelnuovo@uninsubria.it

© The Author(s), under exclusive license to Springer Nature Switzerland AG 2023
G. Bonavolontà et al. (eds.), *Cranio-Orbital Mass Lesions*,
https://doi.org/10.1007/978-3-031-35771-8_11

SEA   Superior eyelid approach
SOF   Superior orbital fissure
SOM   Spheno-orbital meningiomas
TONES   Transorbital neuro-endoscopic surgery

11.1　Introduction

The orbit is a challenging anatomical area which often requires invasive surgical approaches due to its restricted surgical accessibility. Nonetheless, considering its crucial location within the skull, it is a subject of shared interest among several surgical specialties, including neurosurgery, otorhinolaryngology, ophthalmology, and maxillofacial surgery.

A wide range of pathological conditions can involve the orbit as a surgical target, such as congenital or traumatic bony defects, Basedowian ophthalmopathy, vascular malformations, and neoplastic lesions (both intraconal or extraconal, benign or malignant in nature). Moreover, the orbit can act as a corridor to reach adjacent intracranial anatomical areas.

In the wake of a renewed interdisciplinary collaboration, technological advances, and greater experience by the operators, new pioneering techniques have been developed for the management of orbit pathologies [1, 2] . Orbital surgery has recently been revolutionized by the implementation of endoscopic assistance to both transnasal and transpalpebral approaches. According to anatomical studies and clinical experiences, the authors believe that endoscopic techniques can be integrated magnificently in orbital procedures, offering improved outcomes. Moreover, the value of the endoscope as a teaching tool should be overemphasized, considering that all the members of the operating room staff (e.g., nurses, physicians, residents, and students) share the same view of the first surgeon, thus improving the anatomical knowledge and speeding up the learning curve. These procedures, according to contemporary experiences, allow the achievement of optimal results in terms of radicality and aesthetic-functional outcomes [3–7] . The transnasal endoscopic route allows easy access to all the medial orbital compartment, from the lacrimal area to the orbital apex, with-

out the need for any skin incision or retraction of the cerebral parenchyma. In the current state of the art, transphenoidal or transethmoidal endoscopic surgeries to the orbit have become well-codified procedures and have become widespread worldwide. They are often carried out in close cooperation between neurosurgeons and otolaryngologists [7].

As regards the endoscope-assisted transpalpebral approaches, the application in the literature is limited to case series and expert opinions [8]. However, the published experiences seem to demonstrate that these approaches represent a solid option not only to manage intraorbital lesions but also to use the orbit as a surgical corridor for selected skull base and intracranial pathologies [8–10] . Moe et al. have proposed the term "Transorbital Neuro-Endoscopic Surgery" (TONES) to indicate a group of procedures that use this operative corridor to access the skull base. Indeed, considering orbit as a corridor, it is possible to treat several disorders located into both the anterior and middle cranial fossa [10].

Based on these premises, in this chapter, we will present a review of endoscopic-assisted transorbital procedures, with particular emphasis on transpalpebral approaches, considering that transnasal transorbital approaches have been already described in a previous chapter. Indications, preoperative work-up, operating room setting, and surgical technique will be analyzed and valuable surgical tips will be provided in order to avoid complications. The importance of a multidisciplinary collaboration will be stressed out, as the key to guarantee optimal results while minimizing the risks associated with the single surgical procedure. Finally, postoperative work-up and follow-up will be discussed, along with some speculations regarding possible future improvements and evolution of these surgical approaches.

11.2　Preoperative Work-Up

An accurate preoperative work-up is required in the patient candidate for endoscopic transorbital surgical procedures, with particular reference to a precise radiological evaluation for evaluation of several factors (patients' individual anatomy, the relationship of the lesion with the herein located neuro-vascular structures, the invasion of different cranio-orbital compartments) and an accurate ophthalmological assessment.

11.2.1 Radiological Assessment

A head Computed Tomography (CT) scan is usually the first diagnostic exam performed. It allows for an accurate location of the orbital mass and a study of the endo-orbital structures, although with a lower contrast resolution as compared to Magnetic Resonance Imaging (MRI). A CT scan is generally well-tolerated by the patient, as it is fast and provides important clues useful for a presumptive diagnosis [11]. It represents the gold standard exam for traumas, helping to detect foreign bodies or fractures of the orbital frame. CT must be considered an indispensable first-level examination for the diagnosis of orbital malformations since it allows the study of both the bone component and other secondary alterations. Moreover, if an endoscopic intervention via the transnasal route is planned, CT imaging is paramount to highlight the presence of anatomical variants of the paranasal sinuses to properly plan the surgical procedure.

MRI of the orbit and the maxillo-facial region is also warranted before surgery. It provides better details for the orbital compartment due to its superior definition for soft tissues compared to CT scan and may detect finer pathognomonic characteristics of the lesion [12] . T1, T2, and T2*-weighted MRI sequences, along with time-dependent characteristic of the contrast-enhancement of the lesion, the use of diffusion-weighted imaging (DWI) and fat suppression sequences, provide presumptive indications about the nature of the mass, as well as a more precise localization along the intraconical or extraconical spaces, the involvement of the orbital apex, the extension to the intracranial compartments, and the relationship with the optic nerve [11]. MRI can be completed with a Magnetic Resonance Angiography to offer more precise diagnostic information about the vascular anatomy, to some extent comparable to angiography, without the need of invasive arterial catheterization. To conclude, both CT and MRI are complementary diagnostic exams warranted for patients undergoing endoscopic surgery. To note, the two exams can be merged to be used for intra-operative navigation, clinical and ophthalmological evaluation. The current body of literature shows a homogeneous consensus about the fact that an accurate ophthalmological evaluation should precede orbital surgery, as it detects signs of disease that may go unnoticed by non-specialist colleagues [13]. By checking measurable and repeatable parameters, it is possible to classify the severity of the presenting symptoms and compare it to the post-surgical outcomes. The execution of assessments such as visual field test, exophthalmometry, Hess Lancaster test is the cornerstone of ophthalmological consultation. Hertel's exophthalmometer offers an accurate and reproducible measurement of the degree of the proptosis, with the advantage of comparing both eyes in a single measurement. A difference of at least 2 mm in the two eyes or a value greater than 21 mm is considered pathological. A measurement of less than 14 mm is classified as an enophthalmos. The Hess Lancaster test is used to evaluate the binocular vision, and it is indicated for establishing the presence of diplopia or suppression. The advantage consists in the speed of execution. It is carried out with the aid of glasses with red and green filters.

11.2.2 Photographic Documentation

A photographic imaging of the candidate for transorbital surgery can be useful not only for the diagnosis and the treatment plan but also for the control of the results, to improve communication between colleagues, for didactic use and even for medico-legal issues. A standardized approach considering the main variables for the picture (e.g., patient positioning, lighting, exposure, background, depth of field) is suggested in order to have comparable preoperative and postoperative documentation.

Once all the appropriate investigations have been carried out, a multidisciplinary discussion between all members of the skull base team is performed. Finally, the surgical procedure is discussed with the patient, focusing on the risks and benefits of the specific surgery, and consent is obtained.

11.3 Intraoperative Setting

11.3.1 Patient Positioning

A correct positioning of the patient in the operating room is imperative for a safe and effective surgical procedure. The setting is dependent on several factors, mainly represented by the type and duration of surgery, anesthesiologic plan, specific devices required (e.g., intraoperative navigation). A proper placement should provide safety for the procedure to be performed as well as quick and adequate access to airway and circulation for the anesthesiologist, while providing comfort for the surgeons [14]. Transorbital surgery is performed in general anesthesia, with the patient placed in supine position with the occipital-nuchal region lying on a silicon headrest. Anesthesiologists are free to access the airways, venous lines, and other medical devices. The patient's arms are positioned laterally to the body and secured on armboards. The elbows are padded with foam to avoid ulnar neuropathy from pressure contact at the ulnar groove. Padding should also be retained under the heel area, and a pillow is placed behind the knees to reduce tension on the back. Usually, a slight anti-Trendelenburg's position is adopted, in order to reduce bleeding during the procedure. Rigid fixation with the Mayfield head-holder is unnecessary since it can limit manual adjustments to head position during surgery. Furthermore, it removes the discomfort produced by pin fixation. This frameless positioning allows the free usage of neuronavigation with electromagnetic tracking, with the non-invasive patient reference taped nearly 3 cm over the glabella and the flat emitter (StealthStation S8; Medtronic, Minneapolis, USA) positioned under patient's head [15].

11.3.2 Operating Room-Setting and Instrumentation

In the transorbital approach, the operating room is organized with one monitor in front of each surgeon (usually two monitors during standard procedures, sometimes three in case an adjunctive surgeon is needed). The first and second surgeons also have visual access to the intraoperative neuronavigation device for CT and MRI image-guidance, which can be used during various phases of the procedure (Fig. 11.1). The setting also need to take into account the eventual need for special surgical instrumentation such as Ultrasonic Aspirator devices or Cryoprobes [4] . The endoscope is never fixed with a holder, but held by one of the operators and, as a rule, surgical procedures are performed using a three- or four-handed technique [2]. Depending on the preferences of the surgical team, the first surgeon can hold the endoscope and one other instrument, while the other takes care of the second instrument and aspiration/irrigation; alternatively, the first surgeon can work with both hands while the second holds the endoscope. In the superior eyelid procedures, a third surgeon may be useful to maintain an adequate operating space by use of flexible retractors to displace the orbital content. This action has to be dynamic, that is providing alternatively moments of compression and retraction of the orbital content, so as to avoid mechanical or ischemic damages.

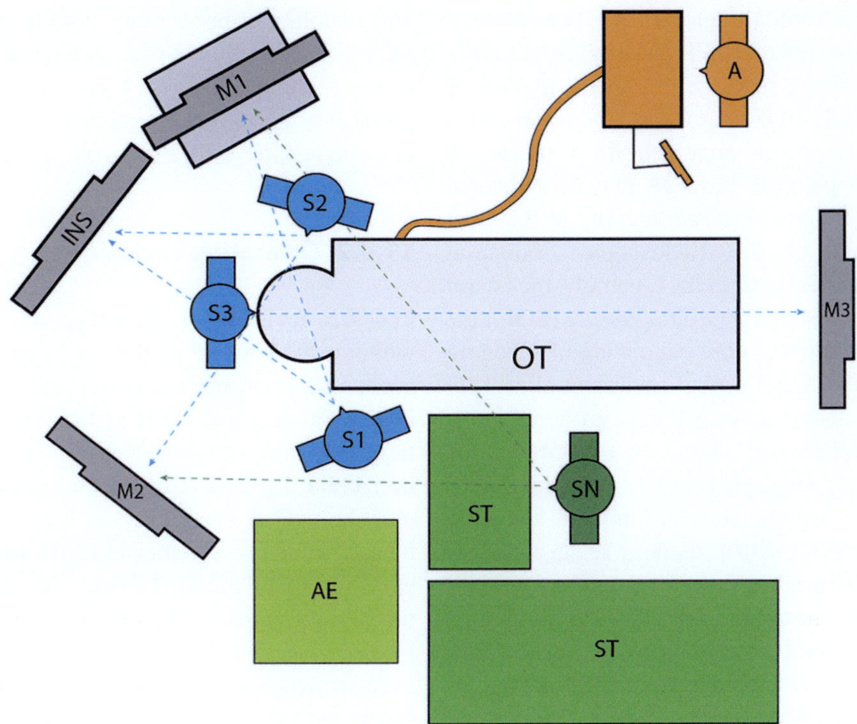

Fig. 11.1 Operating room-setting and instrumentation. Schematic representation of the location of surgeons, nurse, monitors, intraoperative navigation system, and other instrumentation during a standard transorbital procedure. Abbreviations: *A* anesthesiologist, *INS* intraoperative navigation system, *M* monitor, *AE* additional equipment (e.g. Ultrasonic Aspirator devices or Cryoprobes), *OT* operating table, *S* surgeon, *SN* scrub nurse, *ST* serving table; arrows: schematic representation of line of sight of surgeon and scrub nurse toward the monitors in the operating room

11.4 Superior Eyelid Approach

11.4.1 Indications

The Superior Eyelid Approach (SEA) is the real workhorse procedure among the Endoscopic Transpalpebral Approaches (ETA). It allows not only to manage orbital lesions but also to employ the orbit as a surgical corridor for selected skull base regions.

Considering the **orbit as a target**, the SEA can be adopted for lesions located laterally to the optic nerve, both in the extraconal and the intraconal space. This approach can be useful for biopsies, tumoral mass removal, drainage of intraorbital abscesses, and for treating superolateral orbital frame fractures [5] . In this setting, the SEA should be considered as a safe mini-mally invasive approach, alternative to more invasive traditional external procedures, often requiring osteotomies [16].

Considering the **orbit as a corridor**, the SEA represents a highway to reach the far lateral portion of the Frontal Sinus (FS), the Anterior Cranial Fossa (ACF), and the Middle Cranial Fossa (MCF). According to the pneumatization of the Frontal Sinus above the orbital cavity and the location of the disease within it (e.g., inflammatory pathologies, mucoceles, pedicle of benign lesions), traditional endoscopic endonasal approaches are sometimes unable to reach the far lateral portion of the FS itself [17, 18]. Novel techniques have been described, combined with Draf type II and III approaches in order to lateralize the fulcrum of the optics and instrumentation, thus overcoming the limit represented by the supero-medial orbital angle [19, 20]. Nonetheless, in a highly pneumatized FS, the orbit represents a valuable corridor to reach the lateral portion of the sinus, and in these cases the superior eyelid is the most employed approach. If a transdural approach is planned, the SEA may be indicated to manage lesions localized laterally to the most lateral limit of the Endoscopic Endonasal Approach (EEA) to skull base, namely, the lateral portion of the Superior Orbital Fissure (SOF), the retro-orbital region of the great wing of sphenoid bone, and the lateral wall of cavernous sinus [21]. In our clinical practice, we have gathered a significant experience with endoscope-assisted SEA, dealing with Spheno-Orbital Meningiomas [22]. Those tumors arise around the sphenoid ridge and present with a "carpet-like" growth pattern, usually invading the orbital region with their hyperostotic component. Presenting symptoms include unilateral exophthalmos, vision or visual field deficits, extraocular movement palsy, as well as cosmetic deformities. Transorbital approaches can be used in a very effective way to treat the symptoms caused by these neoplasms, instead of the traditional craniotomies (i.e., fronto-temporal, fronto-temporo-orbital, and supraorbital) [23, 24]. Other indications of SEA include the repair of skull base defects, the treatment of anterior and middle cranial fossa fractures, the drainage of epidural abscess or hematoma. Many cadaveric studies have demonstrated indeed the feasibility of an endoscopic amygdalohippocampectomy via a transorbital SEA [25]. If combined with an EEA or with other cranial techniques, the SEA gives rise to a multiportal procedure that overcomes the boundaries of a single approach [26].

11.4.2 Operative Technique

The skin incision for SEA (Fig. 11.2) is made within a hidden fold of the upper eyelid, which accounts for a nearly invisible postoperative scar. Dissection proceeds with sectioning the orbicularis oculi muscle, which is recognized due to the horizontal orientation of its fibers. Utmost care must be paid not to incise the levator palpebrae muscle, which is seen traversing the surgical field with vertically oriented fibers. In order not to damage this muscle, thus causing postoperative ptosis, dissection should be performed delicately in a superficial suborbicularis plane with a supero-lateral direction, until the orbital frame is reached. The decision to spare or to open the orbital septum depends on the purpose of the surgery. In any case, its opening will cause orbital fat herniation into the operating field, which must be managed through the use of retractors [2, 10]. After reaching the orbital rim, the periosteum is incised, and the surgical field enlarged in the same plane to grant a comfortable access for the optics and all the instrumentation needed. Subcutaneous stitches with silicone tubes might

Fig. 11.2 Overview of the superior eyelid approach. The skin incision is made within a hidden fold of the upper eyelid (**a**). Sectioning the orbicularis oculi muscle (**b**). Exposition of the levator palpebrae muscle, recognizable by the vertical orientation of its fibers (**c**). The dissection proceeds in the suborbicular plane, taking care to not damage the levator palpebrae muscle, until the orbital rim is exposed (**d**). 0° endoscopic view of the orbital cavity during subperiosteal dissection, with exposure of the recurrent meningeal branch and the superior orbital fissure (**e**). The critical landmarks in this phase are the optic nerve, the posterior, middle, and the anterior ethmoidal arteries (**f**). Drilling of the orbital roof to enter the frontal sinus (**g**), which is identified with the use of intraoperative image-guidance system (light blue area). Exposure of the anterior cranial fossa and middle cranial fossa dura (**h**). Abbreviations: *OM* orbicularis muscle, *LPM* levator palpebrae muscle, *OR* orbital rim, *PO* periorbit, *RMB* recurrent meningeal branch, *SOF* superior orbital fissure, *ON* optic nerve, *PEA* posterior ethmoidal artery, *MEA* middle ethmoidal artery, *AEA* anterior ethmoidal artery

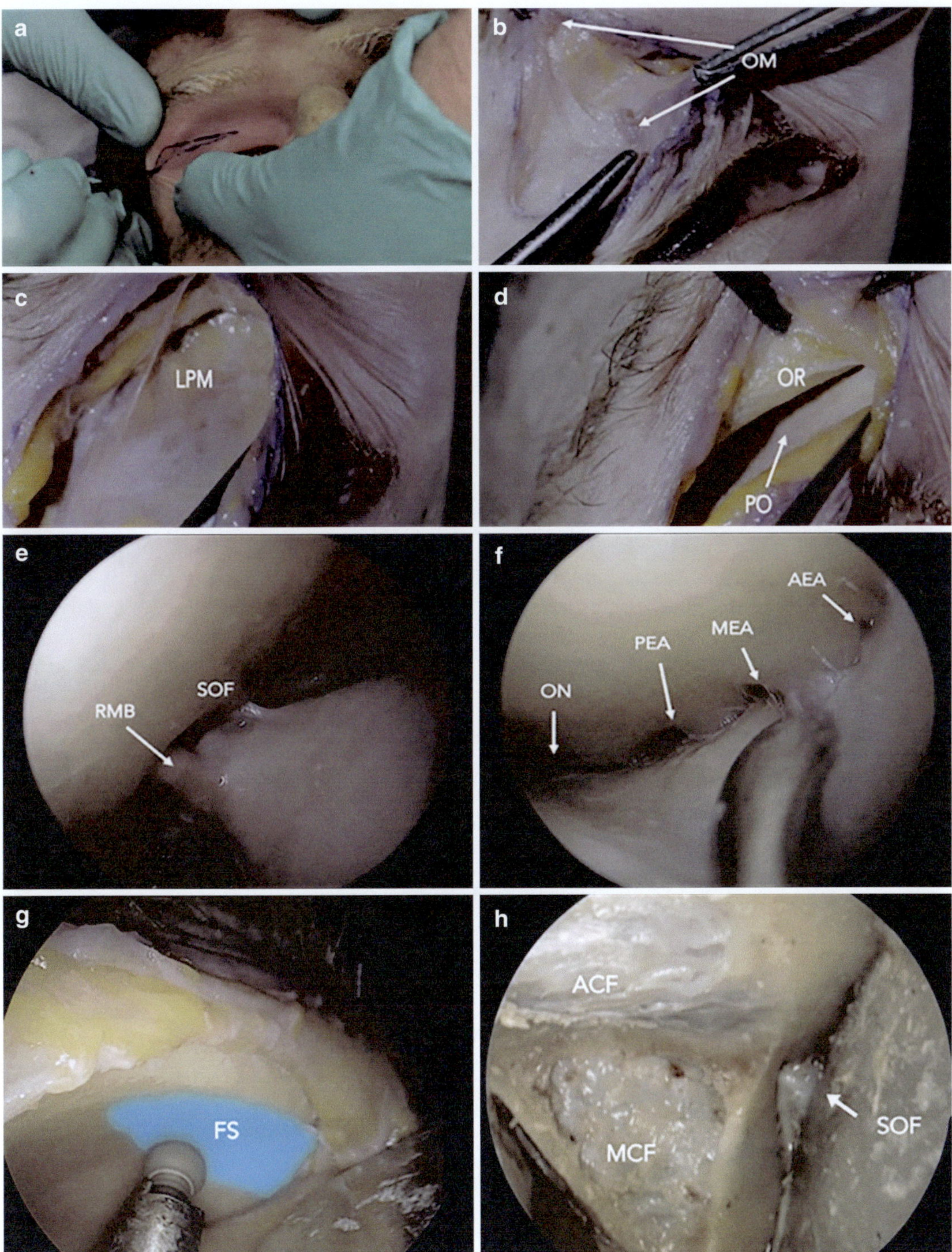
a
b
OM
c
LPM
d
OR
PO
e
SOF
RMB
f
AEA
PEA
MEA
ON
g
FS
h
ACF
MCF
SOF

be helpful to enlarge the skin incision providing more space while reducing the risk of damaging the eyelid [4]. Once sufficient space is available, a 0° endoscope (Karl Storz, Tuttlingen, Germany) is introduced in the surgical cavity and the whole surgery is performed entirely under endoscopic vision. A subperiosteal dissection is advanced in order to visualize the intraorbital anatomical landmarks. The first one to come into view is the Recurrent Meningeal Artery (RMA), which represents an anastomosis between the middle meningeal and the lacrimal artery.

It is seen in most of the cases (about 60–80% of the population) traversing a separate bony canal in the supero-lateral orbital wall, the Hyrtl or meningo-orbital foramen, while in a minority of patients, it is the most supero-laterally located vessel in the SOF. Advancing from above downward and in a latero-medial direction, the SOF is visualized, while the Inferior Orbital Fissure (IOF) is reached extending the dissection infero-laterally. Proceeding from lateral to medial along the roof of the orbital cavity, the Optic Nerve (ON), the Posterior (PEA), and the Anterior Ethmoidal Arteries (AEA) are visualized. Until the identification of the intraorbital landmarks is completed, the surgeon must pay attention to preserve the periorbit, thus avoiding the herniation of the periorbital fat in the surgical fields, which significantly complicates intraorbital dissection.

Orbit as Target. The orbital content is entered with an incision of the periorbit at the approximate depth of the lesion, according to an accurate preoperative evaluation and often with the aid of the image-guidance technologies. The periorbital incision reveals the extraconal fat, which is more represented in the anterior portion of the retrobulbar region, while it is more scarce proceeding toward the orbital apex. After a dissection phase in the periorbital fat, the Lateral Rectus Muscle (LRM) represents the first anatomical landmark during transorbital procedures for lesions located laterally to the ON. Above the LRM, the lacrimal neurovascular "bundle," formed by the nerve, artery and vein, is found, overlying the superior surface of the LRM before its insertion. The RMA can enter the orbit at this level, usually joining the lacrimal artery. It can be spared or

coagulated, according to the need. Near to the superior orbital fissure, posteriorly, the superior branch of the oculomotor cranial nerve is visible. Moreover, the superior ophthalmic vein can be identified more posteriorly, right above the optic nerve and below the superior rectus muscle. Posteriorly, toward the apex and the SOF, the inferior division of the third cranial nerve can be seen. To notice, all these anatomical structures are not always encountered intraoperatively. In fact, once the lesion is identified, surgery proceeds with a gentle pericapsular dissection, with the use of blunt instruments and cottonoid pledges, which are used to isolate the lesion from the surrounding anatomical structures. Once a portion of the lesion is exposed, in case of well circumscribed and encapsulated lesions, such as for example orbital venous malformation type I (OVM, ex cavernous hemangioma), the use of cryoprobes has proven useful to grasp the lesion without the need to further proceed in the dissection in the intraconal space, as dissection can be completed outside the orbital content once the lesion is properly retracted, similarly to medially located intraconal lesions removed via a transnasal route. After removal of the lesion, accurate hemostasis is performed, with the cautious use of bipolar, irrigation with warm saline, and eventually hemostatic agents. In most of the cases, no reconstruction is needed after intraorbital surgery. In case of removal of bulky lesion, the considerable empty space might be filled with autologous fat to reduce the risk of post-operative enophthalmos, but this is rarely needed [23]. Figure 11.3 illustrates a clinical case example of SEA to the orbit for removal of an OVM type I.

Orbit as Corridor. The surgical steps when the orbit is not intended as the target, but the corridor of the approach, are the same as the ones listed in the previous paragraph, up to the visualization of the intraorbital landmarks. Again, it is important to underline that to further proceed with intracranial surgery, dissection is to be performed without accidentally opening the periorbit. During this phase, moments of retraction of the orbital content are realized with malleable retractors and a soft Silastic sheet (Dow Corning, Midland, Michigan, USA) protecting the periorbit.

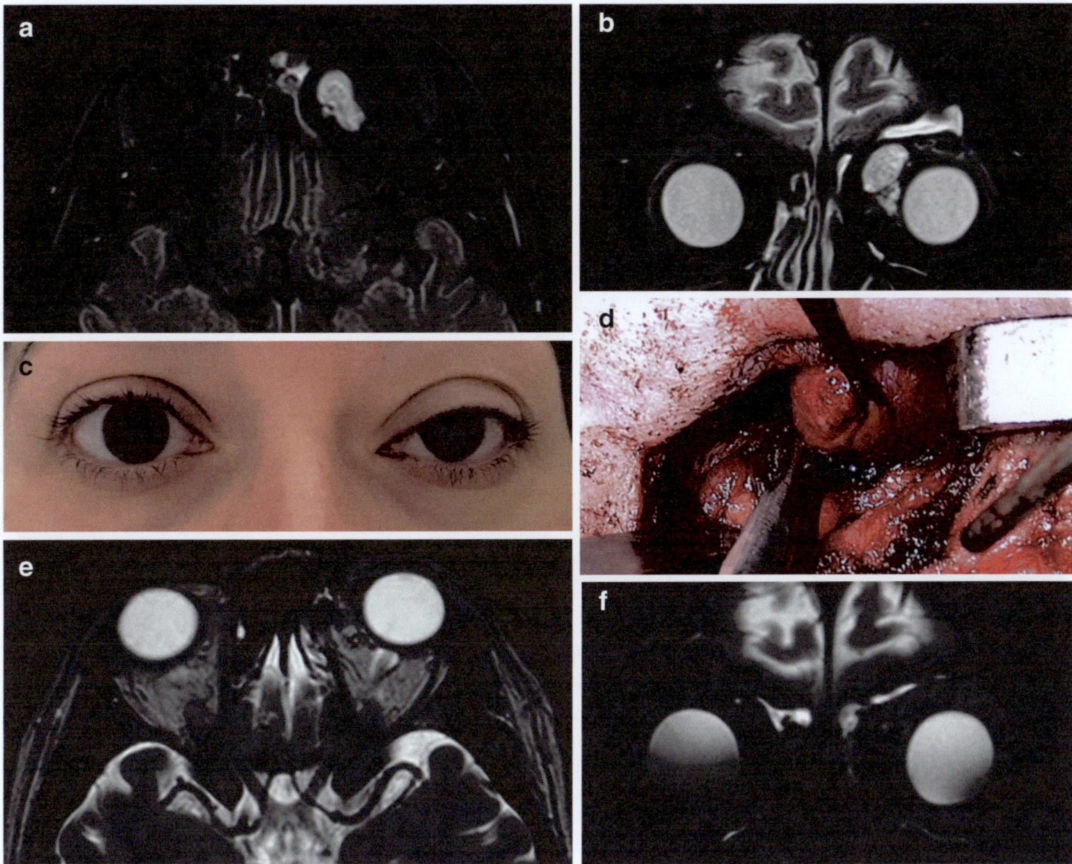

Fig. 11.3 SEA for removal of OVM type I (e.g., cavernous hemangioma). Illustration of a 37-year-old female patient who presented to our department complaining of left periorbital swelling, proptosis, and ocular pain. MRI with contrast was performed, showing a left anterior extraconal supero-medial orbital cavernous neoformation, suspected for OVM type 1, complicated with an ipsilateral frontal mucocele. Preoperative MRI in axial Flair sequence (**a**), coronal T2-weighed (**b**). Periorbital swelling and proptosis (**c**). The patient underwent removal of the neoformation via a SEA (**d**). Postoperative axial (**e**), and coronal T2-weighed MRI (**f**), which demonstrated the complete resection of the orbital hemangioma

For a transorbital access to the frontal sinus, a proper anatomical landmark to safely enter the sinus has not been yet identified. The FS might be variable in pneumatization and is localized very anteriorly along the orbital roof. In most of the cases, the floor has already been interested by the pathology (e.g., orbital complication of frontal sinusitis with orbital wall erosion), so that the sinus can be entered through the pre-existing defect. On the contrary, in case of an intact orbital roof, the intraoperative image-guidance systems are helpful to properly plan the osteotomy [27].

Once entered the sinus, the target of the surgery is usually easily visualized and managed, with the use of either straight or curved instrumentation [28]. The combination of the SEA with an expanded approach to the frontal sinus is usually able to manage the sinus in its entirety [29] (Fig. 11.4).

For an anterior cranial fossa approach, a craniectomy with a diamond-burr is performed by drilling the orbital roof (in the laterobasal frontal bone) and part of the lesser wing of the sphenoid bone. The greater wing is left intact in case of a

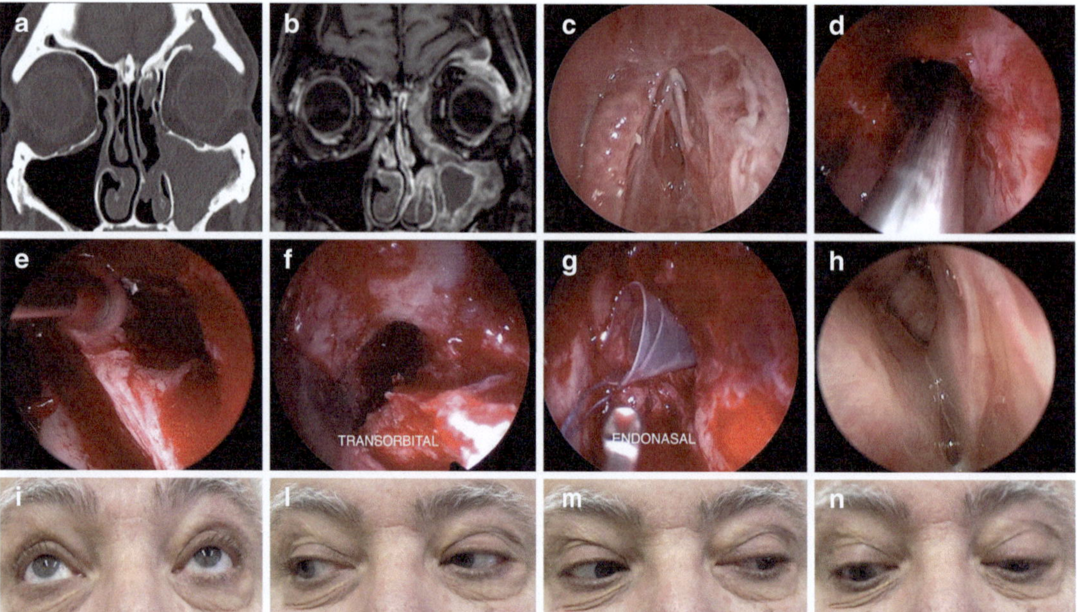

Fig. 11.4 Combined endonasal-transorbital approach for a fronto-orbital abscess. Case illustration of a 76-year-old male who underwent a previous Draf IIA procedure for a left fronto-ethmoidal empyema from Staphylococcus Aureus. After 3 months, he complained of periorbital swelling and tenderness. Coronal CT scan (**a**) and T1-weighed MRI with contrast (**b**), demonstrated a left fronto-ethomoido-maxillary sinusitis with erosion of the orbital roof. He underwent revision surgery by means of a combined endoscopic endonasal and transorbital approach, due to the far lateral location of the inflammatory process within the frontal sinus. Stenosis of left frontal sinusotomy can be seen (**c**). The re-opening is demonstrated under endoscopic view (**d**). Moreover, the frontal ostium was enlarged through drilling via the transorbital approach (**e**, **f**). At the end, a frontal stent was positioned, as seen from the endonasal perspective (**g**). 1-month postoperative endonasal control that demonstrated the patency of left frontal sinus (**h**). The regular eye motility was assessed 1 year after surgery (**i-n**)

pure transorbital exposure of the anterior skull base. The boundary of this surgical approach can be summarized as follows: orbital rim superiorly, lesser sphenoid wing inferiorly, pterional region laterally, lateral aspect of the SOF medially. After the craniectomy, the dural layer of the frontal supraorbital region is unveiled. Dura is divided according to the specific target, and the basal frontal lobe along with the orbital gyri are exposed.

For a transorbital middle cranial fossa approach, the SOF and the IOF have to be fully exposed, as well as the greater wing of the sphenoid until the superolateral orbital wall. The craniectomy is carried on within the greater sphenoid wing, limited supero-medially by the superior orbital fissure and laterally by the temporal muscle (Fig. 11.2). The boundary of this surgical approach can be summarized as follows: SOF superiorly, IOF infero-medially, periosteal layer of the temporalis muscle laterally, and the floor of the middle cranial fossa inferiorly [2, 5]. If more space is needed for the resection, the craniectomy can be enlarged inferiorly to include the floor of the middle cranial fossa and superiorly by removing part of the lesser wing of the sphenoid bone [26]. If an intradural approach is anticipated, the temporal dura is opened, and the polar region of the temporal lobe is reached.

In case of intradural pathology, our experience proves that dural reconstructions is often not needed, because the orbital structures behave like a natural sealant, even if the theoretical risk of Cerebrospinal Fluid Leakage (CSF-L) exists [2, 5]. Nevertheless, several skull base closure techniques have been described in the literature, even for transorbital approaches. Some authors have considered the possibility to perform a multilayer reconstruction, in line with those performed in transnasal endoscopic craniectomy. Alqahtani et al. described a multilayer technique in which they put an intradural layer with synthetic graft, followed by muco-periosteal septal graft overlay covering the superior orbital wall defect [30]. Other possibilities include the use of autologous materials, such as iliotibial tract and fat tissue harvested from patient's thigh [26]. The orbital content dislocated during the intervention is repositioned in its original location. At the end, the wound is closed in layers, and the skin of the upper eyelid is sutured with a running locked intradermal suture (6–0 Fast-Absorbing Surgical Gut Suture). This kind of closure provides excellent functional and cosmetic outcomes since the scar is nearly invisible in the long postoperative period.

11.4.3 Complications

In terms of skin incisions and bone work, the SEA represents a minimally invasive approach. However, surgical site infections, postoperative edema, and diastasis of the cutaneous suture still represent minor concerns that need to be mentioned, even if they are no longer frequently found in clinical practice, as long as strict asepsis is observed.

From a functional standpoint, the SEA involves the risk of damaging the LPM during the phase of subcutaneous dissection in the suborbicularis plane. This complication is extremely uncommon to occur provided that proper training in performing the access is provided. It should nonetheless be openly discussed with every patient before surgery as postoperative ptosis is a significant complication regarding both function and aesthetics.

The risk of ischemic damage to the optic nerve and other intraorbital structure due to compression of the orbital content has already been mentioned. To avoid this, the surgeon should provide moments of relaxation of the orbital content during the surgical procedure [2, 5]. As long as this technical tip is respected, the safety of this type of surgery has been demonstrated by numerous cases, and in the personal experience of the senior authors (P.C. and D.L.), neither intraorbital nor transorbital procedures have been associated with any occurrences of postoperative visual deficit due to ischemic or traumatic damage.

To perform this type of surgery, one must have a thorough understanding of anatomy and exceptional endoscopic abilities, as the majority of potential hazards result from inappropriate maneuvers conducted during the dissection in the intraorbital compartment, which is performed after opening the periorbit. The same can be said about the surgery's intracranial and skull base phases. To prevent damage to critical neurovascular structures, one must have a thorough understanding of the surgical anatomy of the skull base, intracranial, and intraorbital spaces as seen from this novel perspective provided from the SEA.

The danger of postoperative CSF-L can be a concern only during extensive surgeries with resulting large skull base defects, which are not frequently performed via such minimally invasive techniques. These large gaps can be repaired using a variety of procedures (see above), but in the senior authors' personal experience, in the majority of times postoperative CSF-L can be prevented by simply repositioning the orbital content, which acts like an effective sealant for the skull base defect.

In the immediate postoperative period, bleeding represents the most daunting complication to be aware of. The disruption of smaller blood vessels contained in the orbital space might cause a retrobulbar hemorrhage, with collection of blood that can result in the compression of the optic nerve, with consequent optic neuropathy possibly leading to amaurosis or even irreversible vision loss. Indirect signs of increased intraorbital pressures are proptosis (bulging of the globe), increased orbital tension, orbital pain, reduced ocular motility and a change in shape and size of the pupil, with fixed and dilated pupil not responding to light reflex as sign of irreversible damage to the optic nerve and or ciliary ganglion [31], configuring the so-called orbital compartment syndrome. This is more likely to occur during transorbital approaches, because during endoscopic transnasal surgery, the blood drains into the nose. Thorough preoperative assessment, an accurate intraoperative hemostasis, and a regular monitoring of blood pressure are essential measures that should be considered by the surgeon to avoid this complication. This complication can be observed immediately after surgery, it is advisable to return to the operating room to perform orbital decompression. If the complication is observed in the department in a woke patient in the first or second postoperative day, without the possibility for immediate return to the operating room, prompt orbital decompression via lateral canthotomy and inferior cantholysis is an effective maneuver that can be carried out in a local anesthesia setting [32, 33].

11.5 Inferior Eyelid Approach

Inferior Eyelid Approach (IEA) is a surgical route adopted less frequently, compared to the SEA, because orbital lesions rarely occur in the lower quadrants [16], and most of them can be managed with an exclusive endoscopic transnasal approach since the epicenter of the lesion lies inferior to the so-called plane of resectability (POR), which is a plane extending from the contralateral nares through the long axis of the optic nerve [34]. Nonetheless, the IEA can be adopted to manage extraconal and/or intraconal inferiorly located lesions, to achieve an inferior orbital decompression and, most frequently, to repair orbital floor fractures. With transorbital intent, this approach allows the exposure of the floor of the middle cranial fossa as well as to reach the infratemporal fossa, where the main targets are represented by the extracranial segments of the maxillary and mandibular nerves [2].

As far as the technique is concerned, a subtarsal incision located about 3–5 mm below the free edge of the lower eyelid is carried out [5]. The dissection is performed in the plane below the orbicularis muscle and a skin-muscle flap is elevated. Thereafter, the following exposure is accomplished in the pre-septal plane until the orbital frame is reached and the periosteum is clearly visualized. The latter can be incised, so that the dissection continues along a subperiosteal plane, up to the IOF, in order to obtain adequate surgical space for the subsequent operative phases. During the detachment, any venous bridging veins running between the orbital cone and the bone can be coagulated and cut. If the aim of the procedure is to access the orbital structures, the orbital septum is opened and the intraorbital phase of the surgery is carried out with the same principles already exposed in the previous paragraphs. The IEA also allows for a transorbital route to the floor middle cranial fossa. This is possible with the transection of the content of the inferior orbital fissure with an anterolateral to posteromedial direction, to expose the orbital floor and the anterior maxilla as far as the orbital apex [2]. Most encountered complications are related to the suboptimal aesthetic results related to the skin incision and paresthesia of the region of the infraorbital nerve in case of section of the IOF content.

11.6 Medial Conjunctival Approaches

Medial conjunctival approaches comprise a set of surgical techniques employed to address pathologies located in the medial and anterior region of the orbit, via an incision of the conjunctiva of the medial canthal region [35, 36]. They include the precaruncular, transcaruncular, and retrocaruncular approaches, which differ for the site of the incision and the initial phases of dissection. They all address the same anatomical area and, compared to earlier procedures that target the medial orbital region, such as the cutaneous (i.e., Lynch incision), trans-eyelid, trans-fornix, or medial rectus plane approaches, they expose the anatomy in a novel way [37].

When considering transorbital endoscopic procedures to the skull base and the orbit, in the authors' experience, these approaches are used less frequently than the SEA. They find the main indications in the management of medial intraorbital lesions with the epicenter located anteriorly to a coronal plane passing through the mid-orbit. This anatomical region is the least accessible for the SEA, due to its location medial to the sagittal plane passing through the optic nerve, and for the endoscopic transnasal approach, as dealing with anterior lesions can be challenging using the nasal corridor. The technique is also described for orbital fracture repair, and anatomical reports confirm the adequacy of the approach to expose the anterior ethmoidal artery [38, 39]. In case of failure with transnasal endoscopic ligation of the artery, the medial conjunctival approaches potentially allow to manage severe nasal bleeding through the transorbital route, avoiding cosmetic deformities or visible scarring that can occur as a result of a cutaneous approach (i.e., Lynch incision) [40]. To note, the contralateral precaruncular approach was also used to address lesions and defects located in the lateral aspect of well-pneumatized sphenoid sinuses, in a multiportal fashion combined with a transnasal endoscopic approach [41].

As far as technique is concerned, a vertical incision is made at the level of the caruncle and is extended 10 mm superiorly and inferiorly in the conjunctiva to create the surgical corridor. To perform the transcaruncular approach, the incision is made directly through the caruncular tissue and dissection is then carried out in a preseptal plane toward the posterior lacrimal crest; the precaruncular approach uses the same preseptal plane, but the incision is performed anteriorly and medially to the caruncular tissue, whilst for the retrocaruncular approach, the incision is made between the caruncle and the plica semilunaris and dissection is extended to the posterior lacrimal crest in a retro-septal plane [42]. The medial orbital wall is reached 1–2 mm posteriorly to the posterior lacrimal crest, where the periosteum is incised. During this phase of the surgery, the Horner muscle represents the main surgical landmark and is kept anteriorly. Attention must be paid to avoid herniation of the orbital fat in the surgical field to avoid getting disorientated and, inevitably, prolonging the duration of the procedure. After the periosteum is incised, the dissection proceeds in a subperiosteal plane, avoiding fracturing the lamina papyracea medi-

ally while proceeding more posteriorly into the orbit. Surgical access is improved by combining the medial incision with an inferior fornix incision. The medial and anterior portions of the orbital walls are easily exposed with this approach, so that fractures herein located can be managed with these techniques. In case of intraorbital lesions, after exposure of the surgical landmarks, the periorbit can be incised and intraorbital dissection proceeds with the same principles in the previous paragraphs. With these approaches, considering the anterior location of both the surgical corridor and the target, the dissection can be performed either under direct vision or with the aid of magnification devices (e.g., microscopes, exoscope, surgical loupes, or endoscope in case of more posteriorly located lesions). At the end of the procedure, the conjunctiva and caruncle are closed with interrupted 6–0 fast-absorbing gut sutures [37]. The most reported complications include damage to the lacrimal pathway, to the lamina papyracea and, potentially, to the skull base, with resulting CSFL. Minor ones include surgical site infections and, rarely, unpleasant aesthetic results. The precaruncular route puts the lacrimal system in a relatively higher jeopardy; the retrocaruncular one implies a slightly higher risk of injuring the periorbit before reaching the target, while the transcaruncular incision might cause increased risk of postoperative edema and erythema due to the complex histology of the caruncula itself [42]. However, a careful dissection is able to provide adequate access without major risk of complications in most of the cases [40].

11.7 Limits of Endoscopic Transorbital Approaches

11.7.1 Anatomical Limitations

Lesions that are located infero-medially to the optic nerve are the main contraindications to using the transpalpebral corridor. The transnasal route is the gold standard method in these clinical scenarios (see above). Almost all other locations can successfully be managed using transpalpebral corridors, SEA for superiorly positioned lesions and IEA for inferiorly located lesions. Although large dimensions and the apical location of the lesions represent actual concerns for endoscopic transorbital approaches, no specific study has been carried out that explicitly states the characteristics of the lesion that demand for an open orbitotomic approach. On the one hand, radical resection is often not required at all cost and, on the other, it is always possible to revert the approach to an open orbitotomic or craniotomic one, for example, in case of intraoperative finding of intractable adhesions. Lesions that are posteriorly expanded toward the squamous section of the temporal bone or laterally toward the temporal fossa are absolute contraindications to endoscopic transpalpebral approaches to the anterior and middle cranial fossa. A fronto-temporal or pterional craniotomy may be the most effective surgical procedure in these circumstances.

11.7.2 Endoscopic Technical Limitations

Endoscopic surgery has several drawbacks that cannot be neglected, even considering the possibility of magnification and the potential to operate successfully in small anatomical spaces. First of all, it offers bidimensional vision in an unfamiliar anatomical region, which can occasionally lead to disorientation. Second, maintaining clear eyesight is essential for the surgical intervention to be successful, despite the working space's limited width, the possibility of fat herniation, and any bleeding that may occur. Finally, in order to avoid instrumentation conflicts or poor-quality vision, it is imperative to develop a synergistic working habit between the two or three surgeons who are operating simultaneously in the orbital cavity. Some of these limitations might be overcome with the use of technological advancements such as intraoperative lens irrigation devices, cryoprobes, and intraoperative image guidance systems. However, a steep learning curve is nec-

essary, particularly adequate, and in-depth preclinical anatomical training. This is necessary to develop both manual skills and anatomical knowledge, which is the crucial factor preventing the surgeon from getting lost during this particular subset of endoscopic procedures.

11.8 Postoperative Workup and Follow-Up

The postoperative evaluation aims to recognize and treat any surgical complications and to evaluate any clinical issues that might develop immediately or long after the procedure. As for preoperative workup, postoperative care should be performed in a multidisciplinary setting with examinations performed by the whole orbital team (otolaryngologist, neurosurgeon, ophthalmologist, and dedicated radiologist).

During the immediate postoperative period, vision represents the main concern and is to be checked regularly. A universally accepted protocol for elective orbital surgery doesn't exist, but in personal experience, a periodic red saturation test performed every 2 h for 48 h, borrowed from the protocols of orbital trauma management. This appears like an acceptable compromise between what patients can do and the knowledge that irreversible vision loss may be occurring with vascular impairment lasting longer than 90 min. In this phase, controlling pain and nausea is crucial to reduce the likelihood of increased orbital venous pressure and the risk of intraorbital bleeding. However, attention is to be paid not to excessively mask pain, as the patients should be able to report the appearance of orbital pain and/or discomfort, which might represent the red flag for orbital edema or hemorrhage [43].

An early imaging control is usually scheduled during hospitalization. This is not applied in every single case but has become part of the clinical practice. In case of intracranial work after SEA for ACF or MCF lesions, a CT scan is performed in the first or second postoperative day and before discharge in order to monitor the postoperative pneumocephalus and the occurrence of possible intracranial complications (e.g., bleeding). For intraorbital procedures, if feasible, MRI performed in the first 72 h is the preferred imaging method, as it is a highly effective way to detect residual lesions with reduced risk of false-positive, as postoperative edema and scarring are still to develop in this early postoperative phase. Moreover, it provides a useful reference image for subsequent follow-up.

Finally, patients are submitted to adjuvant treatments or to a regular follow-up program. As a general rule, the first clinical examination is performed 10–15 days after the procedure, after the pathologic examination is completed. In this occasion, a multidisciplinary consultation is possible, and the patient is then addressed to a specific follow-up protocol according to the biology of the pathologic condition treated. A detailed examination is out of the aim of this chapter. As a rule, for traumatic or benign conditions, clinical and radiologic examinations are performed twice in the first year and then once every 1 or 2 years or according to the occurrence of symptoms. For malignancies, the follow-up is more strict and follows the principle of sinonasal malignancies surveillance [44, 45].

Two months after surgery, an ophthalmologic and orthoptic examination is performed to assess the patient's visual acuity and field once healing is completed. If any pathological finding is confirmed as outcome of the procedure, the patient is examined for possible correction and following examinations are performed according to ophthalmologic opinion. In case a visual deficit or motility impairment appears as new onset symptoms, imaging is promptly executed in order to rule out possible recurrence of the disease.

Clinical, ophthalmology, and radiologic examination during the surveillance should be recorded and stored in a dedicated database. This should be part of the practice for every kind of surgical intervention but is of utmost importance for orbital surgery considering the rarity of the diseases and the need to collect data in order to progressively improve outcomes.

11.9 Future Perspectives

A profound evolution of skull base surgery was observed in the last decades, with a progressive shift from the more classical extensive transcranial procedures toward minimally invasive approaches. In this setting, the advent of endoscopic techniques has represented a revolution for the management of orbital pathologies, thanks to the magnified view and the possibility to expose the lesion and perform dissection in such a narrow anatomical area, which is the orbital cavity. Neuroanatomical research, mainly intended as cadaver dissections preclinical studies, have played a pivotal role in the refinements of novel approaches "to and through" the orbit. Indications are constantly expanding, and currently include selected intra-orbital, skull base, and even intra-axial lesions, both benign and malignant in nature [46]. In recent years, the development of dedicated medical software, 3D volumetrics evaluation, computer analysis, and machine learning are providing a further effort to the refinement of contemporary orbital surgical approaches. Many contributions demonstrate the importance of medical engineering to perform operations tailored according to the individual's anatomy [47–49].

Guizzardi et al., in a remarkable conceptual paper, reported four main steps for planning patient-tailored transorbital approaches. Starting from the study of bone normal anatomy on a dry skull (step 1), all the relevant orbital structures were exposed during the following cadaveric dissection (step 2). Soon after, authors performed a 3D quantitative and qualitative assessment of the post-dissection data, demonstrating the anatomic targets that can be reached via the endoscopic transorbital SEA. The evaluation of the exposure and the working angles with a volume of safe bone removal was crucial to calculate the working areas and the surgical freedom of the approach (step 3). Finally, the last step consisted in transferring the presurgical planning to the clinical practice (step 4) [50].

Among the possible innovations that could lead to an improvement of transorbital procedures, we can expect the introduction of new kinds of autostatic orbital retractors that could facilitate the divarication of the orbital contents, which sometimes still represents a hindrance during the dissection [51]. Moreover, new image-guidance systems could provide a real-time navigation of intraorbital structures avoiding the brain shift, and dedicated instruments might be capable of increasing the safety and the effectiveness of this type of procedure [46].

Finally, among the most fascinating innovations in orbital operations, we can't forget the robotic systems. In a recent publication, Jeannon et al. have introduced the term Robotic-assisted Orbital Surgery (RAOS). Authors claim that RAOS offers multiple advantages over the conventional techniques, such as high definition 3-dimensional optics, dexterous wristed instruments, motion scaling, and tremor filtration [52]. Wang et al. have reported their experience with robot-assisted orbital decompression in 18 patients affected by Graves' ophthalmopathy. The robot utilized was the da Vinci Xi surgical system (Intuitive Surgical, Inc., Sunnyvale, CA). According to their experience, it provided the stability, dexterity, and good visualization necessary for orbital fat decompression surgery [53].

11.10 Conclusions

For decades, transcranial or craniofacial approaches have represented the mainstay of surgical approaches to address the orbital region, even if burdened by a considerable invasiveness [3, 54].

More recently, a profound evolution in endoscopic approaches have reshaped the panorama of orbital surgery, proved their efficacy while granting a reduced morbidity of the procedure, along with more pleasant aesthetic results [10, 55, 56]. One should be aware that the concept of minimal invasiveness does not depend on the entry wound size, but on the limited impact of the procedure on the patient's quality of life. In this respect, transorbital endoscopic surgery should not be considered as an alternative technique for replacing the classical expanded endoscopic endonasal approaches or traditional external craniotomies, but should be considered as a valid alternative proposed as an additional corridor able to improve visualization while minimizing surgical demolition and maximizing the instruments' maneuverability. As already emphasized, the orbital team should be able to convert to external approaches whenever needed (e.g., inadequate surgical exposure, excessive bleeding, intraoperative complication, or unexpected intraoperative findings).

This chapter was intended to be an introductory lecture to familiarize with a niche of surgical approaches to the orbital region and confining anatomical areas. These approaches require a sound anatomical knowledge, a steep learning curve and, more importantly, a multidisciplinary experienced team, not only during the surgical act but from the time of the diagnosis to the postoperative surveillance.

Acknowledgments A.D.A. is a PhD student of the "Biotechnologies and Life Sciences" course at University of Insubria, Varese, Italy.

References

1. Bleier BS. A shift in the orbit: immediate endoscopic reconstruction after transnasal orbital tumors resection: response. J Craniofac Surg. 2018;29(6):1674–5.
2. Locatelli D, Pozzi F, Turri-Zanoni M, Battaglia P, Santi L, Dallan I, et al. Transorbital endoscopic approaches to the skull base: current concepts and future perspectives. J Neurosurg Sci. 2016;60(4):514–25.
3. Abussuud Z, Ahmed S, Paluzzi A. Surgical approaches to the orbit: a neurosurgical perspective. J Neurol Surg B Skull Base. 2020;81(4):385–408.
4. Castelnuovo P, Arosio AD, Volpi L, De Maria F, Ravasio A, Donati S, et al. Endoscopic transnasal cryo-assisted removal of orbital cavernous hemangiomas: case report and technical hints. World Neurosurg. 2019;126:66–71.
5. Locatelli D, Dallan I, Castelnuovo P. Surgery around the orbit: how to select an approach. J Neurol Surg B Skull Base. 2020;81(04):409–21.
6. Paluzzi A, Gardner PA, Fernandez-Miranda JC, Tormenti MJ, Stefko ST, Snyderman CH, et al. "Round-the-clock" surgical access to the orbit. J Neurol Surgery B Skull Base. 2015;76(01):12–24.

7. Zoli M, Sollini G, Milanese L, La Corte E, Rustici A, Guaraldi F, et al. Endoscopic approaches to orbital lesions: case series and systematic literature review. J Neurosurg. 2021;134(2):608–20.

8. Vural A, Carobbio ALC, Ferrari M, Rampinelli V, Schreiber A, Mattavelli D, et al. Transorbital endoscopic approaches to the skull base: a systematic literature review and anatomical description. Neurosurg Rev. 2021;44:2943.

9. Ciporen JN, Moe KS, Ramanathan D, Lopez S, Ledesma E, Rostomily R, et al. Multiportal endoscopic approaches to the central skull base: a cadaveric study. World Neurosurg. 2010;73(6):705–12.

10. Moe KS, Bergeron CM, Ellenbogen RG. Transorbital neuroendoscopic surgery. Oper Neurosurg. 2010;67(3):ons16–28.

11. Khan SN, Sepahdari AR. Orbital masses: CT and MRI of common vascular lesions, benign tumors, and malignancies. Saudi J Ophthalmol. 2012;26(4):373–83.

12. Nagesh CP, Rao R, Hiremath SB, Honavar SG. Magnetic resonance imaging of the orbit, part 1: basic principles and radiological approach. Indian J Ophthalmol. 2021;69(10):2574–84.

13. Patil SG, Kotwal IA, Joshi U, Allurkar S, Thakur N, Aftab A. Ophthalmological evaluation by a maxillofacial surgeon and an ophthalmologist in assessing the damage to the orbital contents in Midfacial fractures: a prospective study. J Maxillofac Oral Surg. 2016;15(3):328–35.

14. Jellish WS, Murdoch J, Leonetti JP. Perioperative management of complex skull base surgery: the anesthesiologist's point of view. Neurosurg Focus. 2002;12(5):e5.

15. Veiceschi P, Locatelli D, Dario A, Agresta G. Frameless neuronavigation-assisted brain biopsy with electromagnetic tracking: how I do it? Acta Neurochir. 2022;164(12):3317–22.

16. Dallan I, Castelnuovo P, Turri-Zanoni M, Fiacchini G, Locatelli D, Battaglia P, et al. Transorbital endoscopic assisted management of intraorbital lesions: lessons learned from our first 9 cases. Rhinology. 2016;54(3):247–53.

17. Weber R, Draf W, Kratzsch B, Hosemann W, Schaefer SD. Modern concepts of frontal sinus surgery. Laryngoscope. 2001;111(1):137–46.

18. Eloy JA, Vázquez A, Liu JK, Baredes S. Endoscopic approaches to the frontal sinus: modifications of the existing techniques and proposed classification. Otolaryngol Clin N Am. 2016;49(4):1007–18.

19. Karligkiotis A, Pistochini A, Turri-Zanoni M, Terranova P, Volpi L, Battaglia P, et al. Endoscopic endonasal orbital transposition to expand the frontal sinus approaches. Am J Rhinol Allergy. 2015;29(6):449–56.

20. Papatsoutsos E, Kalyvas A, Drosos E, Neromyliotis E, Koutsarnakis C, Komaitis S, et al. Defining the limits and indications of the Draf III endoscopic approach to the lateral frontal sinus and maximizing visualization and maneuverability: a cadaveric and radiological study. Eur Arch Otorhinolaryngol. 2022;279(10):4969–76.

21. Di Somma A, Andaluz N, Cavallo LM, de Notaris M, Dallan I, Solari D, et al. Endoscopic transorbital superior eyelid approach: anatomical study from a neurosurgical perspective. J Neurosurg. 2018;129(5):1203–16.

22. Peron S, Cividini A, Santi L, Galante N, Castelnuovo P, Locatelli D. Spheno-orbital meningiomas: when the endoscopic approach is better. Acta Neurochir Suppl. 2017;124:123–8.

23. Dallan I, Sellari-Franceschini S, Turri-Zanoni M, de Notaris M, Fiacchini G, Fiorini FR, et al. Endoscopic transorbital superior eyelid approach for the management of selected spheno-orbital meningiomas: preliminary experience. Oper Neurosurg. 2018;14(3):243–51.

24. Locatelli D, Restelli F, Alfiero T, Campione A, Pozzi F, Balbi S, et al. The role of the transorbital superior eyelid approach in the management of selected spheno-orbital meningiomas: in-depth analysis of indications, technique, and outcomes from the study of a cohort of 35 patients. J Neurol Surg B Skull Base. 2022;83(2):145–58.

25. Chen HI, Bohman LE, Loevner LA, Lucas TH. Transorbital endoscopic amygdalohippocampectomy: a feasibility investigation. J Neurosurg. 2014;120(6):1428–36.

26. Dallan I, Castelnuovo P, Locatelli D, Turri-Zanoni M, AlQahtani A, Battaglia P, et al. Multiportal combined transorbital transnasal endoscopic approach for the management of selected skull base lesions: preliminary experience. World Neurosurg. 2015;84(1):97–107.

27. Arosio AD, Coden E, Valentini M, Czaczkes C, Battaglia P, Bignami M, et al. Combined endonasal-transorbital approach to manage the far lateral frontal sinus: surgical technique. World Neurosurg. 2021;151:5.

28. Makary CA, Limjuco A, Nguyen J, Ramadan HH. Combined lid crease and endoscopic approach to lateral frontal sinus disease with orbital extension. Ann Otol Rhinol Laryngol. 2018;127(9):637–42.

29. Miller C, Berens A, Patel SA, Humphreys IM, Moe KS. Transorbital approach for improved access in the management of paranasal sinus mucoceles. J Neurol Surg B Skull Base. 2019;80(6):593–8.

30. Alqahtani A, Padoan G, Segnini G, Lepera D, Fortunato S, Dallan I, et al. Transorbital transnasal endoscopic combined approach to the anterior and middle skull base: a laboratory investigation. Acta Otorhinolaryngol Ital. 2015;35(3):173–9.

31. Shaftel SS, Chang S-H, Moe KS. Hemostasis in orbital surgery. Otolaryngol Clin N Am. 2016;49(3):763–75.

32. Kumar S, Blace N. Retrobulbar hematoma. Treasure Island, FL: StatPearls; 2022.

33. Desai NM, Shah SU. Lateral orbital canthotomy. Treasure Island, FL: StatPearls; 2022.

34. Reshef ER, Bleier BS, Freitag SK. The endoscopic Transnasal approach to orbital tumors: a review. Semin Ophthalmol. 2021;36(4):232–40.

35. Garcia GH, Goldberg RA, Shorr N. The transcaruncular approach in repair of orbital fractures: a retrospective study. J Craniomaxillofac Trauma. 1998;4(1):7–12.

36. Shorr N, Baylis HI, Goldberg RA, Perry JD. Transcaruncular approach to the medial orbit and orbital apex. Ophthalmology. 2000;107(8):1459–63.

37. Goldberg RA, Mancini R, Demer JL. The transcaruncular approach: surgical anatomy and technique. Arch Facial Plast Surg. 2007;9(6):443–7.

38. Zhou G, Tu Y, Yu B, Wu W. Endoscopic repair of combined orbital floor and medial wall fractures involving the inferomedial strut. Eye (Lond). 2021;35(10):2763–70.

39. You H-J, Kim D-W, Dhong E-S, Yoon E-S. Precaruncular approach for the reconstruction of medial orbital wall fractures. Ann Plast Surg. 2014;72(6):652–6.

40. Cornelis MMK, Lubbe DE. Pre-caruncular approach to the medial orbit and landmarks for anterior ethmoidal artery ligation: a cadaveric study. Clin Otolaryngol. 2016;41(6):777–81.

41. Lubbe DE, Douglas-Jones P, Wasl H, Mustak H, Semple PL. Contralateral Precaruncular approach to the lateral sphenoid sinus-a case report detailing a new, multiportal approach to lesions, and defects in the lateral aspect of well-pneumatized sphenoid sinuses. Ear Nose Throat J. 2020;99(1):62–7.

42. Kempton SJ, Cho DC, Thimmappa B, Martin MC. Benefits of the retrocaruncular approach to the medial orbit: a clinical and anatomic study. Ann Plast Surg. 2016;76(3):295–300.

43. Roth FS, Koshy JC, Goldberg JS, Soparkar CNS. Pearls of orbital trauma management. Semin Plast Surg. 2010;24(4):398–410.

44. Arosio AD, Bernasconi DP, Valsecchi MG, Pacifico C, Battaglia P, Bignami M, et al. Patterns of recurrences in sinonasal cancers undergoing an endoscopic surgery-based treatment: results of the MUSES* on 940 patients: *MUlti-institutional collaborative study on endoscopically treated Sinonasal cancers. Oral Oncol. 2022;134:106123.

45. Ferrari M, Mattavelli D, Tomasoni M, Raffetti E, Bossi P, Schreiber A, et al. The MUSES∗: a prognostic study on 1360 patients with sinonasal cancer undergoing endoscopic surgery-based treatment: ∗Multi-institutional collaborative study on endoscopically treated Sinonasal cancers. Eur J Cancer. 2022;171:161–82.

46. Dallan I, Cristofani-Mencacci L, Fiacchini G, Turri-Zanoni M, van Furth W, de Notaris M, et al. Endoscopic-assisted transorbital surgery: where do we stand on the scott's parabola? Personal considerations after a 10-year experience. Front Oncol. 2022;12:937818.

47. Agosti E, Turri-Zanoni M, Saraceno G, Belotti F, Karligkiotis A, Rocca G, et al. Quantitative anatomic comparison of microsurgical transcranial, endoscopic endonasal, and transorbital approaches to the spheno-orbital region. Oper Neurosurg. 2021;21(6):E494–505.

48. Agosti E, Saraceno G, Rampinelli V, Raffetti E, Veiceschi P, Buffoli B, et al. Quantitative anatomic comparison of endoscopic transnasal and microsurgical transcranial approaches to the anterior cranial fossa. Oper Neurosurg. 2022;23(4):e256–66.

49. Bly RA, Su D, Hannaford B, Ferreira MJ, Moe KS. Computer modeled multiportal approaches to the skull base. J Neurol Surg B Skull Base. 2012;73(6):415–23.

50. Guizzardi G, Di Somma A, de Notaris M, Corrivetti F, Sánchez JC, Alobid I, et al. Endoscopic transorbital avenue to the skull base: four-step conceptual analysis of the anatomic journey. Front Oncol. 2022;12:988131.

51. Wong Y, Lee P, Sullivan T. Utilising the Alexis retractor for lateral orbital access, a case series. Orbit. 2018;37(6):447–9.

52. Jeannon J-P, Faulkner J, Uddin J, Daniel C, Arora A. Robotic assisted orbital surgery (RAOS)—a novel approach to orbital oncology surgery. Eye. 2022;37:1040.

53. Wang Y, Sun J, Liu X, Li Y, Fan X, Zhou H. Robot-assisted orbital fat decompression surgery: first in human. Transl Vis Sci Technol. 2022;11(5):8.

54. Dandy W. Results following the transcranial operative attack on orbital tumors. Arch Ophthalmol. 1941;25(2):191–216.

55. Balakrishnan K, Moe KS. Applications and outcomes of orbital and transorbital endoscopic surgery. Otolaryngol Head Neck Surg. 2011;144(5):815–20.

56. Castelnuovo P, Dallan I, Locatelli D, Battaglia P, Farneti P, Tomazic PV, et al. Endoscopic transnasal intraorbital surgery: our experience with 16 cases. Eur Arch Otorhinolaryngol. 2012;269(8):1929–35.

Part IV

Diagnosis and Management of Cranio-Orbital Mass Lesions

Tumors of the Optic Nerve and Its Sheath

12

Francesco Maiuri [iD], Fausto Tranfa,
Paola Bonavolontà, Paolo Tini,
and Giuseppe Minniti

12.1 Surgical Anatomy of the Optic Nerve

The optic nerve begins within the eyeball at the optic disc and ends in the suprasellar region, where it continues with the chiasm.

Four different parts of the optic nerve may be distinguished: intraocular, intraorbital, intracanalicular, and intracranial [1, 2].

The **intraocular part** is the most anterior component and is located within the eyeball. The optic nerve head, also defined optic disc, is approximatively 1.5 mm wide. The amyelinated fibers are supplied by the central retinal artery.

The **intraorbital part** courses from the posterior part of the eyeball to the intraorbital

F. Maiuri (✉)
Division of Neurosurgery, Department of
Neurosciences, Reproductive and
Odontostomatological Sciences, University of Naples
"Federico II", Naples, Italy
e-mail: frmaiuri@unina.it

F. Tranfa
Division of Ophthalmology, Department of
Neurosciences, Reproductive and
Odontostomatological Sciences, University of Naples
"Federico II", Naples, Italy

P. Bonavolontà
Department of Clinical Medicine and Surgery,
University of Naples "Federico II", Naples, Italy

P. Tini · G. Minniti
Department of Medicine, Surgery and Neurosciences,
University of Siena, Siena, Italy

opening of the optic canal. Its length is about 25 mm. This segment is myelinated and surrounded by three meningeal layers (dura, arachnoid, and pia mater). The subarachnoid space is rather large and narrows posteriorly at the optic canal. Just before it enters the optic canal, the optic nerve is adjacent to the third and the sixth nerves and superomedial to the ophthalmic artery, thus it is closely related to the anulus of Zinn.

The **intracanalicular part** has a variable length from 4 to 10 mm; the optic nerve travels the canal posteromedially at 35° angle relative to the midsagittal plane. This part of the nerve is also covered by the three meningeal layers.

The **intracranial part** extends from the internal orifice of the optic canal to the optic chiasm. It courses in the parasellar region and lies medial to the internal carotid artery, superomedial to the ophthalmic artery, and below the anterior cerebral artery. This segment of the optic nerve is covered only by the pia mater.

12.2 Classification of Tumors of the Optic Nerve and Its Sheath

Many tumors of different histology may involve the optic nerve and its sheath. Some of them primarily arise from the nerve and its sheath; these tumors are

Table 12.1 Classification of primary tumors of the optic nerve and its sheath

Tumors of the optic nerve
- Benign gliomas
- Malignant gliomas
- Ganglioglioma
- Medulloepithelioma
- Hemangioblastoma

Tumors of the optic nerve sheath
- Meningioma
- Schwannoma

discussed in this chapter. In other cases, tumors of the surrounding structures may secondarily involve the nerve. These include meningiomas of the tuberculum sellae, anterior clinoid, planum sphenoidale, gliomas of the optic chiasm and frontal lobe. These cases are excluded from this chapter.

Several cell types may be present in the optic nerve and its sheath. These include astrocytes, oligodendrocytes, fibroblasts, arachnoid cap cells, ganglion cells, Schwann cells of the sympathetic nerves. Thus, several tumors of different histological origin may be observed. They may be classified as in Table 12.1 according to the WHO Classification [3].

12.3 Primary Tumors of the Optic Nerve

12.3.1 Gliomas

Gliomas of the optic nerve occur in two different forms: the more frequent benign gliomas of the pediatric population and the rare malignant gliomas of adults [4–6].

12.3.1.1 Pediatric Benign Gliomas

Optic nerve gliomas account for 2–5% of the central nervous system neoplasms and 7% of all gliomas in pediatric population [7, 8]. They may occur as sporadic lesions or in association to type I neurofibromatosis (NF1). NF1-related tumors occur at younger age (mean 4, 5 years) and are often bilateral [8]. Sporadic tumors are unilateral and occur later, mostly in the first or less in the second decade [7] (Fig. 12.1).

Histologically, pediatric optic nerve gliomas are WHO I pilocytic astrocytomas, rarely diffuse WHO II astrocytomas. Sporadic tumors show higher values of proliferation markers and more aggressive histopathological features.

The biomolecular studies have shown different features between NF1-related and sporadic tumors. The NF1 gene encodes the neurofibromin protein, which functions as tumor suppressor; NF1 dysfunction causes unregulate Ras and m-TOR activity [9]. On the other hand, BRAF mutations are not evidenced in NF1-associated pilocytic astrocytomas but are identified in many sporadic cases [10].

Most optic nerve gliomas are asymptomatic at diagnosis and detected incidentally. However, the clinical course is rather variable; most cases remain stable for years and never grow, while others show visual worsening and slow or more rapid growth pattern over many years [5, 11].

Sporadic optic nerve gliomas are at higher risk of visual loss than those related to the NF1.

Among the non-visual symptoms and signs, proptosis is the most common presenting sign in symptomatic cases. Limitation of the ocular motility and diplopia occur in about 30% of gliomas confined to the orbit whereas they are rare in gliomas of the intracranial optic nerve.

The high incidence of optic nerve glioma in children with NF1 suggests several recommendations for the screening. Children with NF1 and no evident optic nerve glioma should be examined every year up to the age of 18 years. Those with NF1 and history of optic nerve glioma should be studied every 3 months in the first year and every 6 months in the following years.

The vision loss is the most important factor for deciding to treat the glioma, The optic coherence tomography (OCT) is the best study to assess the optic nerve function [12].

Children with sporadic or NF1 optic nerve gliomas and no visual loss must not be treated.

In pediatric patients with substantial tumor progression on MR and/or worsening of visual acuity, chemotherapy is the first-line treatment, particularly in children below 5 years of age [13]. The combination of vincristine and carboplatin has been the most common first-line treatment for optic nerve gliomas. For patients with NF1 who undergo treatment with vincristine/carboplatin, the 3-year progression-free survival (PFS) rate is 77% [14] and the 5-year PFS is 69%, although these cohorts include gliomas beyond

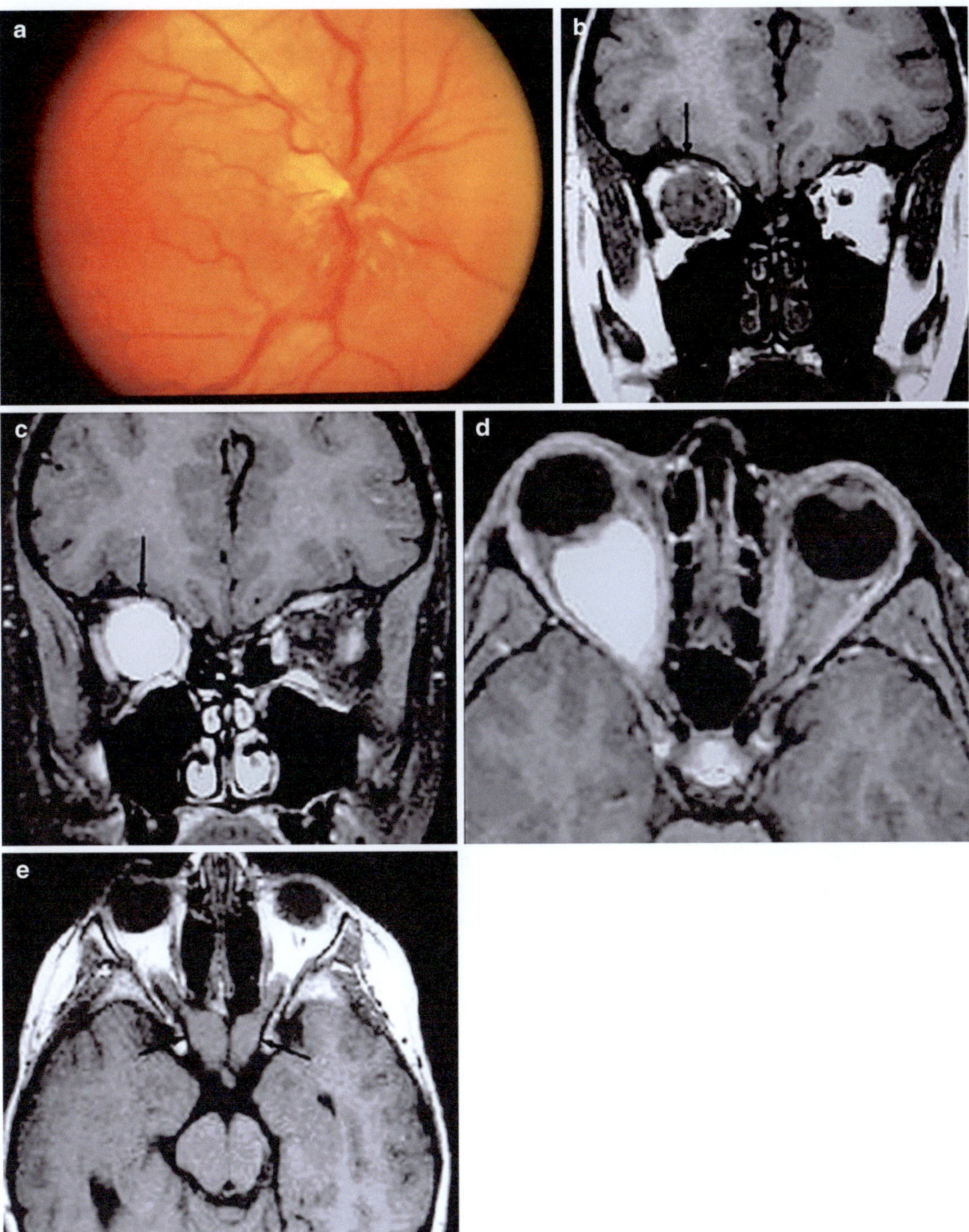

Fig. 12.1 Benign right **optic nerve glioma**. (**a**) Exam of the eye fundus: optic disc with blurred margins. (**b–d**) Preoperative magnetic resonance T1 sequences, before (**b**) and after (**c, d**) gadolinium: large right intraorbital tumor of the optic nerve with regular margins and homogeneous enhancement; right proptosis is evident. (**e**) Postoperative MR: good tumor resection

the optic nerve. Thioguanine, procarbazine, lomustine, and vincristine may represent a treatment alternative to carboplatin/vincristine in NF1 patients with a reported similar survival [15, 16]. More recently, monotherapies with temozolamide [17], vinblastine [18, 19] and vinorelbine [20] have been used for progressive or refractory disease with positive results and low toxicity.

Surgical debulking is reserved to cases with significant mass effect, aesthetic problems, and no or very limited residual vision. On the other hand, radical surgical resection and radiotherapy represent the last management option in a limited number of patients [11].

The prognosis of optic nerve glioma is rather variable. The features associated to worse outcome include younger age at diagnosis, sporadic tumors, greater contrast enhancement, and extension to the chiasm [8, 21, 22].

12.3.1.2 Malignant Gliomas

Malignant optic nerve gliomas are very aggressive neoplasms occurring in middle-aged males and presenting with rapidly progressive visual loss [4, 15, 23].

The radiological aspect is a mass involving the optic nerve and showing intense contrast enhancement. Histologically, these tumors are anaplastic WHO III astocytomas or glioblastomas (WHO IV). The biopsy is advisable to define the diagnosis.

The tumor progression is very rapid. In the orbit, the tumor infiltrates the meninges of the nerve and the surrounding soft tissues. Gliomas arising from the intracranial optic nerve infiltrate the optic chiasm, hypothalamus, and the surrounding brain.

The management includes combined radiation therapy and chemotherapy [23]. Radiation therapy is a treatment option for patients with malignant optic nerve gliomas and can be used as adjunctive therapy or as an alternative to surgery [24]. Historical series of patients treated with radiation therapy with a total dose of 50–54 Gy given in 1.8–2 Gy per fraction [25–29] reported a local control around 62–89% and overall survival 83–100% at 10 years. The treatment is associated with clinical improvement, including shrinkage of tumor mass and subsequent reduction of proptosis, reduction in optic disc swelling, arrest of progressive visual loss, and improvement of vision. Long-term toxicity reported with the use of conventional radiotherapy includes endocrine abnormalities (13–22%) [1, 27, 28, 30], cerebrovascular disease [31–33], poor visual outcomes (15%) [25–29], secondary malignancies [34, 35], and neurocognitive decline [35], particularly in young patients [26, 36]. Modern techniques have been recently employed to minimize long-term complications of radiation, including fractionated stereotactic radiation therapy [37–39], proton beam radiation therapy [40, 41], and stereotactic radiosurgery (Gamma Knife) [42, 43]. Proton beam therapy has been used for patients with malignant optic nerve gliomas [44]. In a series of 101 patients with malignant optic nerve gliomas receiving photon radiotherapy or proton beam radiotherapy with a total dose of 50.4–54.0 Gy (RBE), Indelicato et al. [44] showed similar progression-free survival and overall survival of 88% and 93%, respectively. The total dose has impact on the local control of the tumors; 54 GyRBE showed a better local control and progression-free survival as compared with a dose less than 54 GyRBE. As for other newly diagnosed high-grade astrocytomas, radiotherapy can be given in combination with temozolomide. Recurrence or progression may be treated with re-resection, a second course of radiotherapy, or most commonly, using systemic alkylating agent chemotherapy [45].

12.3.2 Ganglioglioma

The ganglioglioma, a well-differentiated slow-growing tumor composed of a combination of neoplastic ganglion and glial cells, rarely occurs in the optic nerve [4, 46, 47]. The intracranial optic nerve segment is less rarely affected than the intraorbital one [47]. The association with the NF1 is evidenced in half of the reported cases.

The clinical presentation and the imaging characteristics of ganglioglioma are rather like optic nerve glioma; however, ganglioglioma of the optic nerve causes more rapid, progressive visual failure. Thus, the correct diagnosis is possible only by histological studies.

Most reported gangliogliomas of the optic nerve underwent surgical removal because of the progressive visual loss and potential tumor extension. This management option differs from that of the pilocytic astrocytomas of the optic nerve, where the clinical course is more favorable and the surgical resection is rarely necessary.

Given the rarity of optic nerve gangliogliomas, treatment recommendations are based on evidence or results of the treatment of intracranial gangliogliomas. After a gross total resection is achieved, there is no evidence that adjuvant radiation improves tumor control or patient outcome, and therefore radiation is not recommended in this scenario. After subtotal resection, adjuvant radiation appears to improve local tumor control [48].

12.3.3 Medulloepithelioma

The medulloepithelioma is an embryonal neoplasm, considered in the 2021 WHO classification [3] as subtype of the "embryonal tumors with multilayered rosettes." It rarely occurs in the optic nerve, where it arises from the neuroepithelium that lines the optic vescicles and cavities of the optic nerve [49].

Medulloepithelioma of the optic nerve mainly affects young males and is always malignant. Tumors located in the orbital portion present with proptosis and optic disc swelling, as for optic gliomas; those occurring in more posterior segments of the nerve cause progressive retrobulbar optic neuropathy [4]. The radiological aspect is a fusiform enlargement of the nerve, suggesting an optic glioma.

Most reported cases of optic nerve medulloepithelioma have been treated with tumor excision followed by chemotherapy and radiotherapy. However, the mortality rate is high because of recurrence, CSF spread, and brain invasion [49].

12.3.4 Hemangioblastoma

Hemangioblastomas very rarely occur in the optic nerve, with only 37 reported cases included in two recent reviews [50, 51]. They may occur sporadically or more frequently in association with the Von Hippel Lindau (VHL) disease. The tumor is mostly located in the intraorbital portion of the nerve than in the intracranial one. The reduced vision is the most common presenting symptom, followed by slowly progressive axial proptosis; asymptomatic cases are found incidentally on VHL screening. About one-third of the patients show optic atrophy at initial examination.

The diagnosis is rather easy in VHL patients, but it is difficult in sporadic cases. On MR, the presence of a solid or mixed solid-cystic well-defined lesion within the optic nerve, showing vascular flow voids, intense contrast enhancement and peritumoral edema may suggest the hemangioblastoma.

The best management option of optic nerve hemangioblastomas is controversial. Asymptomatic patients with stable vision should be managed conservatively. However, without treatment most patients will probably lose vision of the affected eye. Surgery is indicated in cases with progressive vision loss, significant proptosis, and bilateral visual symptoms due to edema.

The microsurgical tumor resection is possible, because the optic nerve fibers are dislocated rather than infiltrated. However, it is at risk of visual worsening, particularly for tumors with intracanalicular component. No cases were treated by stereotactic radiosurgery; however, it may be used as alternative option to surgery in advanced cases.

12.4 Tumors of the Optic Nerve Sheath

12.4.1 Meningioma

Optic nerve sheath meningiomas are rare tumors accounting for 1% of all meningiomas and about 2% of all orbital tumors [52, 53]; they are the most frequent tumors of the optic nerve after gliomas. Optic nerve meningiomas are predominant in middle age and in female patients, although they may rarely be found in children in association with type II neurofibromatosis (NF2) in one-third of cases. These tumors are usually monolateral (95%) and rarely bilateral (5%) in NF2 patients. The intraorbital portion of the nerve is the most common site of origin (> 90%).

These meningiomas arise from the arachnoid cap cells lining the meningeal optic nerve sheath. They mainly grow circumferentially around the optic nerve and can extent along the entire path of the nerve; other growth patterns include globular, fusiform, and focal enlargement [54]. Histologically, they are benign WHO I, mainly of transitional (50%) or mixed meningothelial-transitional type (30%) [55].

The clinical presentation is characterized by painless and progressive visual loss in the affected eye, which leads to complete blindness, if untreated. Optic disc edema or atrophy are evident. Chronic edema may be associated to posterior tumors causing enlargement of the anterior perioptic subarachnoid space [56]. Visual field defect mainly includes peripheral constriction and enlarged blind spot. Proptosis is inconstant and always follows the visual loss. In pediatric patients, these tumors are more aggressive and result in more rapid visual loss [57].

The diagnosis of optic nerve sheath meningioma is often confirmed by MR with gadolinium-enhanced fat-suppression sequences. The most typical aspect is widening and intense enhancement of the meningeal sheath with central non-enhancing nerve (tram-trak sign) (Fig. 12.2).

The less frequent fusiform enhancement may mimic an optic nerve glioma [54, 58]. Because of the expression of somatostatin receptor subtype 2 by the meningioma cells, the gallium-68 labeled dodecotetracetic acid-tyrosine-3-octreotate positron emission tomography-CT scan may show significant uptake in meningiomas, differently from other tumors [59].

The best management of optic nerve sheath meningiomas depends on the state of visual function and the tumor extension. Cases where the visual function is intact or remains stable should only be observed and closely followed-up by serial ophthalmological examinations and repeated MR every year [58, 60].

The surgical tumor resection results in severe visual loss due to the close tumor relationship to the optic nerve and damage of the pial vascular plexus. Thus, it should be reserved to cases with blind affected eye and disfiguring proptosis or particularly intracranial extension. Patients with blind eye and stable intraorbital tumor may be observed or treated by radiotherapy and operation if the tumor grows. The surgical resection

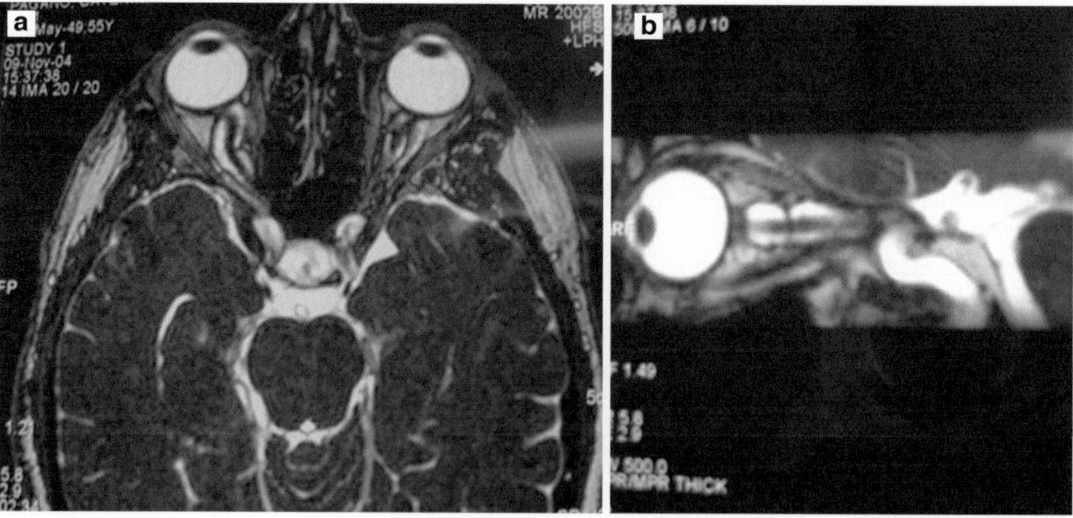

Fig. 12.2 Meningioma of the right intraorbital optic nerve. Magnetic resonance, fat suppression axial (**a**) and post contrast (**b**) sequences: intense contrast enhancement of the meningeal sheath with central non-enhancing nerve (tram-track sign)

may be realized through transcranial approach or lateral orbitotomy [61]. The transnasal endoscopic optic nerve decompression allows to decompress the optic canal and orbital apex, also with the aim to avoid contralateral optic nerve diffusion of the tumor [62, 63]. This less invasive technique shows stabilization of the disease and sometimes improvement of the visual deficit [60, 62, 63].

Radiotherapy is the treatment of choice for most primary optic nerve stealth meningiomas [64]. Current radiation techniques include intensity-modulated radiotherapy [65], stereotactic radiosurgery (SRS) [66], proton beam therapy (PBT) [67], stereotactic fractionated radiotherapy [68]. Such techniques allow better conformal dose to the shape of the tumor significantly reducing the dose to the surrounding healthy organs compared to 3D-conformal RT [69].

A recent meta-analysis comparing different radiotherapy techniques results showed an excellent tumor control rate from 80 to 100% following fractionated radiotherapy using doses of 50–54 Gy in 28–30 fractions of 1.8–2.0 Gy each [70].

Regarding long-term toxicity, three-conformal radiation technique showed a rate of complications higher than more advanced techniques. Reported complication rates using three-conformal radiotherapy, stereotactic fractionated radiotherapy, intensity-modulated radiotherapy, stereotactic radiosurgery, and proton beam radiotherapy were 19% (0–36%), 6% (0–33%), 7% (0–20%), 4.7% (0–4.7%), and 12.5% (0–12.5%), respectively [70]. The most common adverse effect related to RT was retinopathy (44,0.4%), followed by cataract (18%), dry eye (11%), pituitary dysfunction (9%), optic neuritis (6.6%), orbital pain (4.4%), and iritis (4.4%).

12.4.2 Schwannoma

Optic nerve sheath schwannomas are very rare tumors, with only 14 reported cases in recent literature reviews [71–73]. Because the optic nerve is not surrounded by Schwann cells, the origin of these tumors is controversial. The most reliable theory is that they arise from perivascular Schwann cells accompanying the sympathetic nerves innervating the blood vessels of the optic nerve or the central retinal artery. Alternatively, the origin from ectopic Schwann cells may be suggested.

In the reported cases, the clinical presentation is aspecific. At MR, a round homogeneously enhancing tumor in relationship with the optic nerve is evidenced.

Surgery (craniotomy or orbitotomy) has been the primary treatment, allowing large tumor removal; however, the visual prognosis is poor. Fractionated radiotherapy using doses of 45–54 Gy in 28–33 fractions of 1.8 Gy per fraction has been used as complementary treatment in several cases.

12.5 Conclusion

Tumors of the optic nerve and its sheath are mainly gliomas and meningiomas, whereas other oncotypes are exceptional. Most of them are benign and cause slowly progressive visual loss and variable proptosis. The diagnosis of gliomas and meningiomas is usually easy on post-contrast MRI; on the other hand, more rare tumors are diagnosed intraoperatively or at histological examination. Observation is justified in benign tumors with preserved or stable visual function; surgery is often delayed because of the risk of visual worsening, whereas radiation therapy is used in meningiomas and malignant gliomas. However, the visual prognosis is more often poor although with difference according to the tumor type.

References

1. Crumbie L. Optic nerve. https://www.kenhub.com/en/library/anatomy/the-optic-nerve2022.
2. Smith AM. Neuroanatomy, cranial nerve 2 (optic). In: StatPearls [Internet]. Treasure Island, FL: StatPearls Publishing; 2022. https://www.ncbi.nlm.nih.gov/books/NBK507907/.
3. Louis DN, Perry A, Wesseling P, Brat DJ, Cree IA, Figarella-Branger D, et al. The 2021 WHO classifica-

tion of tumors of the central nervous system: a summary. Neuro Oncol. 2021;23(8):1231–51. https://doi.org/10.1093/neuonc/noab106.

4. Miller NR. Primary tumours of the optic nerve and its sheath. Eye (Lond). 2004;18(11):1026–37. https://doi.org/10.1038/sj.eye.6701592.

5. Wladis EJ, Adamo MA, Weintraub L. Optic nerve gliomas. J Neurol Surg B Skull Base. 2021;82(1):91–5. https://doi.org/10.1055/s-0040-1722634.

6. Huang M, Patel J. Optic nerve glioma. In: StatPearls [Internet]. Treasure Island, FL: StatPearls Publishing; 2022. https://www.ncbi.nlm.nih.gov/books/NBK557878/.

7. Beres SJ, Avery RA. Optic pathway gliomas secondary to neurofibromatosis type 1. Semin Pediatr Neurol. 2017;24(2):92–9. https://doi.org/10.1016/j.spen.2017.04.006.

8. Rasool N, Odel JG, Kazim M. Optic pathway glioma of childhood. Curr Opin Ophthalmol. 2017;28(3):289–95. https://doi.org/10.1097/ICU.0000000000000370.

9. Avery RA, Fisher MJ, Liu GT. Optic pathway gliomas. J Neuroophthalmol. 2011;31(3):269–78. https://doi.org/10.1097/WNO.0b013e31822aef82.

10. Yu J, Deshmukh H, Gutmann RJ, Emnett RJ, Rodriguez FJ, Watson MA, et al. Alterations of BRAF and HIPK2 loci predominate in sporadic pilocytic astrocytoma. Neurology. 2009;73(19):1526–31. https://doi.org/10.1212/WNL.0b013e3181c0664a.

11. Farazdaghi MK, Katowitz WR, Avery RA. Current treatment of optic nerve gliomas. Curr Opin Ophthalmol. 2019;30(5):356–63. https://doi.org/10.1097/ICU.0000000000000587.

12. Fard MA, Fakhree S, Eshraghi B. Correlation of optical coherence tomography parameters with clinical and radiological progression in patients with symptomatic optic pathway gliomas. Graefes Arch Clin Exp Ophthalmol. 2013;251(10):2429–36. https://doi.org/10.1007/s00417-013-2394-4.

13. Fisher MJ, Loguidice M, Gutmann DH, et al. Visual outcomes in children with neurofibromatosis type 1-associated optic pathway glioma following chemotherapy: a multicenter retrospective analysis. Neuro Oncol. 2012;14:790–7.

14. Packer RJ, Ater J, Allen J, et al. Carboplatin and vincristine chemotherapy for children with newly diagnosed progressive low-grade gliomas. J Neurosurg. 1997;86:747–54.

15. Ater J, Holmes E, Zhou T, et al. Abstracts from the thirteenth international symposium on pediatric neuro-oncology: results of COG protocol A9952-a randomized phase 3 study of two chemotherapy regimens for incompletely resected low-grade glioma in young children. Neuro-Oncology. 2008;10:451–2.

16. Massimino M, Spreafico F, Cefalo G, et al. High response rate to cisplatin/ etoposide regimen in childhood low-grade glioma. J Clin Oncol. 2002;20:4209–16.

17. Gururangan S, Fisher MJ, Allen JC, et al. Temozolomide in children with progressive low-grade glioma. Neuro Oncol. 2007;9:161–8.

18. Bouffet E, Jakacki R, Goldman S, et al. Phase II study of weekly vinblastine in recurrent or refractory pediatric low-grade glioma. J Clin Oncol. 2012;30:1358–136.

19. Lassaletta A, Scheinemann K, Zelcer SM, et al. Phase II weekly vinblastine for chemotherapy-naive children with progressive low-grade glioma: a Canadian pediatric brain tumor consortium study. J Clin Oncol. 2016;34:3537–43.

20. Cappellano AM, Petrilli AS, da Silva NS, et al. Single agent vinorelbine in pediatric patients with progressive optic pathway glioma. J Neuro-Oncol. 2015;121:405–12.

21. Fisher MJ, Loguidice M, Gutmann DH, Listernick R, Ferner RE, Ullrich NJ, et al. Visual outcomes in children with neurofibromatosis type 1-associated optic pathway glioma following chemotherapy: a multicenter retrospective analysis. Neuro-Oncology. 2012;14(6):790–7. https://doi.org/10.1093/neuonc/nos076.

22. Wan MJ, Ullrich NJ, Manley PE, Kieran MW, Goumnerova LC, Heidary G. Long-term visual outcomes of optic pathway gliomas in pediatric patients without neurofibromatosis type 1. J Neuro-Oncol. 2016;129(1):173–8. https://doi.org/10.1007/s11060-016-2163-4.

23. Alireza M, Amelot A, Chauvet D, Terrier LM, Lot G, Bekaert O. Poor prognosis and challenging treatment of optic nerve malignant gliomas: literature review and case report series. World Neurosurg. 2017;97:751.e1–6. https://doi.org/10.1016/j.wneu.2016.10.083.

24. Marwaha G, Macklis R, Singh AD. Radiation therapy: orbital tumors. Dev Ophthalmol. 2013;52:94–101.

25. Bataini JP, Delanian S, Ponvert D. Chiasmal gliomas: results of irradiation management in 57 patients and review of literature. Int J Radiat Oncol Biol Phys. 1991;21:615–23.

26. Cappelli C, Grill J, Raquin M, et al. Long-term follow up of 69 patients treated for optic pathway tumours before the chemotherapy era. Arch Dis Child. 1998;79:334–8.

27. Grabenbauer GG, Schuchardt U, Buchfelder M, et al. Radiation therapy of optico-hypothalamic gliomas (OHG)–radiographic response, vision and late toxicity. Radiother Oncol. 2000;54:239–45.

28. Horwich A, Bloom HJ. Optic gliomas: radiation therapy and prognosis. Int J Radiat Oncol Biol Phys. 1985;11:1067–79.

29. Jenkin D, Angyalfi S, Becker L, et al. Optic glioma in children: surveillance, resection, or irradiation? Int J Radiat Oncol Biol Phys. 1993;25:215–25.

30. Pierce SM, Barnes PD, Loeffler JS, et al. Definitive radiation therapy in the management of symptomatic patients with optic glioma. Survival and long-term effects. Cancer. 1990;65:45–52.

31. Grill J, Couanet D, Cappelli C, et al. Radiation-induced cerebral vasculopathy in children with neurofibromatosis and optic pathway glioma. Ann Neurol. 1999;45:393–6.

32. Kestle JR, Hoffman HJ, Mock AR. Moyamoya phenomenon after radiation for optic glioma. J Neurosurg. 1993;79:32–5.

33. Tsang DS, Murphy ES, Merchant TE. Radiation therapy for optic pathway and hypothalamic low-grade gliomas in children. Int J Radiat Oncol Biol Phys. 2017;99:642–51.

34. Sharif S, Ferner R, Birch JM, et al. Second primary tumors in neurofibromatosis 1 patients treated for optic glioma: substantial risks after radiotherapy. J Clin Oncol. 2006;24:2570–5.

35. Kim N, Lim DH. Recent updates on radiation therapy for pediatric optic pathway glioma. Brain Tumor Res Treat. 2022;10(2):94–100.

36. Lacaze E, Kieffer V, Streri A, et al. Neuropsychological outcome in children with optic pathway tumours when first-line treatment is chemotherapy. Br J Cancer. 2003;89:2038–44.

37. Combs SE, Schulz-Ertner D, Moschos D, et al. Fractionated stereotactic radiotherapy of optic pathway gliomas: tolerance and long-term outcome. Int J Radiat Oncol Biol Phys. 2005;62:814–9.

38. Marcus KJ, Goumnerova L, Billett AL, et al. Stereotactic radiotherapy for localized low-grade gliomas in children: final results of a prospective trial. Int J Radiat Oncol Biol Phys. 2005;61:374–9.

39. Saran FH, Baumert BG, Khoo VS, et al. Stereotactically guided conformal radiotherapy for progressive low-grade gliomas of childhood. Int J Radiat Oncol Biol Phys. 2002;53:43–51.

40. Fuss M, Hug EB, Schaefer RA, et al. Proton radiation therapy (PRT) for pediatric optic pathway gliomas: comparison with 3D planned conventional photons and a standard photon technique. Int J Radiat Oncol Biol Phys. 1999;45:1117–26.

41. Hug EB, Muenter MW, Archambeau JO, et al. Conformal proton radiation therapy for pediatric low-grade astrocytomas. Strahlenther Onkol. 2002;178:10–7.

42. Liang CL, Lu K, Liliang PC, Chen HJ. Gamma knife surgery for optic glioma. Report of 2 cases. J Neurosurg. 2010;113(Suppl):44–7.

43. El-Shehaby AM, Reda WA, Abdel Karim KM, et al. Single-session gamma knife radiosurgery for optic pathway/hypothalamic gliomas. J Neurosurg. 2016;125:50–7.

44. Indelicato DJ, Rotondo RL, Uezono H, Sandler ES, Aldana PR, Ranalli NJ, et al. Outcomes following proton therapy for pediatric low-grade glioma. Int J Radiat Oncol Biol Phys. 2019;104:149–56.

45. Weller M, van den Bent M, Hopkins K, Tonn JC, Stupp R, Falini A, Cohen-Jonathan-Moyal E, Frappaz D, Henriksson R, Balana C, Chinot O, Ram Z, Reifenberger G, Soffietti R, Wick W. EANO guideline for the diagnosis and treatment of anaplastic gliomas and glioblastoma. Lancet Oncol. 2014;15:e395–403.

46. Wilhelm H. Primary optic nerve tumours. Curr Opin Neurol. 2009;22(1):11–8. https://doi.org/10.1097/WCO.0b013e32831fd9f5.

47. Gacic EM, Skender-Gazibara MK, Gazibara TM, Nagulic MA, Nikolic IM. Intraorbital ganglioglioma of optic nerve in a patient with neurofibromatosis type 1. J Neuroophthalmol. 2012;32(4):350–3. https://doi.org/10.1097/WNO.0b013e318267ff55.

48. Rolston JD, Han SJ, Cotter JA, et al. Gangliogliomas of the optic pathway. J Clin Neurosci. 2014;21:2244–9.

49. Lindegaard J, Heegaard S, Toft PB, Nysom K, Prause JU. Malignant transformation of a medulloepithelioma of the optic nerve. Orbit. 2010;29(3):161–4. https://doi.org/10.3109/01676830903421200.

50. McGrath LA, Mudhar HS, Salvi SM. Hemangioblastoma of the optic nerve. Surv Ophthalmol. 2019;64(2):175–84. https://doi.org/10.1016/j.survophthal.2018.10.002.

51. Darbari S, Meena RK, Sawarkar D, Doddamani RS. Optic nerve hemangioblastoma: review. World Neurosurg. 2019;128:211–5. https://doi.org/10.1016/j.wneu.2019.04.224.

52. Parker RT, Ovens CA, Fraser CL, Samarawickrama C. Optic nerve sheath meningiomas: prevalence, impact, and management strategies. Eye Brain. 2018;10:85–99. https://doi.org/10.2147/EB.S144345.

53. Rassi MS, Prasad S, Can A, Pravdenkova S, Almefty R, Al-Mefty O. Prognostic factors in the surgical treatment of intracanalicular primary optic nerve sheath meningiomas. J Neurosurg. 2018;131(2):481–8. https://doi.org/10.3171/2018.4.JNS173080.

54. Saeed P, Rootman J, Nugent RA, White VA, Mackenzie IR, Koornneef L. Optic nerve sheath meningiomas. Ophthalmology. 2003;110(10):2019–30. https://doi.org/10.1016/S0161-6420(03)00787-5.

55. Jain D, Ebrahimi KB, Miller NR, Eberhart CG. Intraorbital meningiomas: a pathologic review using current World Health Organization criteria. Arch Pathol Lab Med. 2010;134(5):766–70. https://doi.org/10.5858/134.5.766.

56. Arnold AC, Lee AG. Dilation of the perioptic subarachnoid space anterior to optic nerve sheath meningioma. J Neuroophthalmol. 2021;41(1):e100–e2. https://doi.org/10.1097/WNO.0000000000000908.

57. Narayan DS, Traber GL, Figueira E, Pirbhai A, Landau K, Davis G, et al. Natural history of primary paediatric optic nerve sheath meningioma: case series and review. Br J Ophthalmol. 2018;102(8):1147–53. https://doi.org/10.1136/bjophthalmol-2017-310672.

58. Patel BC, De Jesus O, Margolin E. Optic nerve sheath meningioma. In: StatPearls [Internet]. Treasure Island (FL): StatPearls Publishing; 2022. https://www.ncbi.nlm.nih.gov/books/NBK430868/Updated. Accessed 24 May 2022.

59. Al Feghali KA, Yeboa DN, Chasen B, Gule MK, Johnson JM, Chung C. The use of 68 Ga-DOTATATE PET-TC in the non invasive diagnosis of optic nerve sheath meningiomas; a case report. Front Oncol. 2018;8:454. https://doi.org/10.3389/fonc.2018.00454.

60. Hénaux PL, Bretonnier M, Le Reste PJ, Morandi X. Modern management of meningiomas compressing the optic nerve: a systematic review.

World Neurosurg. 2018;118:e677–e86. https://doi.org/10.1016/j.wneu.2018.07.020.

61. Kennerdell JS, Maroon JC, Malton M, Warren FA. The management of optic nerve sheath meningiomas. Am J Ophthalmol. 1988;106:450–7.

62. Zoia C, Bongetta D, Pagella F, Antoniazzi ER, Gaetani P. New surgical option for optic nerve sheath meningiomas: fully endoscopic transnasal approach. Can J Ophthalmol. 2018;53(4):e142–e4. https://doi.org/10.1016/j.jcjo.2017.10.020.

63. Maza G, Subramaniam S, Yanez-Siller JC, Otto BA, Prevedello DM, Carrau RL. The role of Endonasal endoscopic optic nerve decompression as the initial management of primary optic nerve sheath meningiomas. J Neurol Surg B Skull Base. 2019;80(6):568–76. https://doi.org/10.1055/s-0039-1677689.

64. Melian E, Jay WM. Primary radiotherapy for optic nerve sheath meningioma. Semin Ophthalmol. 2004;19(3–4):130–40.

65. Bloch O, Sun M, Kaur G, Barani IJ, Parsa AT. Fractionated radiotherapy for optic nerve sheath meningiomas. J Clin Neurosci. 2012;19:1210–5.

66. Marchetti M, Bianchi S, Milanesi I, et al. Multisession radiosurgery for optic nerve sheath meningiomas: an effective option. Preliminary results from a monoinstitutional experience. Neurosurgery. 2011;69:1116–22.

67. Arvold ND, Lessell S, Bussiere M, Beaudette K, Rizzo JF, Loeffler JS, et al. Visual outcome and tumor control after conformal radiotherapy for patients with optic nerve sheath meningioma. Int J Radiat Oncol Biol Phys. 2009;75:1166–72.

68. Soldà F, Wharram B, Gunapala R, Brada M. Fractionated stereotactic conformal radiotherapy for optic nerve sheath meningiomas. Clin Oncol. 2012;24:e106–12.

69. Augspurger ME, Teh BS, Uhl BM, Lee AG, Grant WH, Butler EB, et al. 2091 conformal intensity modulated radiation therapy for the treatment of optic nerve sheath meningioma. Int J Radiat Oncol. 1999;45:324.

70. de Melo LP, Arruda Viani G, de Paula JS. Radiotherapy for the treatment of optic nerve sheath meningioma: a systematic review and meta-analysis. Radiother Oncol. 2021;165:135–41.

71. Ramey WL, Arnold SJ, Chiu A, Lemole M. A rare case of optic nerve schwannoma: case report and review of the literature. Cureus. 2015;7(4):e265. https://doi.org/10.7759/cureus.265.

72. Kashkouli MB, Abdolalizadeh P, Jafari S, Shahrzad S, Karimi N. Is primary optic nerve sheath schwannoma a misnomer? Report of two cases and literature review. Orbit. 2019;38(5):419–23. https://doi.org/10.1080/01676830.2018.1545239.

73. Sharma A, Singh D, Saran R. Primary optic nerve sheath schwannoma: a case report. Br J Neurosurg. 2021:1–3. https://doi.org/10.1080/02688697.2020.1869181.

Giuseppe Mariniello [ID], Sergio Corvino,
Adriana Iuliano, and Francesco Maiuri [ID]

13.1 Introduction

Since the first definition of spheno-orbital meningiomas (SOM) as en-plaque meningiomas provided by Cushing and Eisenhardt in 1938 [1], several terminologies have been adopted over the years to define these tumors, such as "sphenoid wing meningioma," "en-plaque meningioma," "hyperostosing meningioma of the sphenoid ridge," and "pterional meningioma." They are tumors arising at the sphenoid wing with secondary involvement of the periorbit [2], usually through the lateral wall and roof of the orbit, the superior orbital fissure (SOF), and/or the optic canal (OC) and characterized by an hyperostotic component of various degree and thin, carpet-like soft tissue growth at the dura. This pattern of growth accounts for the classic triad of presenting symptoms and signs of SOMs, consisting of proptosis, visual impairment, and ocular paresis.

There is no unanimous consensus in literature concerning the best treatment strategy, which should be tailored according to the tumor size and extension and the patient's clinical features.

This chapter reports the current knowledge concerning the spheno-orbital meningiomas, mainly focusing on their surgical management.

13.2 Natural History

Spheno-orbital meningiomas account for 2–9% of all intracranial meningiomas [3]. They mainly affect females (82%), who usually are younger than males at diagnosis, with a mean age of 51 ± 6 years old and who more often express the progesterone receptor at histological examination [4, 5]. Furthermore, the spheno-orbital region represents the most frequent location for intracranial meningiomas in sex female [5].

In most cases, these tumors are slow-growing (0.3 cm³ per year) [6] and benign (WHO grade I).

The site of origin and the pattern of growth account for the main presenting signs and symptoms due to the mass effect: proptosis (84%), visual acuity (46%), and visual field (31%) deficits for the involvement of the optic nerve, and ophthalmoplegia (22%) with consequent diplopia due to the involvement of the oculomotor cranial nerves (III 11%, IV 6%, VI 4%). Other less

G. Mariniello (✉) · S. Corvino · F. Maiuri
Division of Neurosurgery, Department of
Neurosciences, Reproductive and
Odontostomatological Sciences, University of Naples
"Federico II", Naples, Italy
e-mail: giumarin@unina.it; frmaiuri@unina.it

A. Iuliano
Division of Ophthalmology, Department of
Neurosciences, Reproductive and
Odontostomatological Sciences, University of Naples
"Federico II", Naples, Italy

frequent clinical manifestations include neurological impairment, such as mental change, memory deficit, and seizures [4].

13.3 Clinical and Neuroradiological Evaluation

A careful clinical and radiological evaluation for the tumor definition and planning of the therapeutic strategy is required and includes.

The clinical evaluation includes: the neurologic examination by a neurologist to evaluate symptoms of intracranial tumor extension; the assessment of proptosis with an ophthalmometer, the ocular motility, the visual acuity, and visual field by an ophthalmologist; the optic coherence tomography (OCT) may be sometimes useful.

The diagnostic imaging by a radiologist must include high-resolution 3D CT scans and MRI. CT scan of the skull must assess the hyperostosis degree of the sphenoid wing and the surrounding structures, mainly the optic canal, superior orbital fissure, and anterior clinoidal process. The contrast-enhanced MRI must define the intracranial and intraorbital components of the tumor, the extent of dura mater involvement, the relationship of the tumor with the surrounding soft tissues and neurovascular structures (Fig. 13.1). Finally, the neurosurgeon and radiotherapist complete the multidisciplinary team for the decision-making process about the treatment strategy.

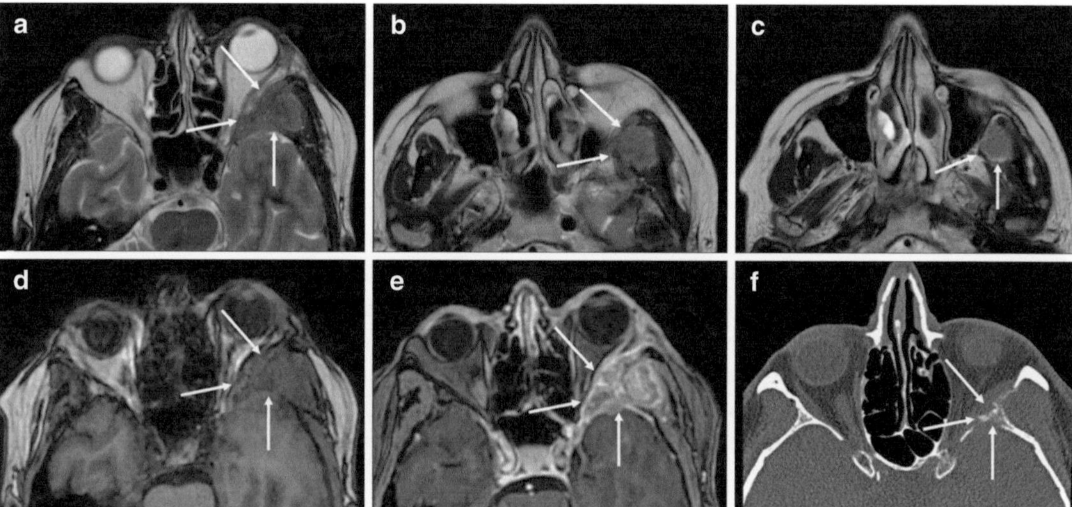

Fig. 13.1 Preoperative axial images of left **spheno-orbital meningioma:** (**a–c**) MRI T2-weighted sequences showing the lesion arising from the dura of greater sphenoid wing, with caudal involvement of the inferior orbital fissure and the insertion of the temporalis muscle; MRI T1-weigthed pre- (**d**) and post- (**e**) contrast sequences; (**f**) bone-window CT scan showing the bone remodeling of the greater sphenoid wing resulting from the lesion

13.4   Treatment Strategies

At the state of the art, there are no defined guidelines in literature concerning the best treatment strategy, which presents several controversies, such as the "wait and see" option, the role of surgery and its timing, the surgical approach, the extension of the tumor resection or decompression of the hyperostosis, the management of the periorbita, the dural and bone reconstruction, the role of radiation therapy and the management of the residual tumor and recurrences, the validity of the Simpson grading system.

13.4.1 The Role of Surgery

The role of surgery was matter of debate in the past for several reasons [7]. The spheno-orbital meningiomas are slow-growing tumors with often long and stable clinical phase; there is involvement of vulnerable and highly functional nervous structures, such as optic and/or oculomotor cranial nerves; the possibility of a total resection is limited and increases the risk of postoperative morbidity.

Some authors are in favor of a "wait and scans" strategy [6], others are oriented toward a gross-total resection with proptosis correction [8, 9], others aim at a symptom-oriented surgery [10].

Nowadays, the surgery represents the first choice when functional impairment occurs, with the aim of an onco-functional balance between the need to achieve a maximal safe resection and the need to preserve/restore a good neurological and ophthalmological function [4, 11, 12]. In this scenario, the subtotal resection followed by radiation therapy for selected locations of residual meningioma, that is, -the cavernous sinus [2], or without adjuvant treatment but with second surgery at regrowth [13] are some of the management strategies.

Surgery of spheno-orbital meningiomas is extremely challenging, due to their anatomical relationship with vulnerable and highly functional neurovascular structures, such as optic and oculomotor nerves, cavernous sinus, trigeminal nerve branches. Therefore, the choice of an aggressive surgical approach might lead to unnecessary peri- and postoperative morbidity; on the other hand, a less invasive and more conservative approach might not provide an adequate exposure of the surgical target area, not guarantee the control of the neurovascular structures, a satisfying bony decompression and tumor removal. It results in no clinical improvement and high rate of recurrence.

Although the extent of resection affects the progression-free survival, the gross-total resection of spheno-orbital meningiomas is achieved in 25%–69% [3] and is burdened by high risk of severe morbidity.

Several surgical approaches have been described for the treatment of spheno-orbital meningiomas, either microsurgical, such as the pterional and its "extended" variant, the lateral orbitotomy [14], the supraorbital-pterional, the frontotemporo-orbitozygomatic (FTOZ), and more recently, endoscopic, via endonasal, transorbital, supraorbital and trans-maxillary, the latter being performed in isolated or combined multiportal manner, based on the tumor size and extension, each of them with related advantages and limits [4, 14–20].

Concerning the transcranial microsurgical routes, our group in the past has proposed an algorithm in the choice of the approach according to the intraorbital tumor extent in relationship with the axis of the optic nerve [19]: in the detail, we suggested the lateral orbitotomy [14] in cases of lateral and superolateral involvement of the orbit, the supraorbital-pterional approach for medial, inferomedial and orbital apex meningiomas, and the fronto-temporo-orbito-zygomatic approach for diffuse meningiomas with invasion of the cavernous sinus and infratemporal fossa.

The endoscopic approaches aim to minimize perioperative and postoperative morbidity and reducing aesthetic disfigurement. The surgical indications of superior eyelid transorbital endoscopic approach for neurosurgical intracranial pathologies are constantly and rapidly increasing, mainly for spheno-orbital meningiomas. This endoscopic technique has concrete advantages, such as the minimally invasive nature, short distance and direct access to the target, reduced bone destruction, minimal brain retraction and manipulation, early tumor deafferentation, satisfactory aesthetic result, short hospital-stay and rapid patient recovery.

From a recent meta-analysis and systematic review on surgical techniques and outcome for SOM [4], which included 38 articles out of 621 identified, the extended pterional resulted the workhorse approach, being the most performed in 37 among 38 surgical series, whereas the endoscopic technique, vie endonasal route, was reported in only three articles. Furthermore, the optic canal was the most frequently decompressed structure (31/38, 82%), followed by the superior orbital fissure (25/38, 66%), while no trend in the extent of decompression or resection of the hyperostotic bone was registered. The data concerning the reconstruction technique was almost heterogeneous: some authors (7/38, 18%) repaired the dural defect with free draft of fascia, others (6/38, 16%) with pericranium, whereas for the bony defect, some authors used the titanium mesh (14/38, 37%), others (11/38, 29%) the inner calvaria graft or polymethylmethacrylate (10/38, 26%). Among the clinical symptoms and signs, proptosis, diplopia, and ophthalmoplegia improved in 96% of cases, visual acuity deficit in 91% and visual field deficit in 87%. Finally, the most common reported complication was trigeminal hypoesthesia (19%), followed by ptosis (17%), cranial nerve deficit (17%), diplopia (17%), ophthalmoplegia (16%), visual acuity deficit (9%), and visual field deficit (4%).

Some authors recommend reconstruction of the orbital walls in order to prevent enophthalmos and/or diplopia; in our experience, we found that partial or complete resection of the orbital roof did not require reconstruction.

The transcranial approach allows wider exposure of the lateral wall and roof of the orbit and the middle cranial fossa but at risk of temporal muscle atrophy and complications related to the brain manipulation [2, 10, 21, 22].

The continue research of the minimal invasiveness to reduce the perioperative and postoperative morbidity and the peculiar advantages demonstrated over the years since its introduction at the beginning of the last century by endoscopic approaches, via endonasal and, more recently transorbital routes, in the management of skull base pathologies, led to progressive expansion of their surgical indication. Nowadays, transorbital endoscopic approaches are used for the management of wide variety of skull base lesions with or without orbit involvement, mainly meningiomas [18].

There is strong evidence of postoperative improvement of the clinical symptoms, mainly proptosis and ocular motility deficits, but also visual acuity and visual field deficits [4]; therefore, the visual outcomes endorse surgery of patients with spheno-orbital meningiomas even with minimal visual impairment or hyperostosis [23], although there are no defined knowledge on the effect of the timing of surgery on visual and neurological outcomes.

At the light of these findings and in agreement with the concept of symptoms-oriented surgery for spheno-orbital meningiomas, we consider that the surgery is primarily directed to the optic nerve decompression in cases of decreased visual acuity; on the other hand, when the proptosis is the main clinical sign without tumor involvement of the optic canal, a lateral orbitotomy may result effective to obtain adequate reduction of the proptosis.

In this scenario, the decompression of the optic canal and nerve, and/or the superior orbital fissure, associated to the maximal safe tumor resection, represent the most appropriated surgical maneuvers.

13.4.2 Adjuvant Treatments

Currently, there is no clear evidence about the indications and the efficacy of the radiation therapy on the treatment of spheno-orbital meningiomas as few studies are focused on this aspect. Some authors suggest performing radiotherapy in WHO grade II tumors and with rapid pattern of growth [10, 21, 24]; or in cases of involvement of the superior orbital fissure and cavernous sinus [2, 9]; or after subtotal resection or WHO grade II and III meningiomas [3, 25].

We recommend the radiation therapy in patients undergone subtotal resection, with ocular muscles infiltration and only a close clinical and radiological follow-up when a gross total resection (Simpson's grades I and II) is achieved, regardless the WHO grade of the tumor.

Concerning the role of the radiosurgery, its application is different among the institutions; its main limit remains the proximity of the optic pathway to the tumor [9].

13.5   Recurrences

13.5.1 Prognostic Risk Factors

Several factors affect the recurrence rate of spheno-orbital meningiomas, including the extent of resection, the tumor location, the WHO grade, and the length of follow-up.

Because of their deep-seated location on the skull base, their pattern of growth, extension, and invasiveness, anatomical relationships with functional neurovascular structures, the gross total resection of spheno-orbital meningiomas is hard to achieve, and this aspect affects the recurrence rate, which ranges from 0 to 56% [13]. In terms of Simpson's grading system [26], the recurrence rate is greater after Simpson's grade III and IV than after grade I [27].

The invasion of the cavernous sinus and intraconal compartment [3], as well as of the orbital apex [13], optic canal [13, 24] and superior orbital fissure [13] are considered unfavorable

prognostic factors of progression free survival; in these conditions, the risk of postoperative morbidity resulting from an aggressive treatment limits the extent of resection in favor of a more conservative approach.

The recurrence rate is also related to the WHO grade, with atypical grade II meningiomas recurring more frequently than the benign grade I (63% vs 18%, respectively) [13].

Finally, the risk of recurrence is affected by the length of follow-up, with a higher recurrence rate after a long follow-up [2, 13].

13.5.2 Management

The management of recurrent spheno-orbital meningiomas is still matter of debated.

We consider the reoperation as the first treatment option in cases of symptomatic tumors at the regrowth and/or recurrence and the "wait and see" strategy for asymptomatic patients with limited regrowth. The aim of the re-surgery, as for the surgery at the first diagnosis, is the relief, restoration/improvement of clinical signs, and symptoms or the arrest of their deterioration. For these purposes, even several reoperations are justified. The role of the radiation treatments on the recurrences is the same for patients at the first diagnosis.

13.6   Conclusion

Spheno-orbital meningioma is a unique skull base tumor representing a challenge of treatment. Although in most cases it is a benign and slow-growth tumor, if underestimated it may lead to highly functional and irreversible neurological deficits. A multidisciplinary team is required for the decision-making concerning the diagnostic and therapeutic processes. The surgery represents the first choice when functional impairment occurs; although the gross total resection is difficult to achieve without severe morbidity, the improvement of the main clinical symptoms is achieved in almost all cases.

References

1. Cushing H, Meningiomas LE. Their classification, regional behaviour, life history, and surgical end results. Springfield, IL: Charles C. Thomas; 1938.

2. Terrier LM, Bernard F, Fournier HD, Morandi X, Velut S, Hénaux PL, et al. Spheno-orbital Meningiomas surgery: multicenter management study for complex extensive tumors. World Neurosurg. 2018;112:e145–e56. https://doi.org/10.1016/j.wneu.2017.12.182.

3. Masalha W, Heiland DH, Steiert C, Krüger MT, Schnell D, Scheiwe C, et al. Progression-free survival, prognostic factors, and surgical outcome of spheno-orbital meningiomas. Front Oncol. 2021;11:672228. https://doi.org/10.3389/fonc.2021.672228.

4. Fisher FL, Zamanipoor Najafabadi AH, Schoones JW, Genders SW, van Furth WR. Surgery as a safe and effective treatment option for spheno-orbital meningioma: a systematic review and meta-analysis of surgical techniques and outcomes. Acta Ophthalmol. 2021;99(1):26–36. https://doi.org/10.1111/aos.14517.

5. Apra C, Roblot P, Alkhayri A, Le Guérinel C, Polivka M, Chauvet D. Female gender and exogenous progesterone exposition as risk factors for spheno-orbital meningiomas. J Neuro-Oncol. 2020;149(1):95–101. https://doi.org/10.1007/s11060-020-03576-8.

6. Saeed P, van Furth WR, Tanck M, Kooremans F, Freling N, Streekstra GI, et al. Natural history of spheno-orbital meningiomas. Acta Neurochir. 2011;153(2):395–402. https://doi.org/10.1007/s00701-010-0878-0.

7. Cophignon J, Lucena J, Clay C, Marchac D. Limits to radical treatment of spheno-orbital meningiomas. Acta Neurochir Suppl (Wien). 1979;28(2):375–80.

8. Bikmaz K, Mrak R, Al-Mefty O. Management of bone-invasive, hyperostotic sphenoid wing meningiomas. J Neurosurg. 2007;107(5):905–12. https://doi.org/10.3171/JNS-07/11/0905.

9. Boari N, Gagliardi F, Spina A, Bailo M, Franzin A, Mortini P. Management of spheno-orbital en plaque meningiomas: clinical outcome in a consecutive series of 40 patients. Br J Neurosurg. 2013;27(1):84–90. https://doi.org/10.3109/02688697.2012.709557.

10. Freeman JL, Davern MS, Oushy S, Sillau S, Ormond DR, Youssef AS, et al. Spheno-orbital meningiomas: a 16-year surgical experience. World Neurosurg. 2017;99:369–80. https://doi.org/10.1016/j.wneu.2016.12.063.

11. Zamanipoor Najafabadi AH, Peeters MCM, Dirven L, Lobatto DJ, Groen JL, Broekman MLD, et al. Impaired health-related quality of life in meningioma patients-a systematic review. Neuro-Oncology. 2017;19(7):897–907. https://doi.org/10.1093/neuonc/now250.

12. Gonen L, Nov E, Shimony N, Shofty B, Margalit N. Sphenoorbital meningioma: surgical series and design of an intraoperative management algorithm. Neurosurg Rev. 2018;41(1):291–301. https://doi.org/10.1007/s10143-017-0855-7.

13. Mariniello G, de Divitiis O, Corvino S, Strianese D, Iuliano A, Bonavolontà G, et al. Recurrences of spheno-orbital meningiomas: risk factors and management. World Neurosurg. 2022;161:e514. https://doi.org/10.1016/j.wneu.2022.02.048.

14. Mariniello G, Maiuri F, de Divitiis E, Bonavolontà G, Tranfa F, Iuliano A, et al. Lateral orbitotomy for removal of sphenoid wing meningiomas invading the orbit. Neurosurgery. 2010;66(6 Suppl Operative):287–92; discussion 92. https://doi.org/10.1227/01.NEU.0000369924.87437.0B.

15. Abou-Al-Shaar H, Krisht KM, Cohen MA, Abunimer AM, Neil JA, Karsy M, et al. Cranio-orbital and Orbitocranial approaches to orbital and intracranial disease: eye-opening approaches for neurosurgeons. Front Surg. 2020;7:1. https://doi.org/10.3389/fsurg.2020.00001.

16. Dallan I, Cristofani-Mencacci L, Fiacchini G, Caniglia M, Sellari-Franceschini S, Berrettini S. When multidisciplinary surgical transorbital approaches should be considered to reach the skull base. Acta Otorhinolaryngol Ital. 2021;41(Suppl. 1):S59–66. https://doi.org/10.14639/0392-100X-suppl.1-41-2021-06.

17. Locatelli D, Restelli F, Alfiero T, Campione A, Pozzi F, Balbi S, et al. The role of the Transorbital superior eyelid approach in the Management of Selected Spheno-orbital meningiomas: in-depth analysis of indications, technique, and outcomes from the study of a cohort of 35 patients. J Neurol Surg B Skull Base. 2022;83(2):145–58. https://doi.org/10.1055/s-0040-1718914.

18. Kong DS, Kim YH, Hong CK. Optimal indications and limitations of endoscopic transorbital superior eyelid surgery for spheno-orbital meningiomas. J Neurosurg. 2020;134(5):1472–9. https://doi.org/10.3171/2020.3.JNS20297.

19. Mariniello G, Maiuri F, Strianese D, Donzelli R, Iuliano A, Tranfa F, et al. Spheno-orbital meningiomas: surgical approaches and outcome according to the intraorbital tumor extent. Zentralbl Neurochir. 2008;69(4):175–81. https://doi.org/10.1055/s-2008-1077077.

20. Lew H, Rootman DB, Nassiri N, Goh A, Goldberg RA. Transorbital approach without craniotomy to orbital tumors with extradural intracranial extension. Orbit. 2014;33(5):343–51. https://doi.org/10.3109/01676830.2014.904374.

21. Cannon PS, Rutherford SA, Richardson PL, King A, Leatherbarrow B. The surgical management and outcomes for spheno-orbital meningiomas: a 7-year review of multi-disciplinary practice. Orbit. 2009;28(6):371–6. https://doi.org/10.3109/01676830903104645.

22. Shrivastava RK, Sen C, Costantino PD, Della RR. Sphenoorbital meningiomas: surgical limitations and lessons learned in their long-term management. J Neurosurg. 2005;103(3):491–7. https://doi.org/10.3171/jns.2005.103.3.0491.

23. Zamanipoor Najafabadi AH, Genders SW, van Furth WR. Visual outcomes endorse surgery of patients with spheno-orbital meningioma with minimal visual impairment or hyperostosis. Acta Neurochir. 2021;163(1):73–82. https://doi.org/10.1007/s00701-020-04554-9.

24. Leroy HA, Leroy-Ciocanea CI, Baroncini M, Bourgeois P, Pellerin P, Labreuche J, et al. Internal and external spheno-orbital meningioma varieties: different outcomes and prognoses. Acta Neurochir. 2016;158(8):1587–96. https://doi.org/10.1007/s00701-016-2850-0.

25. Terpolilli NA, Ueberschaer M, Niyazi M, Hintschich C, Egensperger R, Muacevic A, et al. Long-term outcome in orbital meningiomas: progression-free survival after targeted resection combined with early or postponed postoperative radiotherapy. J Neurosurg. 2019;133:1–11. https://doi.org/10.3171/2019.3.JNS181760.

26. Simpson D. The recurrence of intracranial meningiomas after surgical treatment. J Neurol Neurosurg Psychiatry. 1957;20(1):22–39.

27. Mariniello G, Bonavolontà G, Tranfa F, Maiuri F. Management of the optic canal invasion and visual outcome in spheno-orbital meningiomas. Clin Neurol Neurosurg. 2013;115(9):1615–20. https://doi.org/10.1016/j.clineuro.2013.02.012.

Schwannomas of the Oculomotor Nerves

14

Giuseppe Mariniello, Oreste de Divitiis, Adriana Iuliano, and Francesco Maiuri

14.1 Introduction

Cranial nerves schwannomas are benign slowly growing tumors, most commonly arising from the sensory nerves, mainly from the vestibular, followed by the trigeminal nerve [1]. On the other hand, those arising from the motor nerves, including the oculomotor nerves, are very rare and mostly occur in patients with neurofibromatosis (NF) [2]. Because of their very rare occurrence, the diagnosis of schwannoma of the oculomotor nerves is often difficult, mainly in absence of diplopia and in sporadic cases not associated to NF. Besides, the best management option (conservative versus surgery versus radiosurgery) is controversial, and there are not guidelines of management, as for vestibular schwannomas.

14.2 Surgical Anatomy of the Oculomotor Nerves

The three oculomotor nerves (common oculomotor, trochlear and abducens) arise from the brain stem and end in the orbit to innervate the ocular muscles. For all nerves, three main segments may be recognized: cisternal, cavernous, and orbital.

The **common oculomotor nerve** arises from the anterior surface of mesencephalon, medial to the cerebral peduncle. It courses anteriorly, between the posterior cerebral artery and the superior cerebellar artery, into the interpeduncular cistern. Then, it enters the cavernous sinus, coursing in its wall and crosses the superior orbital fissure to enter the orbit [3]. After coursing in the orbital apex, the nerve divides in two branches (superior and inferior), which cross the anulus of Zinn on its lateral aspect. The superior branch supplies the elevator palpebrae and superior rectus muscles; the inferior branch innervates the inferior rectus, the medial rectus, and the inferior oblique muscles [4, 5].

The **trochlear nerve** originates from the posterior aspect of the mesencephalon, then it courses into the quadrigeminal cistern in lateral and anterior direction around the cerebral peduncle. In the ambient cistern, the nerve courses below the free edge of the tentorium to reach the cavernous sinus, then it enters the orbit through the superior orbital fissure near its medial wall,

G. Mariniello (✉) · O. de Divitiis · F. Maiuri
Division of Neurosurgery, Department of Neurosciences, Reproductive and Odontostomatological Sciences, University of Naples "Federico II", Naples, Italy
e-mail: giumarin@unina.it; frmaiuri@unina.it

A. Iuliano
Division of Ophthalmology, Department of Neurosciences, Reproductive and Odontostomatological Sciences, University of Naples "Federico II", Naples, Italy

outside the anulus of Zinn. In the orbit, it reaches and innervates the superior oblique muscle.

The **abducens nerve** originates from the bulbo-pontine sulcus, courses anteriorly in the ambient cistern up to the petrous apex to reach the cavernous sinus. The nerve passes through the superior orbital fissure, it crosses the anulus of Zinn lateral to the fibers of the oculomotor nerve, and runs in the lateral orbital region to reach the lateral rectus muscle.

14.3 Schwannomas of the Oculomotor Nerves

14.3.1 Demographic and Clinical Aspects

14.3.1.1 Schwannomas of the Common Oculomotor Nerve

Schwannomas of the common oculomotor nerve are very rare, with only 84 well-documented cases collected in several literature reviews [6–8]. They are mainly located in the cisternal segment (40%), followed by the cavernous segment, whereas pure intraorbital tumors are exceptional (10%). The median duration of symptoms before the diagnosis is 10 months. The clinical presentation depends on the affected segment. Diplopia and ptosis are the most frequent complaints; headache and periorbital pain are also referred. Exceptional asymptomatic incidental cases are misdiagnosed [9]. Intraorbital schwannomas may cause proptosis and visual loss [10, 11].

14.3.1.2 Schwannomas of the Trochlear Nerve

Schwannomas of the trochlear nerve (45 reported cases in the literature reviews) [12–14] are almost exclusively located in the cisternal (84%) and cisternal-cavernous (14%) segments, with no intraorbital cases. This is probably due to the longer course of this nerve in the quadrigeminal, ambient, and crural cisterns. Most cases present with diplopia and headache; at examination,

paralyses of the superior oblique muscle was evidenced in half of the patients. The median duration of the symptoms before the diagnosis is 10 months.

14.3.1.3 Schwannomas of the Abducens Nerve

Schwannomas of the abducens nerve are even more rare than those of the third and fourth nerves (30 reported cases) [15–17]. The tumor location was cisternal (34%), cavernous (34%), or both (20%); four pure intraorbital tumors are also reported. Diplopia and paresis of the sixth cranial nerve are the most frequent complaint (80%); headache (60%) and symptoms of involvement of the third, fourth, and fifth cranial nerves (40%) are also referred.

14.3.2 Imaging Studies

On preoperative magnetic resonance (MR), almost all schwannomas are isointense or isohypointense on T1-weighted sequences and all are hyperintense on T2-weighted sequences; a homogenous contrast enhancement is evident, although cystic components may be present [8, 18]. Thin section (1–2 mm) post-contrast MR may define the exact tumor extension in the skull base cisterns or along the course of the nerve in the parasellar spaces or in the cavernous sinus (Fig. 14.1). The 3D gradient echo steady-state sequences are more useful; with this imaging technique, the neural structures, vessels, and dura are visualized as low-signal intensity in the CSF hyperintensity [19]. Thus, small and middle-sized schwannomas are well evidenced as hypo- or isointense masses in the high signal CSF hyperintensity; besides the correct relationship of the tumor with the dura mater (preserved versus transgressed, or extradural versus extra-intradural) may be defined in parasellar schwannomas [18]. Unfortunately, these tumor relationships may not be visible in larger tumors. MR with diffusor tensor tractography is a very useful technique for identifying the schwannoma's origin nerve [20, 21].

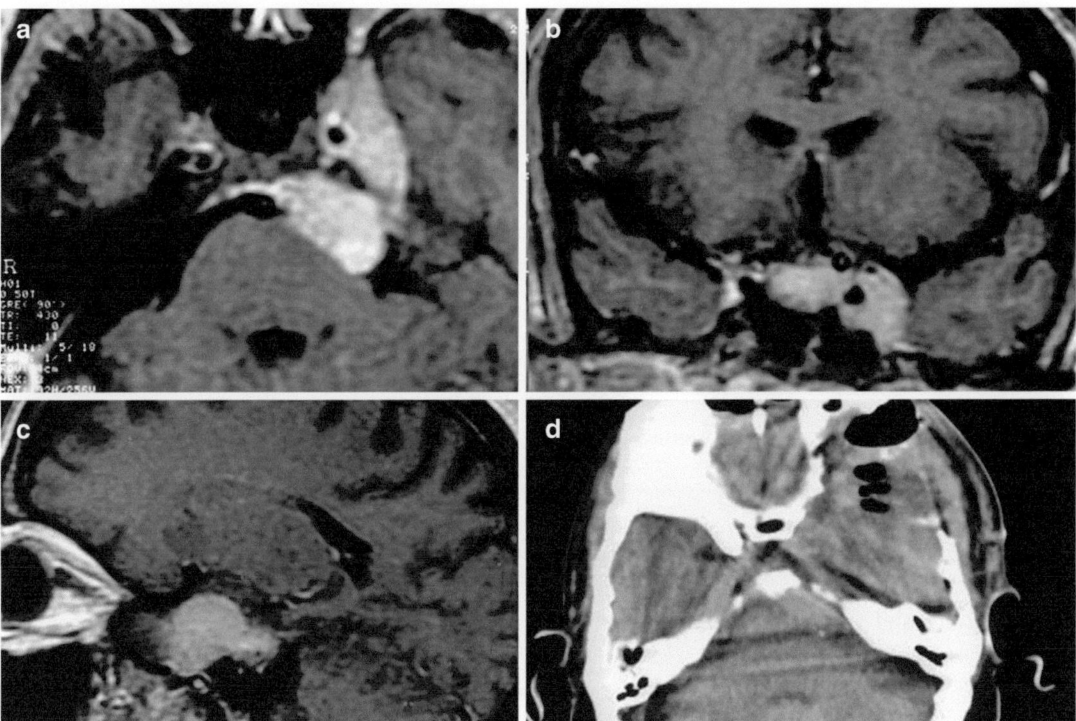

Fig. 14.1 (a–c) Post-contrast cranial magnetic resonance: **schwannoma of the left oculomotor nerve** located in the interpenducular cistern and parasellar region. (d) Post-operative CT scan: removal of the tumor

14.3.3 Management and Outcome

The management options for schwannomas of the oculomotor nerves include wait and see, surgery, and radiosurgery. The choice mainly depends upon entity of the deficit of the eye movements, patient age, size, and growth tendency of the tumor. Patients with large tumors and symptoms and signs of mass effect must be operated on. On the other hand, the management of small schwannomas is controversial. The surgical intervention is at high risk of complete nerve palsy, because of the small nerve size and need for intraoperative manipulation. Thus, some suggest a less aggressive management by stereotactic radiosurgery [22, 23].

The surgical approach depends on tumor location. Schwannomas located in the ambiens, crural, and interpeduncular cisterns are approached through subtemporal, transtentorial, suboccipital, and pterional approaches. Parasellar schwanno-mas may be located in the cavernous sinus or may extend from the cavernous sinus to the cisternal space (cisternal-cavernous). Tumors of the cavernous sinus may be approached by pterional extradural route coupled by anterior clinoidectomy; on the other hand, tumors located in the cisterns or extending from the cavernous sinus to the cisternal space also require an intradural exploration to obtain sufficient exposure of the cisternal portion of the tumor, as in our previously reported cases [18] (Fig. 14.2).

The maximum safe resection of the tumor should be the surgical goal; however, this is at risk of nerve damage. In cases of intraoperative nerve transection, the surgical repair may be realized by direct end-to-end anastomosis [24, 25] or by nerve graft [26].

The stereotactic radiosurgery (SRS) is a good management option for small schwannomas, mainly with preserved nerve function and as adjuvant treatment after partial resection [22,

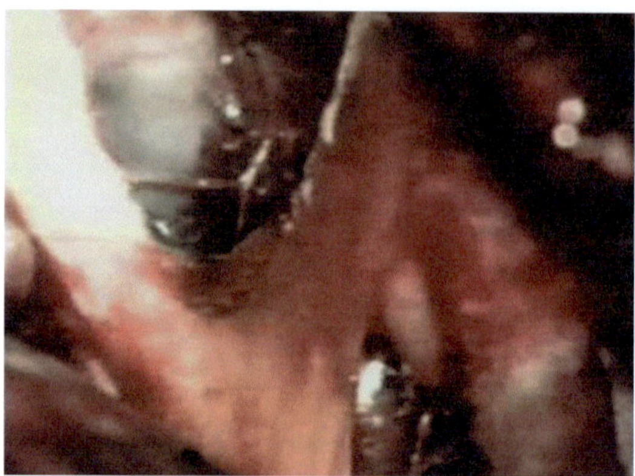

Fig. 14.2 Intraoperative view of a **schwannoma of the right oculomotor nerve** approached by pterional approach

23, 27, 28]. It results in most cases in good tumor control, with stable or decreased size, and no worsening and sometimes improvement of diplopia [23].

14.4 Conclusion

Schwannomas of the oculomotor, trochlear, and abducens nerves are very rare tumors, occurring in the cisterns or cavernous sinus, exceptionally in the orbit, and mainly presenting with variable deficit of the involved nerve. The surgical resection is indicated for larger tumors; however, postoperative worsening of the nerve function occurs in almost half of the patients. Small asymptomatic tumors must only be observed. In cases where symptoms occur or progression is evidenced on MR, stereotactic radiosurgery is the best option; it results in good tumor control and good outcome of the nerve function.

References

1. Sarma S, Sekhar LN, Schessel DA, Malis LI, Day JD. Nonvestibular schwannomas of the brain: a 7-year experience. Neurosurgery. 2002;50(3):437–49. https://doi.org/10.1097/00006123-200203000-00002.
2. Celli P, Ferrante L, Acqui M, Mastronardi L, Fortuna A, Palma L. Neurinoma of the third, fourth, and sixth cranial nerves: a survey and report of a new fourth nerve case. Surg Neurol. 1992;38(3):216–24. https://doi.org/10.1016/0090-3019(92)90172-J.
3. Natori Y, Rhoton AL. Microsurgical anatomy of the superior orbital fissure. Neurosurgery. 1995;36(4):762–75. https://doi.org/10.1227/00006123-199504000-00018.
4. Martins C, E Silva CIE, Campero A, et al. Microsurgical anatomy of the orbit: the rule of seven. Anat Res Int. 2011;2011:1–14. https://doi.org/10.1155/2011/468727.
5. Bernardo A, Evins AI, Mattogno PP, Quiroga M, Zacharia BE. The orbit as seen through different surgical windows: extensive anatomosurgical study. World Neurosurg. 2017;106:1030–46. https://doi.org/10.1016/J.WNEU.2017.06.158.
6. el Asri AC, Arnaout MM, Gerges MM, Gazzaz M, el Mostarchid B, Schwartz TH. Prognosis factor in oculomotor schwannoma: a case of endoscopic Endonasal approach and systematic review of the literature. World Neurosurg. 2019;129:72–80. https://doi.org/10.1016/J.WNEU.2019.05.170.
7. Muhammad S, Niemelä M. Management of oculomotor nerve schwannoma: systematic review of literature and illustrative case. Surg Neurol Int. 2019;10(40):1–6. https://doi.org/10.25259/SNI-75-2019.
8. Douglas VP, Flores C, Douglas KA, Strominger MB, Kasper E, Torun N. Oculomotor nerve schwannoma: case series and literature review. Surv Ophthalmol. 2022;67(4):1160–74. https://doi.org/10.1016/J.SURVOPHTHAL.2021.11.008.
9. Katoh M, Kawamoto T, Ohnishi K, Sawamura Y, Abe H. Asymptomatic schwannoma of the oculomotor nerve: case report. J Clin Neurosci. 2000;7(5):458–60. https://doi.org/10.1054/JOCN.1999.0240.
10. Shamim MS, Bari ME, Chisti KN, Abbas A. A child with intra-orbital oculomotor nerve schwannoma without neurofibromatosis. Can J Neurol Sci. 2008;35(4):528–30. https://doi.org/10.1017/S0317167100009288.
11. Scheller C, Rachinger JC, Prell J, et al. Intraorbital oculomotor nerve schwannoma affecting only the parasympathetic fibers. J Neurol Surg A Cent Eur Neurosurg. 2013;74(2):120–3. https://doi.org/10.1055/S-0032-1313641.
12. Samadian M, Farzin N, Bakhtevari MH, Hallajnejad M, Rezaei O. Isolated trochlear nerve schwannoma presenting with diplopia: a case report and literature review. Interdiscip Neurosurg. 2015;2(2):111–4. https://doi.org/10.1016/J.INAT.2015.03.006.
13. Cunha M, Miranda M, Cecconello G. Trochlear nerve schwannoma: case report and literature review. Arq Bras Neurocir. 2017;36(03):178–84. https://doi.org/10.1055/S-0037-1603919.
14. Ozoner B, Gungor A, Ture H, Ture U. Surgical treatment of trochlear nerve schwannomas: case series and systematic review. World Neurosurg. 2022;162:e288–300. https://doi.org/10.1016/J.WNEU.2022.03.006.
15. Li X, Li J, Li J, Wu Z. Schwannoma of the 6th nerve: case report and review of the literature. Chin

Neurosurg J. 2015;1(1):1–7. https://doi.org/10.1186/S41016-015-0004-5/TABLES/2.

16. Nakamizo A, Matsuo S, Amano T. Abducens nerve schwannoma: a case report and literature review. World Neurosurg. 2019;125:49–54. https://doi.org/10.1016/J.WNEU.2019.01.123.

17. Alhussain ZM, Alharbi SK, Farrash F. Abducens nerve schwannoma of the cavernous sinus: a case report and literature review. Surg Neurol Int. 2020;11:11. https://doi.org/10.25259/SNI_362_2020.

18. Mariniello G, de Divitiis O, Caranci F, Dones F, Maiuri F. Parasellar schwannomas: extradural vs extra-Intradural surgical approach. Oper Neurosurg (Hagerstown). 2018;14(6):627–38. https://doi.org/10.1093/ONS/OPX174.

19. Seitz J, Held P, Strotzer M, et al. MR imaging of cranial nerve lesions using six different high-resolution T1- and T2(*)-weighted 3D and 2D sequences. Acta Radiol. 2002;43(4):349–53. https://doi.org/10.1034/J.1600-0455.2002.430401.X.

20. Hodaie M, Quan J, Chen DQ. In vivo visualization of cranial nerve pathways in humans using diffusion-based tractography. Neurosurgery. 2010;66(4):788–95. https://doi.org/10.1227/01.NEU.0000367613.09324.DA.

21. Wei PH, Qi ZG, Chen G, et al. Identification of cranial nerves around trigeminal schwannomas using diffusion tensor tractography: a technical note and report of 3 cases. Acta Neurochir. 2016;158(3):429–35. https://doi.org/10.1007/S00701-015-2680-5.

22. Kim IY, Kondziolka D, Niranjan A, Flickinger JC, Lunsford LD. Gamma knife surgery for schwannomas originating from cranial nerves III, IV, and VI. J Neurosurg. 2008;109(Suppl(Supplement)):149–53. https://doi.org/10.3171/JNS/2008/109/12/S23.

23. Langlois AM, Iorio-Morin C, Faramand A, et al. Outcomes after stereotactic radiosurgery for schwannomas of the oculomotor, trochlear, and abducens nerves. J Neurosurg. 2021;135(4):1044–50. https://doi.org/10.3171/2020.8.JNS20887.

24. Sekhar LN, Lanzino G, Sen CN, Pomonis S. Reconstruction of the third through sixth cranial nerves during cavernous sinus surgery. J Neurosurg. 1992;76(6):935–43. https://doi.org/10.3171/JNS.1992.76.6.0935.

25. Park JH, Cho YH, Kim JH, Lee JK, Kim CJ. Abducens nerve schwannoma: case report and review of the literature. Neurosurg Rev. 2009;32(3):375–8. https://doi.org/10.1007/S10143-009-0203-7.

26. Mariniello G, Horvat A, Dolenc V, v. En bloc resection of an intracavernous oculomotor nerve schwannoma and grafting of the oculomotor nerve with sural nerve. Case report and review of the literature. J Neurosurg. 1999;91(6):1045–9. https://doi.org/10.3171/JNS.1999.91.6.1045.

27. Pollock BE, Foote RL, Stafford SL. Stereotactic radiosurgery: the preferred management for patients with nonvestibular schwannomas? Int J Radiat Oncol Biol Phys. 2002;52(4):1002–7. https://doi.org/10.1016/S0360-3016(01)02711-0.

28. Peciu-Florianu I, Tuleasca C, Comps JN, et al. Radiosurgery in trochlear and abducens nerve schwannomas: case series and systematic review. Acta Neurochir. 2017;159(12):2409–18. https://doi.org/10.1007/S00701-017-3348-0.

Primary Cranio-Orbital Bone Tumors

Giulio Bonavolontà [iD], Paola Bonavolontà, and Francesco Maiuri [iD]

15.1 Introduction

Primary bone tumors of the orbit are a group of bone lesions, both neoplastic and reactive, arising from the bone walls of the orbit. They are rare, accounting for 0.6–2% of all orbital tumors [1, 2].

This chapter discusses the clinical and diagnostic aspects and the management of the different tumor types.

15.2 Topographic and Pathological Classifications

Bone tumors may arise from all orbital walls. Those occurring in the superior wall arise from the frontal bone and frontal sinus wall; those occurring in the medial wall originate from the ethmoidal sinus and nasal cavities. Tumors of the

lateral orbital wall are extension of sphenoid wing tumors; those of the inferior wall arise from the maxillary bone and sinus. Besides, bone tumors may exceptionally be located within the orbital cavity, with no relationship with the orbital walls (extraskeletal tumors) [3]. Thus, most bone lesions involving the orbit are really cranio-orbital tumors that arise from cranial structures.

According to their histological origin and pathology, the primary orbital bone tumors may be classified into dance groups (Table 15.1). The group of benign fibro-osseous and cartilaginous lesions includes the benign tumors and the fibrous dysplasia [4]. The group of reactive lesions

Table 15.1 Classifications of primary orbital bone pathologies

1. Benign Fibro-osseous and Cartilaginous Lesions
Osteoma
Osteoblastoma
Ossifying fibroma
Chondroma
Fibrous dysplasia
2. Reactive Bone Lesions
Aneurysmal bone cyst
Giant cell granuloma
3. Neoplasms
Osteosarcoma
Ewing sarcoma
Chondrosarcoma
Hemopoietic and histiocytic lesions
Giant cell tumor
4. Vascular Lesions
Osseous hemangioma

G. Bonavolontà
Department of Neuroscience, University of Naples Federico II, Naples, Italy

P. Bonavolontà (✉)
Department of Clinical Medicine and Surgery, University of Naples, Federico II, Naples, Italy
e-mail: paola.bonavolonta@unina.it

F. Maiuri
Division of Neurosurgery, Department of Neurosciences, Reproductive and Odontostomatological Sciences, University of Naples "Federico II", Naples, Italy
e-mail: frmaiuri@unina.it

includes the aneurysmal bone cyst and the giant cell granuloma. In the group of neoplasms are listed malignant tumors of bone, cartilaginous and hemopoietic origin, and benign lesions such as histiocytosis and giant cell tumor. Osseous hemangioma is the unique vascular lesion.

15.3 General Clinical and Diagnostic Aspects

The clinical presentation and evolution of primary orbital tumors mainly depend on their type and growth rate. Benign bone cartilaginous and reactive lesions may often be asymptomatic. Symptomatic cases present with slow progressive mass effect over years [4], causing gradual proptosis and eye displacement. Sudden increase of the mass effect due to hemorrhage causing worsening of the proptosis may be observed for several reactive bone lesions. Malignant tumors present with signs of mass effect and infiltration within weeks or months, including pain, decrease of the vision, and impairment of the eye movements.

Diagnostic imaging studies include computerized tomography (CT) and magnetic resonance (MR). CT with bone window and particularly 3D CT define the tumor components (compact bone versus cartilaginous, fibrous and soft components), the intraorbital tumor extension, the involvement of the optic canal and superior orbital fissure, the osteolysis of the surrounding involved bone, the tumor extension into the paranasal sinus cavities. MR better defines the compression and displacement of the intraorbital structures, mainly the optic nerve.

15.4 General Surgical Management

The surgical approach to orbital bone tumors mainly depends on their location and size. Endoscopic endonasal and orbital, external orbital and combined cranio-orbital approaches may be used. The endoscopic endonasal approach is mainly used for tumors arising in the frontal, ethmoid, and sphenoid sinuses and located in the medial orbital compartment [5, 6]. The traditional external orbital approach is represented by the orbitotomy that can be performed through a mininvasive eyelid anterior incision or through antero-lateral incision if an osteoplasty is needed. The orbital endoscopic approach, as unique procedure or combined with the endonasal endoscopic one, allows to resect even large bone tumors [7]; in these instances, the endoscopic endonasal and orbital approaches may be combined with a microsurgical external orbitotomy [8, 9]. On the other hand, the cranio-orbital approaches may be limited to cases with significant cranial extension.

15.5 Specified Pathological Entities

15.5.1 Benign Fibro-Osseous and Cartilaginous Lesions

15.5.1.1 Osteoma

Osteomas are benign bone tumors which frequently occur in the cranial sinuses. The frontal sinus is most frequently involved (58–68%) followed by the ethmoidal sinus [10]. The orbital involvement results from extension from the frontal bone and frontal and ethmoid sinuses. Obstruction of the sinus ostia by the tumor may result in a mucocele.

Most sinus osteomas are asymptomatic; those arising from the frontal bone may present with a palpable mass. In symptomatic cases, gradual proptosis is the main complaint, with globe displacement. Posterior osteomas arising from the sphenoid sinus may cause compression of the apical structures.

Osteomas are classically associated with Gardner syndrome, an autosomal-dominant disease that presents with intestinal polyposis, osteomas and other cutaneous soft tissue tumors [11]. Thus, patients with multiple skull osteomas must be investigated with gastrointestinal studies due to risk of colon cancer [12].

On CT scan osteomas appear as hyperdense bone masses with regular margins within the involved sinus and orbit (Figs. 15.1 and 15.2).

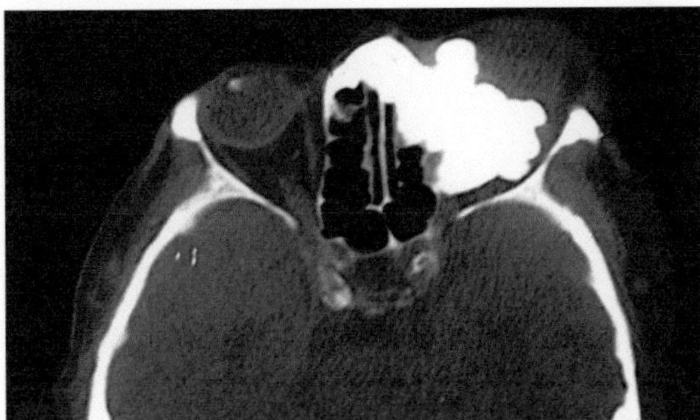

Fig. 15.1 CT of the skull: large lobulated osteoma of the ethmoid sinus largely extending in the left orbit and causing lateral globe displacement and proptosis

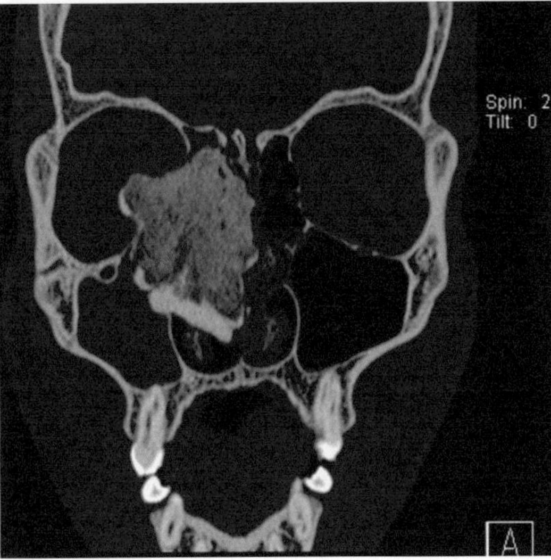

Fig. 15.2 CT of the skull, coronal section with bone window: **osteoma** of the right ethmoid and maxillary sinus extending into the inferomedial compartment of the right orbit

This imaging technique well defines the tumor size and degree of extension.

Some osteomas may be observed only because of their slow growth rate.

The surgical removal is warranted for enlarging and/or symptomatic tumors, for those with intracranial extension [5, 13, 14] or sinus outflow obstruction resulting in mucocele [4]. Many osteomas may be treated by endoscopic endonasal or/ and orbital approach [6, 9]. Larger tumors require an external orbital or combined approach [14]. The cranio-orbital approach may be reserved to

large posterior osteomas involving the orbital apex and optic canal [15]. The complete resection by drill cavitation up to the tumor attachment is the goal of surgery. The tumor attachment is more often with a large base, although a narrow pedicle may sometimes be found.

15.5.1.2 Osteoblastoma

Osteoblastoma is a rare benign bone tumor (1% of all bone neoplasms). Cranio-maxillo-facial locations account for about 15% and mainly involve the mandible and temporal bone. The endo-orbital location is exceptional, with a few reported cases [2, 16–20].

The orbital involvement arises from the orbital roof or ethmoid sinus and causes gradual globe displacement and proptosis.

CT scan shows a lesion with well-demarcated sclerotic borders, bone destruction, mottled calcifications, and variable contrast enhancement.

The complete surgical resection is suggested, because of the high recurrence rate after incomplete resection and the risk of malignant transformation (16–20%) [20].

15.5.1.3 Ossifying Fibroma

Ossifying fibroma is a rare distinct fibro-osseous neoplasm, characterized by fibrous tissue intermixed with a mineralized component. It is most frequently found in the mandible in young individuals. The orbital location is very rare [1, 2, 4, 21, 22] and occurs from tumors of the frontal, ethmoidal, and maxillary bones. It manifests with slow, painless proptosis, and globe displacement.

The radiological aspect is a well-circumscribed round mass with central osteoblastic and osteolytic areas. The tumor mass is often large.

Complete surgical excision is indicated.

15.5.1.4 Chondroma

Chondromas can arise in the intracranial and extracranial portions of the skull base (10% of all chordomas). They mostly occur in the parasellar region, middle fossa and ethmoid sinus [23–26]. Those involving the orbit are exceptional (0.07–0.15% of all mesenchymal orbital tumors) [1,

21]. These tumors occur in adolescents and young adults and present with a slowly growing mass near the orbital rim and trochlea [23, 27].

The CT aspect is a well-circumscribed hyperdense inhomogeneous sessile or pedunculated mass.

MR allows to differentiate the pure cartilaginous components from those variably mineralized; the high-water content in non-mineralized portions provides low T1 signal and high T2 signal [24].

Because of the risk of malignant degeneration, wide surgical resection is the treatment of choice.

15.5.1.5 Fibrous Dysplasia

Fibrous dysplasia is a benign congenital skeletal condition characterized by bone thin cortex and fibrous replacement with bone marrow [28]. It exists in two forms: monostotic and polyostotic.

The craniofacial involvement occurs in 10% of the monostotic forms and in 50–100% of the polyostotic forms. It presents with swelling and deformities of the affected bone areas. The orbital involvement occurs in fibrous dysplasia affecting the frontal, sphenoid, and ethmoid bones. The clinical presentation includes facial asymmetry, proptosis, and globe displacement, often lasting for years at the diagnosis and slowly worsening during the life [29–33]. Other symptoms, according to the location, are diplopia, cranial nerve palsies, intracranial hypertension. Decrease of the visual function due to optic nerve compression may also be present. Malignant sarcomatous degeneration is rare and associated to pain and rapid symptoms progression [34].

The radiological aspect of the fibrous dysplasia is often rather typical. The involved bone appears to be expanded with distorted anatomical form. CT scan shows an inhomogeneous density due to the ratio of fibrous and bone areas (Fig. 15.3); cystic and more sclerotic areas may be present [35]. This bone structure may also be evident on the skull radiograms. On MR, fibrous dysplasia shows low T1 intensity and heterogeneous T2 signal [30, 36].

Most patients with fibrous dysplasia may be treated conservatively, due to the very slow progression of the disease and long stable periods

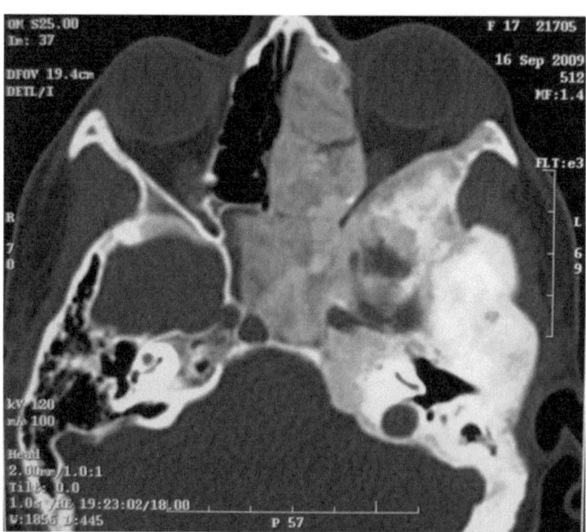

Fig. 15.3 CT scan: extensive **fibrodysplasia** of the skull base involving the sphenoid sinus, the left ethmoid sinus, and the left sphenoid wing; the left orbit is invaded and narrowing with conseguent proptosis

[37]. Bisphosphonates are the initial medical treatment and may result in pain relief, cosmetic improvement, and normalization of the bone turnover [38]. Indications to surgery include significant deformity, ophthalmological and neurological deficits, and the rare malignant degeneration.

Complete resection of the involved bone is often difficult and sometimes impossible; thus partial resection may be advisable. The surgery may require combined cranio-facial approaches with the cooperation of neurosurgeon, ophthalmic, and maxillofacial surgeons. The reconstruction is realized in one-step operation.

The optic nerve decompression is advised in patients with initial visual deficit; on the other hand, the prophylactic decompression of the optic canal is at risk of postoperative blindness and should be avoided [39].

15.5.2 Reactive Bone Lesions

15.5.2.1 Aneurysmal Bone Cyst

The aneurysmal bone cyst is a benign reactive lesion consisting in a red-brown friable mass containing blood-filled cysts separated by septa of trabecular bone and surrounded by fibrous tissue and reactive bone. The mass of variable size often causes extensive osteolysis.

Aneurysmal bone cysts of the orbit are exceptional with only 33 reported cases [40–45]. Most are located in the orbital roof or lesser in the sphenoid-ethmoid bone. They may cause symptoms of chronic mass effect, such as proptosis and diplopia; sudden symptoms may result from intralesional hemorrhage. Some aneurysmal bone cysts are associated to the other bone pathologies, such as several tumours and fibro-dysplasia [1, 4].

The radiological aspect on CT and MR is a round destructive bone lesion with irregular contrast enhancement and cyst with hemorrhagic component (Fig. 15.4) [44–46]. The biomolecular studies of detection of ubiquitin-specific peptidase 6/tre-2 gene may allow to confirm the diagnosis [45].

The surgical resection and curettage result in clinical remission. The preoperative embolization is useful for large cysts with high vascular flow. Recurrences may be observed, usually within 2 years. The medical treatment with receptor activator of nuclear factor kappa-b ligand (RANKL) inhibitors may improve the outcome [45].

15.5.2.2 Giant Cell Granuloma

Giant cell granuloma is a non-neoplastic reactive bone lesion which may result from trauma,

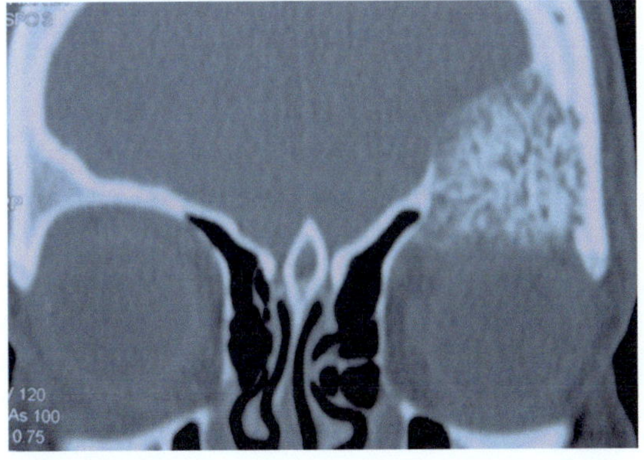

Fig. 15.4 CT in coronal scan: large hyperdense inhomogeneous mass lesion of the left frontal bone and left orbital roof causing diffuse osteolysis and invading the cranial cavity and the orbit (**aneurysmal bone cyst**)

inflammation, or infectious processes [47]. It consists in uniform cell stroma with fibroblasts, spindle-shaped and mononuclear infiltrative, and giant cells [48]. This reactive bone lesion mostly occurs in maxilla, mandible, and cranial bones; on the other hand, the orbital location is very rare [2, 4, 48–50]. The lesion occurs in the supero-lateral orbital compartment and causes variable bone erosion. It tends to be silent and relatively stable and may present with painless deformation of the involved bone and intraorbital mass lesion with proptosis [51].

The radiological aspect on CT is a high density mass with mildly enhancement and bone destruction. Surgical excision and additional curettage is indicated for large and symptomatic lesions.

The giant cell granuloma must be differentiated from other granular lesions, including giant cell tumor, cholesterol granuloma, Langherans cell histiocytosis, aneurysmal bone cyst, Brown's tumor of hyperparathyroidism [48].

15.5.3 Neoplasms

15.5.3.1 Osteosarcoma

Although osteosarcoma is the most common primary bone malignant tumor, the orbital involvement is rare and mainly occurs from a maxillary location. Orbital osteosarcomas may arise "de novo" or may be secondary to Paget disease, fibrous dysplasia, or radiotherapy [1, 2, 21, 52–55].

Orbital osteosarcomas present with a several month history of progressive mass lesion and infiltrative effects consisting in orbital pain, diplopia and decreased vision.

The radiological appearance is an irregular lytic and sclerotic bone mass with infiltrating soft tissue component [53, 54]. Exceptional cases of primary orbital osteosarcomas without connection to the bone have been reported [3, 56]; they are malignant mesenchymal neoplasms with osteoid matrix.

The treatment protocol includes preoperative chemotherapy, surgical resection, and postoperative chemotherapy. These tumors are resistant to radiotherapy, which is reserved to residual and recurrent cases. The prognosis is poorer than osteosarcomas of other skeletal regions, because of the often incomplete resection.

15.5.3.2 Ewing's Sarcoma

Ewing's sarcoma is a highly malignant, small round cell neoplasms derived from primitive neuroectodermal cells with variable grades of differentiation. The two primary forms are skeletal and extraskeletal. Ewing's sarcoma accounts for 10% of all primary bone neoplasms and 4% of head and neck tumors. Skull neoplasms are mainly located in the maxillary bone and sinus, followed by ethmoid and frontal bones [57, 58]. Primary Ewing's sarcomas of the orbit are rare and mainly arise from the ethmoid sinus wall [58–62].

The clinical presentation occurs in the first two decades of life with non-axial proptosis of short duration and orbital pain. The infiltrative tumor mass causes bone destruction and is associated with a soft tissue component (Fig. 15.5).

Patients with orbital Ewing sarcoma must carefully be investigated for the possible presence of a primary tumor because the orbital locations are more often metastatic.

The treatment protocol first includes chemotherapy followed by surgery and adjuvant chemotherapy and eventually radiotherapy and proton beam therapy [62]; it may result in more favorable outcomes. Complete resolution followed by chemotherapy and radiotherapy alone has been reported.

15.5.3.3 Chondrosarcoma

Chondrosarcomas occurring in the orbit originate in the sinuses and nasal cavities [63–68]. The orbital extension causes medial or inferior mass effect with pain, proptosis, and globe displacement associated to symptoms of nasal sinus obstruction. CT and MR show a well-defined mottled lesion with calcified areas and moderate contrast enhancement associated to variable and often extensive osteolysis. The presence of areas of bone metaplasia may cause more hyperdense aspect on CT (Fig. 15.6).

Surgery through endoscopic endonasal approach [68, 69] or external route is the treatment of choice. The entity of surgical resection is the most important factor affecting overall survival. However, complete resection is often not possible, because of the extensive bone involvement. Adjuvant radiotherapy and chemotherapy are usually indicated. The 5-year survival is very variable (44–87%) and recurrence is estimated at 40–60% [68].

15.5.3.4 Hematopoietic and Histiocytic Lesions

Multiple myeloma and more rarely solitary plasmocytoma may involve the orbital bone [2, 52, 70]. The clinical presentation includes pain and

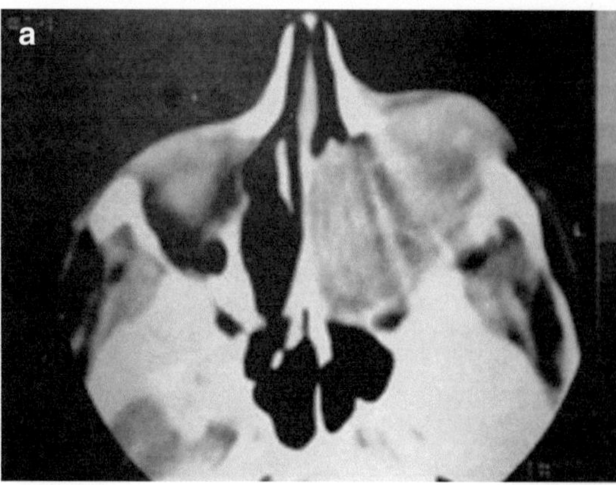
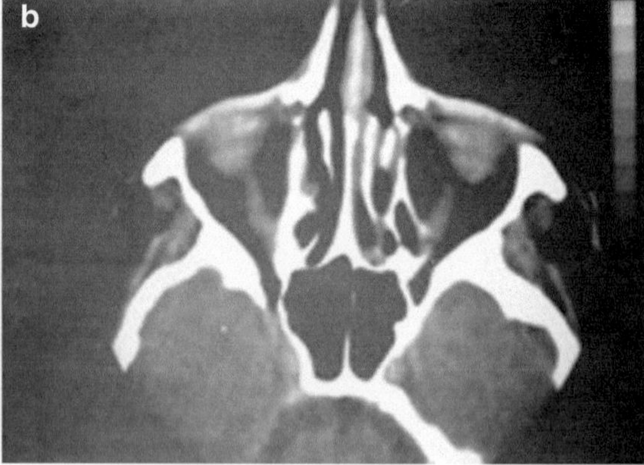

Fig. 15.5 (a) Post-contrast axial CT of the skull: mass lesion of the left ethmoid sinus invading the left orbit and causing moderate proptosis (**Ewing's sarcoma**); (b) Postoperative CT shows resection of the tumor and resolution of the proptosis

subacute proptosis. Symptoms and signs of systemic involvement may be present.

The Langerhan's cell histiocytosis, also defined eosinophilic granuloma, is a benign lesion which may rarely occur in the orbit [2, 71, 72], mainly in the supero-lateral orbital wall and in children. It causes osteolysis and intraorbital extension resulting in proptosis. The CT finding of central hypodensity with enhancing rim is rather typical (Fig. 15.7). The surgical curettage is curative.

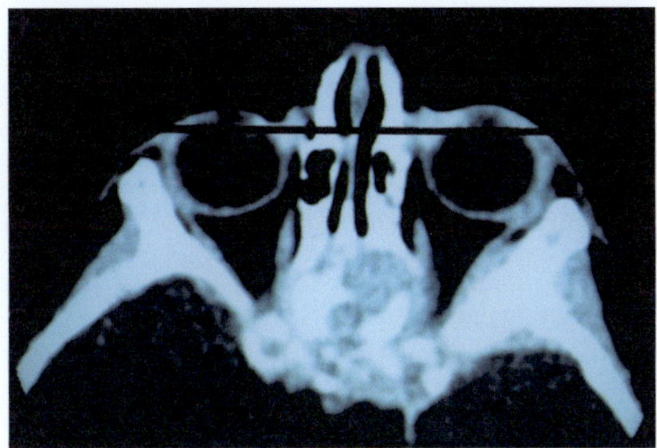

Fig. 15.6 CT of the skull base: large round hyperdense mass lesion of the sphenoid sinus, extending in both orbits, mainly on the left (**chondrosarcoma** with bone metaplasia)

15.5.3.5   Giant Cell Tumor

Giant cell tumor is a benign neoplasm of mesenchymal origin accounting for 15–20% of all benign bone tumors. It presents as a soft mass that erodes the bone and is surrounded by shell of reactive bone. The craniofacial location is exceptional (1%); the orbital involvement may occur from the temporal bone and sphenoid and ethmoid sinuses [2, 4, 73–77].

The orbital locations present as lytic or soft tissue masses causing headache, decrease of vision, or cranial nerve palsies. CT shows a lytic lesion with thin cortex; however, this radiological finding is aspecific [76].

The surgical treatment with wide resection is the recommended treatment, whereas radiotherapy should be reserved to inoperable cases. However, the recurrence rate ranges from 7% to 60% according to the extent of resection.

15.5.4 Vascular Lesions

15.5.4.1   Hemangioma

Intraosseous hemangiomas of the skull are rare (5% of all locations) [78, 79] and most frequently occur in the frontal bone; the orbital

Fig. 15.7 CT of the orbits: large lesion of the right orbit associated to osteolysis of the lateral orbital wall; the lesion shows central hypodensity and enhancing rim (**eosinophilic granuloma**)

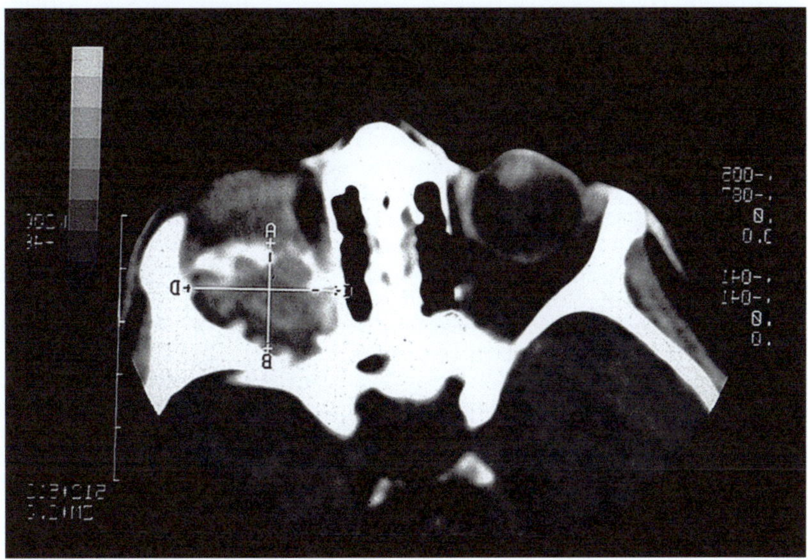

involvement is exceptional and mostly at the orbital rim [79–82].

Orbital cavernous haemangioma causes a painful or painless mass resulting in proptosis and visual impairment.

The radiographic aspect is a typical circumscribed area with pattern of trabeculation radiating from a common center [82]. CT clearly defines the typical trabecular pattern and stippled matrix [79]. On MR, the intensity signal varies according to the venous blood flow and the bone marrow.

The complete surgical resection is the treatment of choice in symptomatic cases; however, it may be difficult due to the profuse bleeding.

References

1. Shields JA, Bakewell B, Augsburger JJ, Flanagan JC. Classification and incidence of space-occupying lesions of the orbit. A survey of 645 biopsies. Arch Ophthalmol. 1984;102(11):1606–11. https://doi.org/10.1001/ARCHOPHT.1984.01040031296011.
2. Selva D, White VA, O'Connell JX, Rootman J. Primary bone tumors of the orbit. Surv Ophthalmol. 2004;49(3):328–42. https://doi.org/10.1016/j.survophthal.2004.02.011.
3. Hui J, Zhao Y, Zhang L, Lin J, Zhao H. Primary orbital extraskeletal osteosarcoma and review of literature. BMC Ophthalmol. 2020;20(1):425. https://doi.org/10.1186/S12886-020-01690-9.
4. Waldman S, Shimonov M, Yang N, et al. Benign bony tumors of the paranasal sinuses, orbit, and skull base. Am J Otolaryngol. 2022;43(3):103404. https://doi.org/10.1016/J.AMJOTO.2022.103404.
5. Turri-Zanoni M, Dallan I, Terranova P, et al. Frontoethmoidal and intraorbital osteomas: exploring the limits of the endoscopic approach. Arch Otolaryngol Head Neck Surg. 2012;138(5):498–504. https://doi.org/10.1001/ARCHOTO.2012.644.
6. Khoueir N, Ismail S, Cherfane P. Exclusive endoscopic excision of a large ethmoido-orbital osteoma with video. Eur Ann Otorhinolaryngol Head Neck Dis. 2021;138(Suppl 4):129–30. https://doi.org/10.1016/J.ANORL.2021.02.015.
7. Jafari A, von Sneidern M, Lehmann AE, et al. Exclusively endoscopic endonasal resection of benign orbital tumors: a systematic review and meta-analysis. Int Forum Allergy Rhinol. 2021;11(5):924–34. https://doi.org/10.1002/ALR.22745.
8. Rimmer RA, Graf AE, Fastenberg JH, et al. Management of orbital masses: outcomes of endoscopic and combined approaches with no orbital reconstruction. Allergy Rhinol (Providence). 2020;11:215265671989992. https://doi.org/10.1177/2152656719899922.
9. Chung SY, Kazim M, Gudis DA. Minimally invasive surgery for massive orbital osteomas. Eur Ann Otorhinolaryngol Head Neck Dis. 2021;138(Suppl 4):125–7. https://doi.org/10.1016/J.ANORL.2021.04.011.
10. Georgalas C, Goudakos J, Fokkens WJ. Osteoma of the skull base and sinuses. Otolaryngol Clin N Am. 2011;44(4):875–90. https://doi.org/10.1016/J.OTC.2011.06.008.
11. Alexander AAZ, Patel AA, Odland R. Paranasal sinus osteomas and Gardner's syndrome. Ann Otol Rhinol Laryngol. 2007;116(9):658–62. https://doi.org/10.1177/000348940711600906.
12. Avila SA, Nguyen G, Wojno T, Kim HJ. Orbital osteomas associated with Gardner's syndrome: a case presentation and review of literature. Orbit. 2022:1. https://doi.org/10.1080/01676830.2022.2080231.
13. Wolf A, Safran B, Pock J, Tomazic PV, Stammberger H. Surgical treatment of paranasal sinus osteomas: a single center experience of 58 cases. Laryngoscope. 2020;130(9):2105–13. https://doi.org/10.1002/LARY.28299.
14. Giotakis E, Sofokleous V, Delides A, et al. Gigantic paranasal sinuses osteomas: clinical features, management considerations, and long-term outcomes. Eur Arch Otorhinolaryngol. 2021;278(5):1429–41. https://doi.org/10.1007/S00405-020-06420-X.
15. Ciappetta P, Delfini R, Iannetti G, Salvati M, Raco A. Surgical strategies in the treatment of symptomatic osteomas of the orbital walls. Neurosurgery. 1992;31(4):628–35. https://doi.org/10.1227/00006123-199210000-00003.
16. Batay F, Savas A, Uğur HC, Kanpolat Y, Kuzu I. Benign osteoblastoma of the orbital part of the frontal bone: case report. Acta Neurochir. 1998;140(7):729–30. https://doi.org/10.1007/S007010050172.
17. Akhaddar A, Gazzaz M, Rimani M, Mostarchid B, Labraimi A, Boucetta M. Benign fronto-orbital osteoblastoma arising from the orbital roof: case report and literature review. Surg Neurol. 2004;61(4):391–7. https://doi.org/10.1016/S0090-3019(03)00455-5.
18. Nielsen GP, Rosenberg AE. Update on bone forming tumors of the head and neck. Head Neck Pathol. 2007;1(1):87. https://doi.org/10.1007/S12105-007-0023-4.
19. Novelli G, Gramegna M, Tonellini G, et al. Orbital osteoblastoma: technical innovations in resection and reconstruction using virtual surgery simulation. Craniomaxillofac Trauma Reconstr. 2016;9(3):271–6. https://doi.org/10.1055/S-0036-1584397.
20. Wang K, Yu F, Chen K, et al. Osteoblastoma of the frontal bone invading the orbital roof: a case report. Medicine. 2018;97(42):e12803. https://doi.org/10.1097/MD.0000000000012803.

21. Jack R. Diseases of the orbit: a multidisciplinary approach, vol. 628. Philadelphia, PA: Lippincott; 1988. Accessed 4 Jan 2023. https://books.google.com/books/about/Diseases_of_the_Orbit.html?hl=it&id=lKBsAAAAMAAJ.

22. Nakagawa K, Takasato Y, Ito Y, Yamada K. Ossifying fibroma involving the paranasal sinuses, orbit, and anterior cranial fossa: case report. Neurosurgery. 1995;36(6):1192–5. https://doi.org/10.1227/00006123-199506000-00021.

23. Pasternak S, O'Connell JX, Verchere C, Rootman J. Enchondroma of the orbit. Am J Ophthalmol. 1996;122(3):444–5. https://doi.org/10.1016/S0002-9394(14)72081-1.

24. Murphey MD, Choi JJ, Kransdorf MJ, Flemming DJ, Gannon FH. Imaging of osteochondroma: variants and complications with radiologic-pathologic correlation. Radiographics. 2000;20(5):1407–34. https://doi.org/10.1148/RADIOGRAPHICS.20.5.G00SE171407.

25. Harrison A, Loftus S, Pambuccian S. Orbital chondroma. Ophthalmic Plast Reconstr Surg. 2006;22(6):484–5. https://doi.org/10.1097/01.IOP.0000240808.50566.87.

26. Hongo H, Oya S, Abe A, Matsui T. Solitary osteochondroma of the skull base: a case report and literature review. J Neurol Surg Rep. 2015;76(1):e13–7. https://doi.org/10.1055/S-0034-1387189.

27. Kabra R, Patel S, Shanbhag S. Orbital Chondroma: a rare mesenchymal tumor of orbit. Indian J Ophthalmol. 2015;63(6):551–4. https://doi.org/10.4103/0301-4738.162638.

28. DiCaprio MR, Enneking WF. Fibrous dysplasia. Pathophysiology, evaluation, and treatment. J Bone Joint Surg Am. 2005;87(8):1848–64. https://doi.org/10.2106/JBJS.D.02942.

29. Bibby K, McFadzean R. Fibrous dysplasia of the orbit. Br J Ophthalmol. 1994;78(4):266. https://doi.org/10.1136/BJO.78.4.266.

30. Katz BJ, Nerad JA. Ophthalmic manifestations of fibrous dysplasia: a disease of children and adults. Ophthalmology. 1998;105(12):2207–15. https://doi.org/10.1016/S0161-6420(98)91217-9.

31. Ricalde P, Horswell BB. Craniofacial fibrous dysplasia of the fronto-orbital region: a case series and literature review. J Oral Maxillofac Surg. 2001;59(2):157–67. https://doi.org/10.1053/JOMS.2001.20487.

32. Cruz AAV, Constanzi M, De Castro FAA, dos Santos AC. Apical involvement with fibrous dysplasia: implications for vision. Ophthalmic Plast Reconstr Surg. 2007;23(6):450–4. https://doi.org/10.1097/IOP.0B013E318158E9A8.

33. Rahman AMA, Madge SN, Billing K, et al. Craniofacial fibrous dysplasia: clinical characteristics and long-term outcomes. Eye (Lond). 2009;23(12):2175–81. https://doi.org/10.1038/EYE.2009.6.

34. Mardekian SK, Tuluc M. Malignant sarcomatous transformation of fibrous dysplasia. Head Neck Pathol. 2015;9(1):100–3. https://doi.org/10.1007/S12105-014-0567-Z.

35. Lee JS, Fitzgibbon EJ, Chen YR, et al. Clinical guidelines for the management of craniofacial fibrous dysplasia. Orphanet J Rare Dis. 2012;7(Suppl 1(Suppl 1)):S2. https://doi.org/10.1186/1750-1172-7-S1-S2.

36. Kushchayeva YS, Kushchayev SV, Glushko TY, et al. Fibrous dysplasia for radiologists: beyond ground glass bone matrix. Insights Imaging. 2018;9(6):1035–56. https://doi.org/10.1007/S13244-018-0666-6.

37. Valentini V, Cassoni A, Marianetti TM, Terenzi V, Fadda MT, Iannetti G. Craniomaxillofacial fibrous dysplasia: conservative treatment or radical surgery? A retrospective study on 68 patients. Plast Reconstr Surg. 2009;123(2):653–60. https://doi.org/10.1097/PRS.0B013E318196BBBE.

38. Mäkitie AA, Törnwall J, Mäkitie O. Bisphosphonate treatment in craniofacial fibrous dysplasia—a case report and review of the literature. Clin Rheumatol. 2008;27(6):809–12. https://doi.org/10.1007/S10067-008-0842-Z.

39. Edelstein C, Goldberg RA, Rubino G. Unilateral blindness after ipsilateral prophylactic transcranial optic canal decompression for fibrous dysplasma. Am J Ophthalmol. 1998;126(3):469–71. https://doi.org/10.1016/S0002-9394(98)00118-4.

40. Ronner HJ, Jones IS. Aneurysmal bone cyst of the orbit: a review. Ann Ophthalmol. 1983;15(7):626–9. Accessed Jan 4 2023. https://europepmc.org/article/med/6571346.

41. Henderson JW. Fibro-osseous, osseous, and cartilaginous tumors of orbital bone: orbital tumors. Trans Indiana Acad Ophthalmol Otolaryngol. 1963;46:1–8.

42. Bilyk JR, Lucarelli MJ, Shore JW, Rubili PAD, Yaremchuk MJ. Aneurysmal bone cyst of the orbit associated with fibrous dysplasia. Plast Reconstr Surg. 1995;96(2):440–5. https://doi.org/10.1097/00006534-199508000-00029.

43. Citardi MJ, Janjua T, Abrahams JJ, Sasaki CT. Orbitoethmoid aneurysmal bone cyst. Otolaryngol Head Neck Surg. 1996;114(3):466–70. https://doi.org/10.1016/S0194-59989670220-6.

44. Senol U, Karaali K, Akyüz M, Gelen T, Tuncer R, Lüleci E. Aneurysmal bone cyst of the orbit. AJNR Am J Neuroradiol. 2002;23(2):319. https://doi.org/10.2214/ajr.100.3.526.

45. Phan T, Tong J, Krivanek M, Graf N, Dexter M, Tumuluri K. Aneurysmal bone cyst of the orbit with USP6 gene rearrangement. Ophthalmic Plast Reconstr Surg. 2022;20:206. https://doi.org/10.1097/IOP.0000000000002287.

46. Hermann AL, Polivka M, Loit MP, Guichard JP, Bousson V. Aneurysmal bone cyst of the frontal bone—a radiologic-pathologic correlation. J Radiol Case Rep. 2018;12(7):16–24. https://doi.org/10.3941/JRCR.V12I7.3344.

47. Mombaerts I, Ramberg I, Coupland SE, Heegaard S. Diagnosis of orbital mass lesions: clinical, radiological, and pathological recommendations. Surv Ophthalmol. 2019;64(6):741–56. https://doi.org/10.1016/J.SURVOPHTHAL.2019.06.006.

48. Zhu Y, Wang Y, He W. Locally aggressive orbital giant cell reparative granuloma in an infant: case report and literature review. Int J Clin Exp Pathol. 2021;14(6):776. Accessed 4 Jan 2023. /pmc/articles/PMC8255204/.

49. D'Ambrosio AL, Williams SC, Lignelli A, et al. Clinicopathological review: Giant cell reparative granuloma of the orbit. Neurosurgery. 2005;57(4):773–8. https://doi.org/10.1227/01.NEU.0000181346.81156.69.

50. Chawla B, Khurana S, Kashyap S. Giant cell reparative granuloma of the orbit. Ophthalmic. Plast Reconstr Surg. 2013;29(4):e94. https://doi.org/10.1097/IOP.0B013E31827BDAC3.

51. Gupta M, Gupta M, Singh S, Kaur R. Central giant cell granuloma of the maxilla. BMJ Case Rep. 2013;2013:bcr2013009102. https://doi.org/10.1136/BCR-2013-009102.

52. Dahlin DC, Unni KK. Bone tumors: general aspects and data on 8,547 cases. 4th ed. Springfield: Charles C. Thomas; 1986.

53. Mark RJ, Sercarz JA, Tran L, Dodd LG, Selch M, Calcaterra TC. Osteogenic sarcoma of the head and neck. The UCLA experience. Arch Otolaryngol Head Neck Surg. 1991;117(7):761–6. https://doi.org/10.1001/ARCHOTOL.1991.01870190073015.

54. el Quessar A, Boumedin H, Chakir N, El Hassani MR, Jiddane M, Boukhrissi N. Primary osteosarcoma of the skull. Medicine (Baltimore). 1997;96(51):e9392. Accessed 4 Jan 2023. https://pubmed.ncbi.nlm.nih.gov/9303947/.

55. Garrity JA, Henderson JW, Cameron JD. Henderson's orbital tumors. 4th ed. Philadelphia, PA: Lippincott Williams & Wilkins; 2007. p. 104–8. Accessed 5 Jan 2023. https://books.google.com/books/about/Henderson_s_Orbital_Tumors.html?hl=it&id=8luD6T3LEqcC

56. de Maeyer VMDS, Kestelyn PAFA, Shah A, van den Broecke C, Denys HGN, Decock C. Extraskeletal osteosarcoma of the orbit: a clinicopathologic case report and review of literature. Indian J Ophthalmol. 2016;64(9):687–9. https://doi.org/10.4103/0301-4738.97555.

57. Whaley JT, Indelicato DJ, Morris CG, et al. Ewing tumors of the head and neck. Am J Clin Oncol. 2010;33(4):321–6. https://doi.org/10.1097/COC.0B013E3181AACA71.

58. Kasturi N, Sarkar S, Gokhale T, Ganesh RN. Primary Ewing's sarcoma of the ethmoid sinus with orbital extension in a young child: a rare case and review of literature. Indian J Ophthalmol. 2022;70(7):2741–4. https://doi.org/10.4103/IJO.IJO_236_22.

59. Woodruff P, Thorner G, Skarf AB. Primary Ewing's sarcoma of the orbit presenting with visual loss. Br J Ophthalmol. 1988;72:786–92.

60. Gray ST, Chen YL, Lin DT. Efficacy of proton beam therapy in the treatment of Ewing's sarcoma of the paranasal sinuses and anterior Skull Base. Skull Base. 2009;19(6):409–16. https://doi.org/10.1055/S-0029-1220207.

61. Li M, Hoschar AP, Budd GT, Chao ST, Scharpf J. Primary Ewing's sarcoma of the ethmoid sinus with intracranial and orbital extension: case report and literature review. Am J Otolaryngol. 2013;34(5):563–8. https://doi.org/10.1016/J.AMJOTO.2013.04.007.

62. Meccariello G, Merks JHM, Pieters BR, et al. Endoscopic management of Ewing's sarcoma of ethmoid sinus within the AMORE framework: a new paradigm. Int J Pediatr Otorhinolaryngol. 2013;77(1):139–43. https://doi.org/10.1016/J.IJPORL.2012.09.023.

63. Potts MJ, Rose GE, Milroy C, Wright JE. Dedifferentiated chondrosarcoma arising in the orbit. Br J Ophthalmol. 1992;76(1):49–51. https://doi.org/10.1136/BJO.76.1.49.

64. Ruark DS, Schlehaider UK, Shah JP. Chondrosarcomas of the head and neck. World J Surg. 1992;16(5):1010–5. https://doi.org/10.1007/BF02067021.

65. Stapleton SR, Wilkins PR, D J Archer DU. Chondrosarcoma of the skull base: a series of eight cases. Neurosurgery. 1993;32(3):529–41. https://doi.org/10.1227/00006123-199303000-00003.

66. Jacobs JL, Merriam JC, Chadburn A, Gamin J, Housepian E, Hilal SK. Mesenchymal chondrosarcoma of the orbit report of three new cases and review of the literature. Cancer. 1994;73(2):399–405. https://doi.org/10.1002/1097-0142.

67. Khan MN, Husain Q, Kanumuri VV, et al. Management of sinonasal chondrosarcoma: a systematic review of 161 patients. Int Forum Allergy Rhinol. 2013;3(8):670–7. https://doi.org/10.1002/ALR.21162.

68. Bouhafs K, Lachkar A, Bouamama T, Miry A, Benfadil D, Ghailan MR. Nasosinusal chondrosarcoma with orbito-cerebral extension. J Surg Case Rep. 2022;2022(6):rjac286. https://doi.org/10.1093/JSCR/RJAC286.

69. Shin M, Kondo K, Hanakita S, et al. Endoscopic transnasal approach for resection of locally aggressive tumors in the orbit. J Neurosurg. 2015;123(3):748–59. https://doi.org/10.3171/2014.11.JNS141921.

70. L Mewis-Levin, C A Garcia. Plasma cell myeloma of the orbit.(1981). 13(4):477–481. Accessed 4 Jan 2023. https://pubmed.ncbi.nlm.nih.gov/7247194/.

71. Jordan DR, McDonald H, Noel LN. Eosinophilic granuloma. Arch Ophthalmol. 1994;111:134.

72. Herwig MC, Wojno T, Zhang Q, Grossniklaus HE. Langerhans cell histiocytosis of the orbit: five clinicopathologic cases and review of the literature. Surv Ophthalmol. 2013;58(4):330–40. https://doi.org/10.1016/J.SURVOPHTHAL.2012.09.004.

73. Abdalla MI, Hosni F. Osteoclastoma of the orbit. Case report. Br J Ophthalmol. 1966;50(2):95–8. https://doi.org/10.1136/BJO.50.2.95.

74. Suster S, Porges R, Nanes M. Giant-cell neoplasm of the sphenoid sinus. Mt Sinai J Med. 1989;56(2):118–22.

75. Tandon DA, Deka RC, Chaudhary C, Misra NK. Giant cell tumour of the temporosphenoidal

region. J Laryngol Otol. 1988;102(5):449–51. https://doi.org/10.1017/S0022215100105316.

76. Borges BBP, Fornazieri MA, De Bezerra APCA, Martins LAL, de Pinna FR, Voegels RL. Giant cell bone lesions in the craniofacial region: a diagnostic and therapeutic challenge. Int Forum Allergy Rhinol. 2012;2(6):501–6. https://doi.org/10.1002/ALR.21050.

77. Mavrogenis AF, Igoumenou VG, Megaloikonomos PD, Panagopoulos GN, Papagelopoulos PJ, Soucacos PN. Giant cell tumor of bone revisited. SICOT J. 2017;3:3. https://doi.org/10.1051/SICOTJ/2017041.

78. Heckl S, Aschoff A, Kunze S. Cavernomas of the skull: review of the literature 1975-2000. Neurosurg Rev. 2002;25(1–2):56–62. https://doi.org/10.1007/S101430100180.

79. Yang Y, Guan J, Ma W, et al. Primary intraosseous cavernous hemangioma in the skull. Medicine. 2016;95(11):e3069. https://doi.org/10.1097/MD.0000000000003069.

80. Zucker JI, Levine MR, Chu A. Primary intraosseous hemangioma of the orbit. Report of a case and review of literature. Ophthalmic Plast Reconstr Surg. 1989;5(4):247–55. https://doi.org/10.1097/00002341-198912000-00004.

81. Relf SJ, Bartley GB, Unni KK. Primary orbital intraosseous hemangioma. Ophthalmology. 1989;98(4):541–6.

82. Banerji D, Inao S, Sugita K, Kaur A, Chhabra DK. Primary intraosseous orbital hemangioma: a case report and review of the literature. Neurosurgery. 1994;35(6):1131–4. https://doi.org/10.1227/00006123-199412000-00017.

Soft Tissue Orbital Tumors

16

Giulio Bonavolontà ⓘ and Paola Bonavolontà

16.1 Introduction

The orbital cavity may harbor many types of mass lesions of neoplastic, vascular, congenital, and inflammatory origin. They may arise from different complex of vascular, neurogenic, mesenchymal, and secretory structures and are in close anatomical relationship with the eyelids, nasal sinuses, and brain [1–4].

Some lesions are benign and well differentiated and show slow clinical course; others are malignant and undifferentiated, with infiltrative aspect and rapid growth and can lead to death.

16.2 Classification

According to their initial location and growth, the lesions involving the orbit may be divided into three main groups: (1) Primary lesions arising in the orbital cavity; (2) Secondary lesions arising from adjacent structures; (3) Metastatic tumors to the orbit. The proposed classification is listed in Table 16.1.

Table 16.1 Classification of orbital mass lesions

1. Primary orbital lesions	Vascular
	Cystic
	Neurogenic
	Mesenchymal
	Lacrimal gland
	Lymphoproliferative and histiocytic
2. Secondary tumors arising from adjacent structures	Spheno-orbital meningioma
	Basal cell carcinoma
	Squamous cell carcinoma
	Melanoma
	Carcinoma of paranasal sinuses and nasopharynx
	Retinoblastoma
	Eccrine histiocytoid carcinoma
	Esthesioneuroblastoma
	Sebaceous carcinoma
	Lacrimal sac origin
	Unspecified origin
3. Metastatic tumors to the orbit	

This chapter discusses the tumors primary arising in the orbital cavity. Bone tumors are treated in Chap. 15 in this book. Tumors of the surrounding structures secondarily invading the orbit are excluded. On the other hand, we also discuss the metastatic tumors to the orbit because they are frequent and often indistinguishable at the initial diagnosis from primary tumors and cystic lesions.

G. Bonavolontà
Department of Neuroscience, University of Naples Federico II, Naples, Italy

P. Bonavolontà (✉)
Department of Clinical Medicine and Surgery, University of Naples Federico II, Naples, Italy
e-mail: paola.bonavolonta@unina.it

© The Author(s), under exclusive license to Springer Nature Switzerland AG 2023
G. Bonavolontà et al. (eds.), *Cranio-Orbital Mass Lesions*,
https://doi.org/10.1007/978-3-031-35771-8_16

## 16.3	Clinical Overview

Patients with an intraorbital mass must undergo a detailed diagnostic process, including clinical history, ophthalmological examination, correct selection of diagnostic tests, and finally a biopsy. Intraorbital lesions can present with different clinical symptoms and signs due to different mechanisms: mass effect, inflammation, infiltration, vascular, and functional mechanisms. The mass effect is characterized by compression and displacement of structures leading to functional deficits and proptosis. The inflammatory effect is characterized by orbital pain, redness, warmth, functional deficit and can be acute, subacute, or chronic. In case of tissue infiltration, a tumor can cause functional deficit such as limitation of the eye movements causing diplopia and sensory changes such as dysesthesias and hypo- and hyperesthesia. Finally, a neoplasia can cause loss of visual acuity and deficits of the visual field and color vision.

The type of eye displacement may aid to define the tumor location and the functional changes. Medial and inferior lesions mainly cause ocular displacement superiorly or laterally. Tumors that involve the lacrimal gland can cause an infero-medial displacement. Apical or intra-conal lesions present with axial exophthalmos. The type of intra-orbital mass lesion may vary according to its anterior to posterior location. Anterior lesions are most commonly lymphopro-liferative. The mid-orbit mainly harbors vascular malformations and different tumor types. Posterior lesions are most commonly neurogenic tumors.

The clinical onset may also be variable. The most common symptoms and signs of orbital lesions are due to the mass and infiltrative effect. Particularly, the neurogenic neoplasms are mostly associated with visual loss and mass effect. Lymphoproliferative lesions present with propto-sis, orbital oedema, palpable mass, and ptosis. In cystic lesions, a palpable swelling is evident and the mass causes proptosis, followed by pain.

When the orbit is involved secondarily from adjacent structures, the neoplasia can cause pain, dysesthesia, proptosis, and globe displacement.

Metastatic tumors to the orbit can present with diplopia, local swelling, ptosis, and pain.

## 16.4	Ophthalmological and Imaging Studies

Patients with orbital mass lesions must undergo a complete ophthalmological evaluation including eyelid malposition, orbital edema, swelling and palpable mass, visual acuity, fundus, globe displacement, exophthalmos, enophthalmos, color test; visual field examination and OCT are useful in selected cases. The extraocular muscle evaluation with Hess scheme is necessary in cases of muscular restriction.

The imaging studies must include orbital echography, computer tomography (CT), and magnetic resonance (MR).

The orbital echography is a rapid and easy noninvasive diagnostic technique [5]; it evidences the intra-orbital lesion and particularly defines the diameter of the optic nerve, which may increase as a result of increase of peri-optic CSF space, as occurs in several intra-orbital masses.

CT and MR with contrast administration are essential to diagnosis of orbital mass lesions [6, 7]. They allow to define the intra-orbital location, the size and margins of the lesion, its type of con-trast enhancement, its relationship with the optic nerve, and other intra-orbital structures. Patients harboring orbital metastases or malignant lym-phoproliferative and bone tumors must also be investigated by Positron Emission Tomography (PET, PET-CT) to staging the neoplastic disease.

## 16.5	Management Options

The management options for patients with intra-orbital mass lesions include biopsy, surgical exci-sion, radiotherapy, chemotherapy and, in rare cases, orbital exenteration.

The biopsy is often necessary to obtain the histopathological diagnosis, with the aim to decide the further management [8]. Different type of biopsy may be used, including fine needle agobiopsy, incisional, or excisional biopsy. The excisional biopsy should be preferred, when possible.

The **surgical excision** of intra-orbital mass lesions may be realized by different approaches, orbital or cranio-orbital [9–11]. The less invasive orbital approaches include the anterior orbitotomy, the lateral orbitotomy (with or without lateral osteoplasty), the medial orbitotomy, and the trans-conjunctival approach [11, 12].

The cranio-orbital microsurgical approaches include the supraorbital-pterional [13], minipterional, orbito-zygomatic, lateral-supra-orbital, and supraorbital key-hole approaches [11].

More recently, the minimally invasive endoscopic approaches (trans-orbital, trans-eyelid, trans-sphenoidal endonasal, and combined endonasal-transorbital) have gained consensus [14–16]. The choice of the surgical approach depends on several factors, including intra-orbital location, size, and eventual intracranial or endonasal extension. The **orbital exenteratio** is the last surgical option in blind patients with very invasive orbital malignant tumors, mainly after multiple recurrences followed by radiotherapy; the severe proptosis with significant disfiguring change is an important indication. However, this radical and very invasive surgical procedure is associated with significant functional and psychological disability and is refused by several patients. Thus, the eye sparing surgery followed by radiotherapy is more widely considered [17].

The **radiotherapy and chemotherapy** are mainly indicated for malignant primary or metastatic orbital tumors as adjuvant or alternative treatments to surgery. Among benign intra-orbital tumors, the radiotherapy is indicated for optic nerve sheath meningiomas and the chemotherapy for benign optic nerve gliomas.

16.6 Specific Pathological Entities

16.6.1 Vascular Lesions

The group of vascular lesions includes proliferative lesions and arterial flow, venous flow, and no flow malformations (Table 16.2).

Table 16.2 Classification of intraorbital vascular lesions

1. Proliferative lesions
Cavernous malformation capillary hemangioma
Hemangioendothelioma
Intravascular papillary endothelial hyperplasia
2. Arterial flow lesions
Shunt/fistula carotid cavernous fistula
Arterial malformation
3. Venous flow lesions
Varix
Combined lymphangioma-varix
4. No flow malformations
Venous lymphatic malformation (lymphangioma)

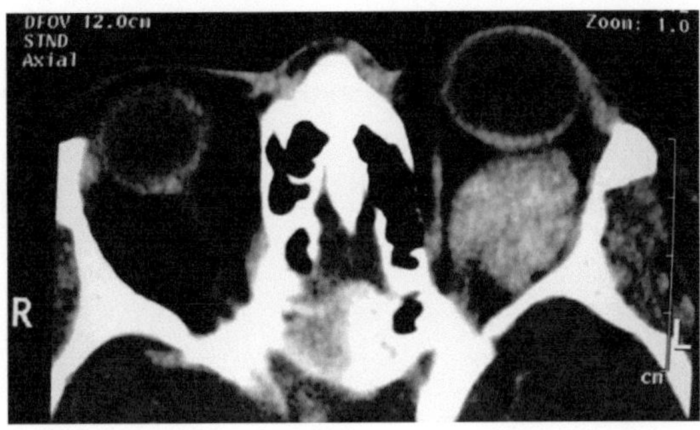

Fig. 16.1 CT scan of the orbits showing a large left **orbital venous malformation** causing axial displacement of the globe

The orbital venous malformation, also known as "cavernous malformation," is the most common vascular orbital lesion and the third more frequent after lymphoid tumors and orbit inflammatory syndrome [18, 19]. It accounts for approximately 5–15% of all vascular abnormalities of the central nervous system and 9% of orbital lesions, and usually occurs in middle age, with females more affected than males. Histologically, it is composed of endothelial-lined spaces surrounded by a well-delineated fibrous capsule.

The clinical presentation is variable. Many cases are asymptomatic and are incidentally discovered during radiological exams performed for other causes. In symptomatic patients, the onset is more often gradual, over years. The axial proptosis is the most common sign (about 70%) (Fig. 16.1). Other symptoms and signs include diplopia, visual field alterations, and rarely visual loss due to optic nerve compression. The diagnosis is performed by CT and MR.

The surgical resection is the gold standard treatment [19, 20]. Different surgical approaches can be used, from minimally invasive approaches to lateral orbitotomy (Fig. 16.2).

16.6.2 Cystic lesions

The cystic intraorbital lesions may be congenital or acquired (Table 16.3).

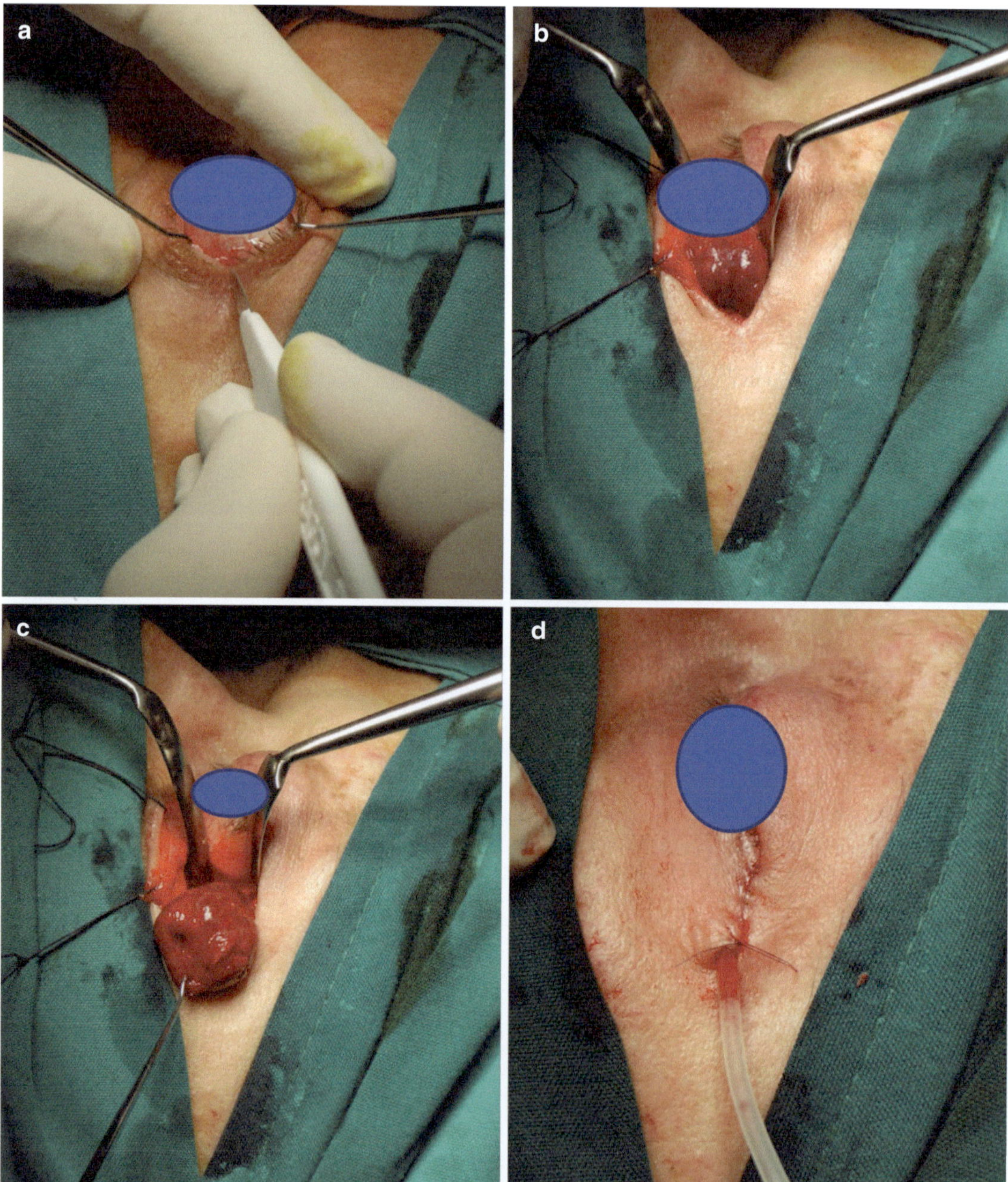

Fig. 16.2 Surgical resection of an **orbital venous malformation** through left orbitotomy: (**a**) Lateral canthotomy. (**b**) Orbital exploration and exposure of the lesion. (**c**) Resection of the malformation. (**d**) Suture and drainage

Table 16.3 Classification of orbital cystic lesions

1. Congenital lesions
Dermoid and epidermoid cyst
Dermolipoma
Sweat gland cyst
Hematic pseudocyst
Arachnoid cyst
Microphthalmos with muscle cyst
2. Acquired lesions
Mucocele
Encephalocele
Lacrimal sac mucocele
Implantation

Orbital epidermoid and dermoid cysts have been classified into juxtasutural, sutural, and soft tissue types and further subdivided according to their relationship to bone [21, 22]. Dermoid cysts arising from congenital rests of epithelial and subepithelial tissue are commonly located in the supero-temporal quadrant of the orbit, near the zygomatic-frontal suture, although they can also occur at other bony sutures. They are present at birth and can rarely remain asymptomatic. They tend to become symptomatic during the first decade [22] or more rarely at a later age. The first clinical manifestation is a slow-growing painless mass, which develops progressively over time and occupies the supero-external quadrant of the orbit. It is most commonly located deep to the epidermis and is fixed to the underlying bone. Only large cysts can cause downward and medial displacement of the globe. In case of perforation of the cyst wall, a strong inflammation can be triggered due to the extravasation of the cystic material in the neighboring tissues. In these cases, the diagnosis can be more complex, mimicking a primary inflammation of the orbit.

Histologically, the cyst wall is composed by epithelial-lined structure with dermal tissue; the cyst contains keratin and hairs in its lumen.

The diagnosis should include ultrasound and CT to better define the cyst relationship. At CT, the cyst usually appears as a well-defined round lesion with enhancing wall and non-enhancing lumen.

Small cysts may be treated conservatively with serial follow up, since they can remain sta-ble for a long time and may even become smaller. Most commonly, however, the cyst enlarges and tends to break, thus requiring a prompt surgical treatment.

The goal of the treatment should be the complete surgical excision of the cyst, while preserving the integrity of its wall. The anterior orbital epidermal-dermoid cysts are best removed by an anterior approach (Fig. 16.3).

16.6.3 Neurogenic Tumors

Neurogenic orbital tumors include more common types, such as the benign optic nerve glioma (described in Chap. 12 of this book), neurofibroma, and schwannoma (approximately 1% of all orbital tumors) and more rare types such as ganglioma, neuroblastoma, and malignant peripheral nerve sheath tumors [23] (Table 16.4).

Schwannomas are benign peripheral nerve sheath tumors that may occur as sporadic forms or associated with neurofibromatosis. They usually arise from superior ciliary nerves or more rarely from smaller peripheral nerves [24]. The tumor typically appears as a globular and encapsulated enlargement of the involved nerve causing nerve displacement (Figs. 16.4 and 16.5).

The schwannoma clinically manifests with slow-growing exophthalmos in young or middle-aged patients; when the lesion occurs in the orbital apex (Fig. 16.6), the symptoms appear early.

The treatment consists in the radical surgical resection (Fig. 16.5) [25].

16.6.4 Mesenchymal Tumors

Primary mesenchymal tumors of the orbit are relatively rare despite the high prevalence of mesenchyme in this region. These include the meningioma of the optic nerve sheath (described in Chap. 12 of this book), several fibrocytic and fibro-osseous lesions, malignant bone tumors and myogenic tumors, mainly the rhabdomyosarcoma (Table 16.5).

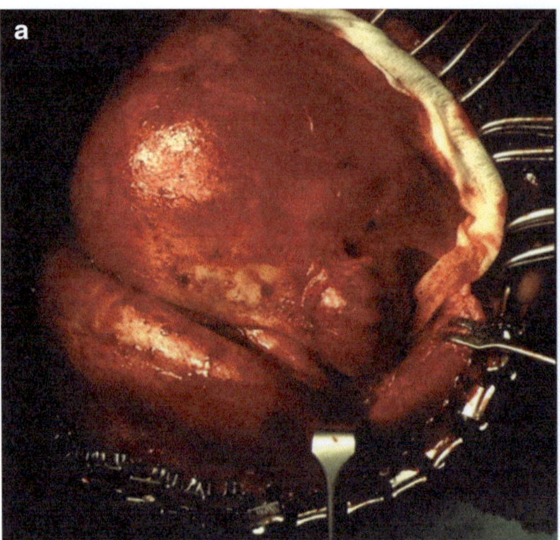
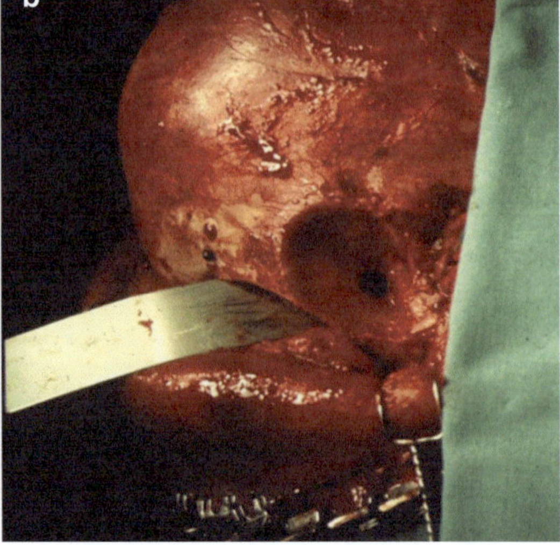

Fig. 16.3 Patient with a large **dermoid cyst** of the left orbit located supero-laterally near the zygomatic-frontal suture (**a**) Coronal approach used to completely remove the large cyst with bony involvement of the temporal fossa. (**b**) At the end of resection, the bony erosion due to the lesion is evident

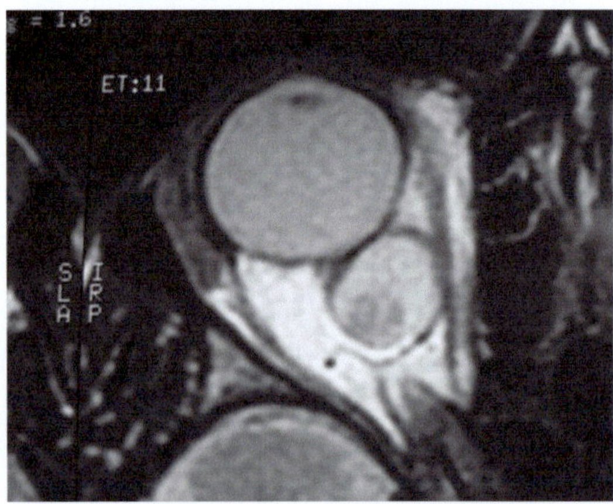

Fig. 16.4 MR of the right orbit: retrobulbar **schwannoma** located between the medial rectus and the optic nerve, causing nerve displacement

Table 16.4 Classification of orbital neurogenic lesions

Optic nerve glioma
Schwannoma
Neurofibroma
Glioneural tumor
Neuroblastoma

The rhabdomyosarcoma is a highly malignant tumor, most commonly found in children; the orbit is involved in 10% of cases.

Three variants of rhabdomyosarcoma are recognized: embryonal, alveolar, and pleomorphic. The embryonal variant is the most common in childhood, ranging between 50 and 70% of the orbital rhabdomyosarcomas [26]. The alveolar subtype accounts for approximately 20–30% of cases. The pleomorphic subtype almost exclusively occurs in adults [27].

Histologically, the embryonal subtype shows bipolar cells with tapered cytoplasmic processes and less commonly cells "tadpole-like" with long cytoplasmic extensions.

The alveolar subtype is a highly cellular tumor composed of a monotonous population of small round primitive cells; they form solid sheets or nests separated by thin fibrous septa. The nests classically show loss of cohesion centrally.

The rhabdomyosarcoma of the orbit clinically presents with rapidly progressive exophthalmos within a few weeks, impairment of extraocular movements, visual deficit, pain, and globe displacement. Parameningeal tumors can cause headache as well as focal neurologic symptoms related to mass effect. If cranial nerve palsies occur, they can indicate skull base erosion and intracranial extension.

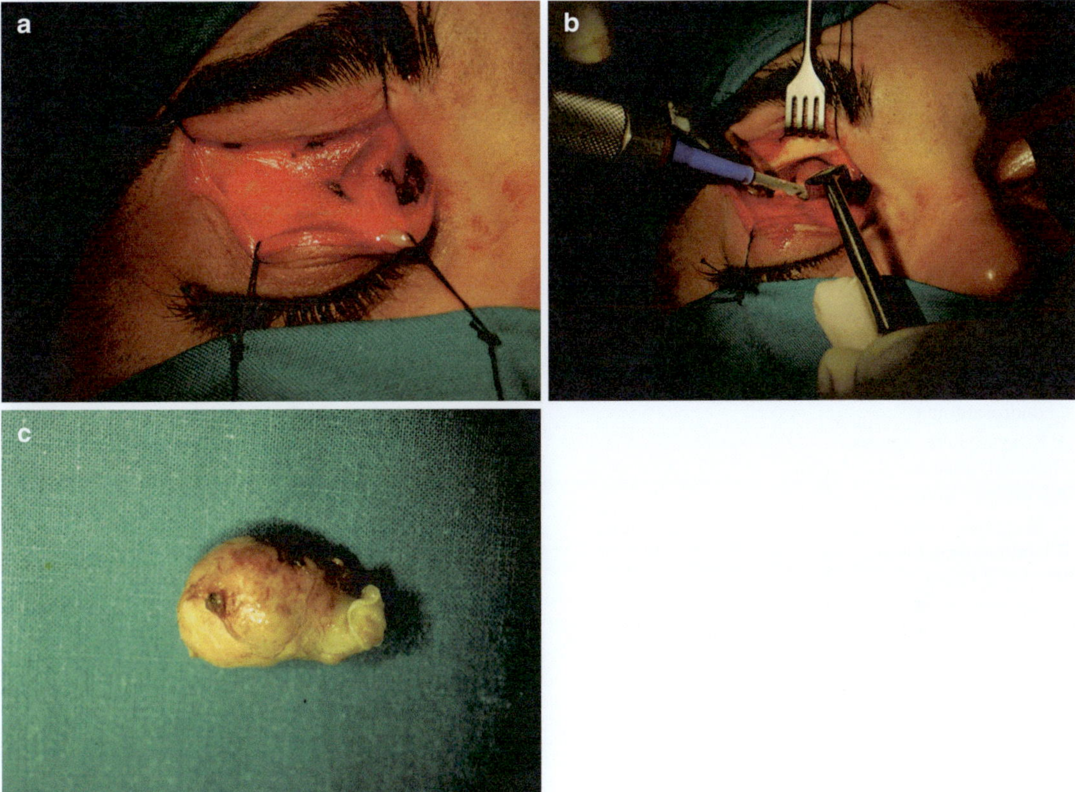

Fig. 16.5 Operative images of the patient of fig. 16.4. (**a**) Anterior orbitotomy by skin crease incision. (**b**) The tumor is easily removed with the aid of Cryo probe without damage of optic nerve and extraocular muscles. (**c**) Surgical specimen

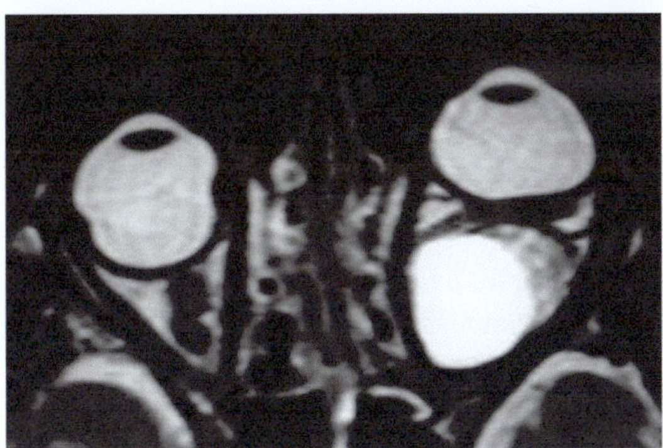

Fig. 16.6 MRI of a patient with severe left exophthalmos showing large apical lesion of the left orbit between optic nerve and lateral rectus muscle (**orbital schwannoma**)

CT and MR are important for the diagnosis and tumor staging. MR with multiplanar reconstructions, using routine spin-echo pre- and post-contrast T1 and T2 sequences, can provide excellent tumor definition (Fig. 16.7).

The treatment of rhabdomyosarcoma includes surgery, chemotherapy, and irradiation depending on its stage.

Complete excision of the primary tumor should be performed when it can be done safely. On the other hand, in patients with aggressive tumor, the radical surgery is not recommended.

Vincristine, actinomycin D, cyclophosphamide, doxorubicin, isofosfamide, and etoposide are the most used chemotherapy drugs; topotecan and irinotecan are also active against this type of cancer.

Radiation is used with doses of 3600–5400 cGy over 4–5 weeks. In cases with parameningeal extension, the irradiation must be extended to the perilesional tissues for at least 2 cm.

Table 16.5 Classification of orbital mesenchymal lesions

1. Fibrocytic lesions
Benign fibrous histiocytoma/solitary fibrous tumor
Fibroma
Fibrosarcoma
Angiofibroma
2. Benign fibro-osseous lesions
Osteoma
Fibrous dysplasia
Ossifying fibroma
3. Malignant bone lesions
Ewing sarcoma
Osteosarcoma
Chondrosarcoma
4. Reactive bone tumors
Giant cell granuloma
Aneurysmal bone cyst
5. Myogenic lesions
Rhabdomyosarcoma
Rhabdoid tumor
6. Lipocytic or myxoid lesions
Lipoma
Liposarcoma
Dermolipoma
Epithelioid sarcoma

Table 16.6 Classification of lacrimal gland lesions

1. Benign neoplastic lesions
Adenoma (monomorphic and pleomorphic)
Warthin tumor
Oncocytoma
2. Non-neoplastic lesions
Nonspecific inflammation
Atypical lymphoid hyperplasia
Lacrimal cyst
3. Malignant tumors
Adenoid cystic carcinoma
Non-Hodgkin lymphoma
Carcinoma ex-pleomorphic adenoma
Adenocarcinoma
Mucoepidermoid carcinoma
Squamous cells carcinoma
Ductal cell carcinoma
Acinic cell carcinoma
Unclassified carcinomas

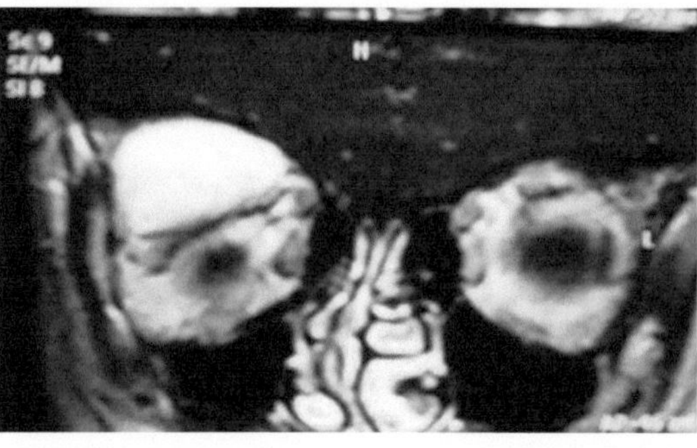

Fig. 16.7 Post-contrast coronal MR of a patient with orbital **rhabdomyosarcoma**: large enhancing lesion occupying the superior part of the right orbit and causing inferior displacement of the globe

16.6.5 Lacrimal Gland Lesions

Lacrimal gland lesions can originate from different cell types [28] (Table 16.6).

The neoplasms are classified into two types: epithelial and non-epithelial. Non-epithelial tumors are the most common, accounting for 70–80% of solid lacrimal gland masses; lymphomas are the most common tumors of this group. Epithelial lacrimal gland tumors mainly include the adenoid cystic carcinoma (60% of cases), followed by pleomorphic adenocarcinoma (20%), and adenocarcinoma -ex-pleomorphic adenoma (10%). Other types of lacrimal gland carcinomas (mucoepidermoid, primary squamous cell, sebaceous gland carcinoma, basal cell adenocarcinoma) are extremely rare.

Histologically, the adenoid cystic carcinoma is characterized by solid areas or cords of bland-appearing malignant epithelial cells. The infiltrative borders of the epithelial areas can be distinguished from the surrounding connective tissue and typically show perineural invasion.

The pleomorphic adenocarcinoma is characterized by myoepithelial cells in the surrounding connective tissue.

The adenocarcinoma (ex-pleomorphic adenoma) is characterized by areas of malignant degeneration in a pleomorphic adenoma, with variable amount of myxoid and chondroid structures; the epithelial cells also show carcinomatous changes.

Clinically, the tumor causes enlargement of the lacrimal gland; it results in "S-shaped" deformity of the eyelid margin, globe displacement, and limited ocular motility causing diplopia (Fig. 16.8).

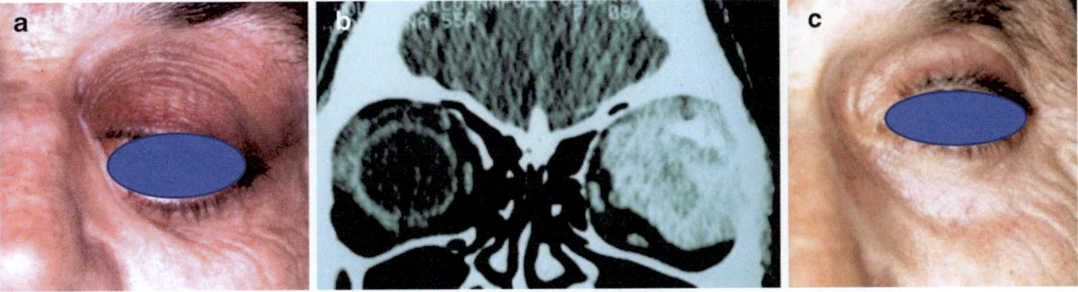

Fig. 16.8 (**a**) Patient with **adenocarcinoma ex pleomorphic adenoma** of the left lacrimal gland showing left orbital proptosis with inferior globe displacement. (**b**) Post-contrast coronal CT: large enhancing lacrimal gland tumor. (**c**) Aspect of the patient after the treatment (surgical excision and radiation therapy): remission of orbital proptosis and displacement

MR is important for the tumor definition and for evaluation of soft tissue involvement. CT is necessary for the evaluation of the bony changes.

Malignant epithelial tumors of the lacrimal gland are characterized by aggressive biological behavior. Thus, also aggressive local surgical treatments, such as the orbital exenteration, do not result in better long-term survival [17]. Perineural and bone invasion are frequently observed; the recurrence and metastases rates are high. The best treatments for malignant tumors of the lacrimal gland seems to be eye-sparing procedures and radiotherapy.

16.6.6 Lymphoproliferative and Histiocytic Lesions

Lymphoproliferative orbital lesions frequently present as orbital masses (24%–49%) in the adult and include a wide spectrum of benign and malignant lesions [29, 30] (Table 16.7).

Lymphoma is the most common orbital neoplasm (55% of the cases in adults). Most orbital lymphomas are primary, low-grade, B-cell, non-Hodgkin lymphomas; the extranodal marginal zone lymphoma of mucosa-associated lymphoid tissue (MALT) is the most common subtype.

In recent years, the classification of lymphoproliferative lesions is considerably changed; several benign, noninfectious, chronic inflammatory diseases have been added, such as IgG4-related ophthalmic disease, reactive lymphoid hyperpla-

Table 16.7 Classification of orbital lymphoproliferative and histiocytic lesions

Lymphoma	Plasmacytoma
Diffuse lymphoma	Histiocytic lymphoma
MALT-type lymphoma	Burkitt lymphoma
Marginal zone lymphoma	Unknown histology lymphoma
Small lymphocytic lymphoma	Atypical lymphoid hyperplasia
Follicular lymphoma	Xanthogranuloma
Mantle cell lymphoma	Eosinophilic granuloma

sia, and idiopathic orbital inflammation [31, 32]. In particular, the IgG4-related ophthalmic disease is increasingly recognized and accounts for 50% of benign lymphoproliferative orbital lesions. Therefore, obtaining a correct diagnosis and differentiating orbital lymphomas from the different lymphoproliferative lesions are fundamental steps to decide the correct therapy, since the clinical behavior of the various pathologies is very different.

The therapy of orbital lymphomas consists of low-dose radiation therapy, whereas others lymphoproliferative lesions are expected to show good response to corticosteroid therapy.

The primary orbital lymphoma originates from the eyelids, extraocular muscles, soft tissue orbital adnexa, conjunctiva, or lacrimal glands. It is typically located in the anterior orbital compartment or beneath the conjunctiva in the extraconal space. It presents with proptosis, slowly growing palpable mass, or painless swelling of the eyelids, with a "salmon-patch appearance" beneath the conjunctiva (Fig. 16.9).

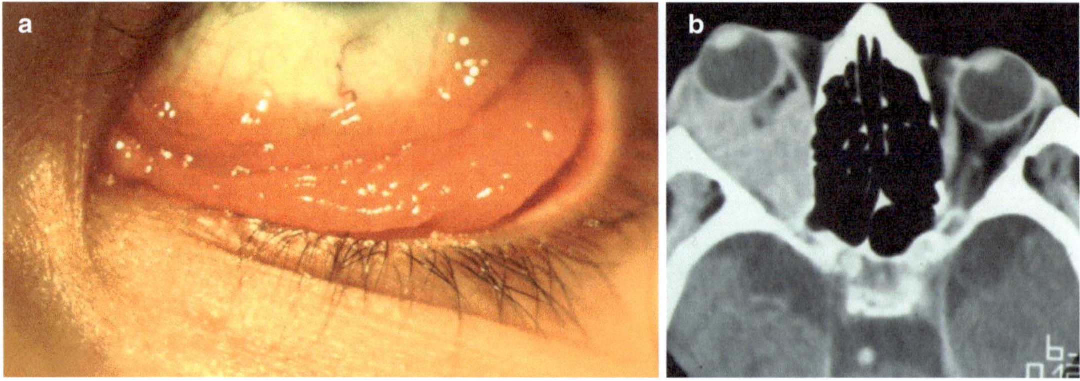

Fig. 16.9 Patient with right **orbital lymphoma**. (**a**) Typical "salmon-patch appearance". (**b**) CT: large right orbital involvement

The occurrence of orbital lymphoproliferative lesions in immuno-compromised patients, such as those affected by AIDS or those who have undergone immunosuppressive therapies, is an important problem. Some studies of the recent literature have confirmed the involvement of some pathogens, such as Chlamydia psittaci, H. pylori, and some viruses in association with orbital lymphoma.

The correct diagnosis by open biopsy is necessary. The staging of the disease must also include the FDG-PET/CT of chest, abdomen and pelvis, the cranial MRI, and the bone marrow biopsy [33].

16.6.7 Metastatic Tumors to the Orbit

Orbital metastases are rare, accounting for 1–13% in the reported series of orbital tumors and for 2–5% among patients with systemic cancers [34] (Table 16.8).

The breast and the lung are the most frequent sites of primary tumors causing orbital metastases, followed by the prostate. Although the prevalence of colorectal cancer is rather similar to breast and lung cancers, its tendency to develop orbital metastases is significantly lower, maybe due to a different metastatic pathway. On the other hand, metastases arising from tumors of the gastrointestinal tract, kidney, and from skin melanoma occur rarely [34].

Table 16.8 Metastatic tumors to the orbit

Breast carcinoma	Prostate carcinoma
Renal cell carcinoma	Bladder carcinoma
Lung carcinoma	Gastric carcinoma
Nasopharyngeal carcinoma	Hepatocarcinoma
Melanoma	Adrenal neuroblastoma
Parotid gland carcinoma	Carcinoma of the penis
Squamous cell carcinoma	Undetermined primary site
Neuroendocrine carcinoma	

Patients who develop orbital metastases may have extremely, rapidly growing exophthalmos followed by double vision due to extraocular muscle involvement, decreased vision, and pain. The diplopia can be caused by direct muscle infiltration or by mass effect. When the metastasis involves the orbital apex, ophthalmoplegia and blindness can occur.

The diagnostics imaging protocol must include ultrasound, CT, and MRI of the orbit. Orbital metastases from breast cancer present diffuse and irregular infiltration along the rectus muscles and fascial planes. Standardized B- and A-scan echography can be used to obtain a fast and accurate differential diagnosis in cases of muscle involvement or more superficial lesions. CT commonly shows a solid enhancing mass often located within the orbital fat and/or the muscles associated with bone erosion. MRI may provide a more accurate definition of the mass (Fig. 16.10).

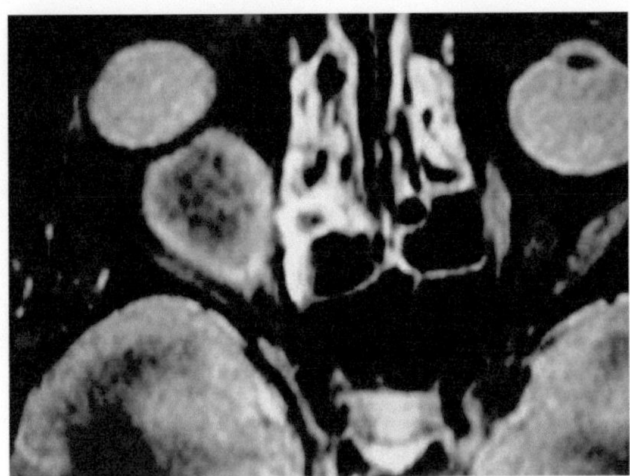

Fig. 16.10 MR of the orbits, T2 -weighted axial sequence: hyperintense right orbital mass involving the inferior rectus muscle (**metastasis** from undifferentiated breast cancer)

The definitive diagnosis of orbital metastases is made by biopsy and histopathological examination. The fine needle aspiration biopsy is a valid procedure in patients with systemic malignancy or in poor condition and when the mass is located deeply within the orbit. When the lesion is in the anterior orbital compartment, an incisional biopsy through transconjunctival or transcutaneous approach should be preferred. In cases with well circumscribed tumor, an excisional biopsy can be performed.

The therapy of orbital metastases is closely linked to the patient's general condition, the clinical staging of the neoplastic disease, the type of primary tumor, as well as the use of radiotherapy and chemotherapy protocols [35].

The mass effect can lead to worsening of vision; thus, the surgical removal or debulking of lesion could be a valid strategy. The exenteration orbitae, which was once considered the first-choice treatment, is currently no longer used, as it does not significantly affect the survival.

Unfortunately, despite all the efforts in the management of orbital metastases, the therapies are effective for local palliation and disease control, but the systemic prognosis remain poor.

References

1. Henderson JW. Orbital tumors. 3rd ed. New York, NY: Raven Press; 1994.
2. Bonavolontà G, Strianese D, Grassi P, et al. An analysis of 2,480 space-occupying lesions of the orbit from 1976 to 2011. Ophthalmic Plast Reconstr Surg. 2013;29(2):79–86. https://doi.org/10.1097/IOP.0B013E31827A7622.
3. Rootman J. Disease of the orbit. A multidisciplinary approach. 2nd ed. Philadelphia, PA: Lippincott Williams and Wilkins; 2002.
4. Louis DN, Perry A, Wesseling P, et al. The 2021 WHO classification of tumors of the central nervous system: a summary. Neuro Oncol. 2021;23(8):1231–51. https://doi.org/10.1093/NEUONC/NOAB106.
5. Nasr AMCG. Ultrasonography in orbital differential diagnosis. In: Karcioglu Z, editor. Orbital tumors. Cham: Springer; 2015.
6. Medel R, Balaguer Ó. Approach to diagnosis of orbital tumours, vol. 5. Basel: Karger; 2014. p. 46–72. https://doi.org/10.1159/000363716.
7. Lee WWEB. Imaging in orbital differential diagnosis. In: Karcioglu A, editor. Orbital tumors: diagnosis and management, vol. 10. Cham: Springer; 2015.
8. Bourne TDKZ. Orbital biopsy. In: Karcioglu A, editor. Orbital tumors: diagnosis and management, vol. 12. Cham: Springer; 2015.
9. Paluzzi A, Gardner PA, Fernandez-Miranda JC, et al. "Round-the-clock" surgical access to the orbit. J Neurol Surg B Skull Base. 2015;76(1):12–24. https://doi.org/10.1055/S-0033-1360580.
10. Abussuud Z, Ahmed S, Paluzzi A. Surgical approaches to the orbit: a neurosurgical perspective. J Neurol Surg B Skull Base. 2020;81(4):385–408. https://doi.org/10.1055/S-0040-1713941.
11. Abou-Al-Shaar H, Krisht KM, Cohen MA, et al. Cranio-orbital and Orbitocranial approaches to orbital and intracranial disease: eye-opening approaches for neurosurgeons. Front Surg. 2020;7:1. https://doi.org/10.3389/FSURG.2020.00001.
12. Mariniello G, Maiuri F, de Divitiis E, et al. Lateral orbitotomy for removal of sphenoid wing meningiomas invading the orbit. Neurosurgery. 2010;66(6 Suppl Operative):287. https://doi.org/10.1227/01.NEU.0000369924.87437.0B.
13. Andrade-Barazarte H, Jägersberg M, Belkhair S, et al. The extended lateral supraorbital approach and extradural anterior clinoidectomy through a frontopterio-orbital window: technical note and pilot surgical series. World Neurosurg. 2017;100:159–66. https://doi.org/10.1016/J.WNEU.2016.12.087.

14. Dallan I, Sellari-Franceschini S, Turri-Zanoni M, et al. Endoscopic transorbital superior eyelid approach for the management of selected spheno-orbital meningiomas: preliminary experience. Oper Neurosurg (Hagerstown). 2018;14(3):243–51. https://doi.org/10.1093/ONS/OPX100.
15. Zoia C, Bongetta D, Gaetani P. Endoscopic transorbital surgery for spheno-orbital lesions: how I do it. Acta Neurochir. 2018;160(6):1231–3. https://doi.org/10.1007/S00701-018-3529-5.
16. Vitulli F, D'Avella E, Solari D, et al. Primary ectopic orbital craniopharyngioma. Acta Neurochir. 2022;164(7):1979–84. https://doi.org/10.1007/S00701-021-04969-Y.
17. Bonavolontà P, Esmaeli B, Donna P, et al. Outcomes after eye-sparing surgery vs orbital exenteration in patients with lacrimal gland carcinoma. Head Neck. 2020;42(5):988–93. https://doi.org/10.1002/HED.26073.
18. Harris GJ, Jakobiec FA. Cavernous hemangioma of the orbit. J Neurosurg. 1979;51(2):219–28. https://doi.org/10.3171/JNS.1979.51.2.0219.
19. Bonavolontà P, Fossataro F, Attanasi F, Clemente L, Iuliano A, Bonavolontà G. Epidemiological analysis of venous malformation of the orbit. J Craniofac Surg. 2020;31(3):759–61. https://doi.org/10.1097/SCS.0000000000006095.
20. Strianese D, Bonavolontà G, Iuliano A, Mariniello G, Elefante A, Liuzzi R. Risks and benefits of surgical excision of orbital cavernous venous malformations (so-called cavernous hemangioma): factors influencing the outcome. Ophthalmic Plast Reconstr Surg. 2021;37(3):248–54. https://doi.org/10.1097/IOP.0000000000001767.
21. Shields JA, Kaden IH, Eagle RC, Shields CL. Orbital dermoid cysts: Clinicopathologic correlations, classification, and management the 1997 Josephine E Schueler Lecture. Ophthalmic Plast Reconstr Surg. 1997;13(4):265–76. https://doi.org/10.1097/00002341-199712000-00007.
22. Shields JA, Shields CL. Orbital cysts of childhood—classification, clinical features, and management. Surv Ophthalmol. 2004;49(3):281–99. https://doi.org/10.1016/j.survophthal.2004.02.001.
23. Roberts F, MacDuff EM. An update on mesenchymal tumours of the orbit with an emphasis on the value of molecular/cytogenetic testing. Saudi J Ophthalmol. 2018;32(1):3–12. https://doi.org/10.1016/J.SJOPT.2018.02.010.
24. Grover AK, Rastogi A, Chaturvedi KU, Gupta AK. Schwannoma of the orbit. Arch Craniofac Surg. 2015;16(2):128–9. https://doi.org/10.7181/ACFS.2015.16.2.67.
25. Mariniello G, de Divitiis O, Caranci F, Dones F, Maiuri F. Parasellar schwannomas: extradural vs extra-Intradural surgical approach. Oper Neurosurg (Hagerstown). 2018;14(6):627–38. https://doi.org/10.1093/ONS/OPX174.
26. National Cancer Institue. Childhood Rabdomyosarcoma Treatment- NCI, cancer.gov.
27. Jurdy L, Merks JHM, Pieters BR, et al. Orbital rhabdomyosarcomas: a review. Saudi J Ophthalmol. 2013;27(3):167–75. https://doi.org/10.1016/J.SJOPT.2013.06.004.
28. Goto H. Review of ocular tumor. In: Practical ophthalmology, vol. 24. Tokyo: Bunkodo; 2008.
29. Jenkins C, Rose GE, Bunce C, et al. Histological features of ocular adnexal lymphoma (REAL classification) and their association with patient morbidity and survival. Br J Ophthalmol. 2000;84(8):907–13. https://doi.org/10.1136/BJO.84.8.907.
30. Diagnosis and Management of Orbital Lymphoma—American Academy of Ophthalmology. Accessed 6 Dec 2022. https://www.aao.org/eyenet/article/diagnosis-management-of-orbital-lymphoma.
31. Espinoza GM. Orbital inflammatory pseudotumors: etiology, differential diagnosis, and management. Curr Rheumatol Rep. 2010;12(6):443–7. https://doi.org/10.1007/S11926-010-0128-8.
32. Takahira M, Ozawa Y, Kawano M, et al. Clinical aspects of IgG4-related orbital inflammation in a case series of ocular adnexal lymphoproliferative disorders. Int J Rheumatol. 2012;2012:635473. https://doi.org/10.1155/2012/635473.
33. Valvassori GE, Sabnis SS, Mafee RF, Brown MS, Putterman A. Imaging of orbital lymphoproliferative disorders. Radiol Clin N Am. 1999;37(1):135–50. https://doi.org/10.1016/S0033-8389(05)70083-X.
34. Magliozzi P, Strianese D, Bonavolontà P, et al. Orbital metastases in Italy. Int J Ophthalmol. 2015;8(5):1018. https://doi.org/10.3980/J.ISSN.2222-3959.2015.05.30.
35. Allen R. Orbital metastases: when to suspect? When to biopsy? Middle East Afr J Ophthalmol. 2018;25(2):60. https://doi.org/10.4103/MEAJO.MEAJO_93_18.

Mucoceles of the Sinuses and Orbit 17

Antonio Romano, Giovanni Audino,
and Luigi Califano

17.1 Definition

The first description of the mucocele was reported by Langenbeck, back in 1820, who first defined it as "hydatid" [1]. The term "mucocele" was used for the first time in 1896 by Rollet [2]. It defines a benign cystic lesion characterized by a slow growth and expansive nature to the detriment of the surrounding structures. The cystic lesion usually contains sterile mucus that can get infected resulting in a mucopyocele. When the etiopathogenetic factor is not recognized, it is defined "primary mucocele." Contrarily, when there is a possible cause, the mucocele is defined as "secondary". Mucoceles are often secondary to paranasal sinus surgery and develop usually in the fourth year after surgery [3]. In a recent meta-analysis, the recurrence rates of frontal mucoceles are between 3 and 10%, whereas complication rates are between 2 and 5%. In 2001, Har-El [4] proposed to classify frontal sinus mucoceles as follows:

1. Type 1. Limited to the frontal sinus (with or without orbital extension).
2. Type 2. Frontoethmoid mucocele (with or without orbital extension).
3. Type 3. Erosion of the posterior wall.
   (a) Minimal or no intracranial extension.
   (b) Major intracranial extension.
4. Type 4. Erosion of the anterior wall.
5. Type 5. Erosion of both posterior and anterior walls.
   (a) Minimal or no intracranial extension.
   (b) Major intracranial extension.

17.2 Epidemiology

Mucoceles are more frequent in patients between 40 and 60 years, with no gender prevalence. In children, mucoceles are rare and are commonly found in association with cystic fibrosis [5]. Frontal sinus is the most frequently affected (65%), followed by the ethmoid (25%), maxillary (10%), and sphenoid (2–5%) sinuses. The anterior ethmoid is more frequently involved than the posterior for several reasons (including a smaller ostium and a higher number of cells); the mucocele can be confined to the ethmoid labyrinth unilaterally or may extend into adjacent ethmoid sinuses, a supraorbital ethmoid cell or bilaterally. Frontal and ethmoid sinuses are often involved together (fronto-ethmoidal mucocele). According to the literature, the mucocele develops 4–5 years after fronto-ethmoidal sinus surgery, about 17 years after a maxillofacial trauma and about 18 years after open paranasal sinus surgery [6]. The bone erosion mechanism of the

A. Romano (✉) · G. Audino · L. Califano
Maxillofacial Surgery Unit, Department of
Neurosciences, Reproductive and
Odontostomatological Sciences, School of Medicine,
University "Federico II", Naples, Italy

mucocele leads to ophthalmic involvement in 30–50% of the cases. The common oculomotor nerve is affected in 70% of the cases.

17.3 Etiopathogenesis

Mucoceles are the result of a persistent or intermittent obstruction of the drainage ostium of the involved sinus together with inflammatory processes. This event causes the accumulation of mucus leading to increase of the internal pressure and size of the cystic lesion that erodes the surrounding bones; it results in bone remodeling with osteolysis, due to a reduced blood supply, and new bone formation. The equilibrium in this bone remodeling promotes the bone resorption with a consequent expansion of the mucocele beyond the involved sinus toward other sinuses, the orbits, the anterior cranial fossa, or the skin, presenting a forehead mass.

Several etiopathogenetic factors may cause ostia obstruction. Even if in almost a third of the cases, the mucocele lacks of a clear trigger factor (idiopathic mucocele), the most common risk factors are a history of sinus surgery (post-surgical scarring) or of maxillofacial trauma (NOE fractures, Le Fort II fractures, frontal bone fractures that can lead to the interruption of the frontal recess and stagnation of the sinus secretions) [3]. Less frequent risk factors include sinus anatomical variations, acute infections, chronic rhinosinusitis, nasosinusal polyposis, and neoplasms such as osteoma, ossifying fibromas, and fibrous dysplasia. Malignant tumors may cause the obstruction of one or more ostia in rare cases.

Nowadays, it is clear that the inflammatory reaction plays an important role in the etiopathogenesis of mucoceles. Histological examination of mucocele lining mainly reveals fibroblasts with cell infiltrate of lymphocytes and monocytes. These cells produce cytokines such as IL-1 and TNFα that can stimulate osteoclastic activity. It has also been demonstrated increased synthesis of PGE2 (over twice as much as the normal mucosa) that directly reflects the levels of inflammatory cytokines produced as a result of the inflammation.

Many cases of iatrogenic mucoceles are reported in literature, most of them related to sinus surgery (both endoscopic and external); the obstruction of an ostium can also follow an ophthalmologic surgical procedure such as a dacryocystorhinostomy; lateralization of the middle turbinate can get in the way of the fronto-ethmoidal outflow. Even cranioplasty surgery in early months of life can arrange for future mucoceles. The advancement or displacement of the fronto-orbital bandeau is achieved after saw cuts that can interfere with the path of the ethmoid air cell pneumatization in to the frontal bone. Moreover, the normal pneumatization of the frontal sinus is inhibited by the gap of the displacement as well as the scar formation.

Many variations in the sinuses anatomy may be observed. One of the most important variation to consider when an endoscopic sinus surgery is planned involves the uncinate process, a thin part of the ethmoid bone extending from the frontal recess to the ethmoid process of the inferior turbinate. Anatomical variation of the superior attachment of the uncinate process changes the size of the frontal sinus ostium, the frontal beak, the skull base. Following the Landsberg-Friedman classification [7] (Fig. *17.1*), some authors studied how the different anatomical variants of the uncinate process may increase the risk of developing a fronto-ethmoidal mucocele. However, they did not find statistically significant relationship between the type of anatomical variation and the development of frontal mucoceles [8].

A case of mucocele following intranasal abuse of cocaine has recently been reported [9]. The cocaine abuse leads to symptoms such as epistaxis, nasal septal perforation, saddle nose deformity, hard palate necrosis in advanced diseases. This substance not only impairs the local vascularization but it negatively influences the mucociliary transport. In the reported case, an extensive scar tissue formation blocked the sinus drainage pathways determining the development of a giant frontoethmoidal mucocele [9].

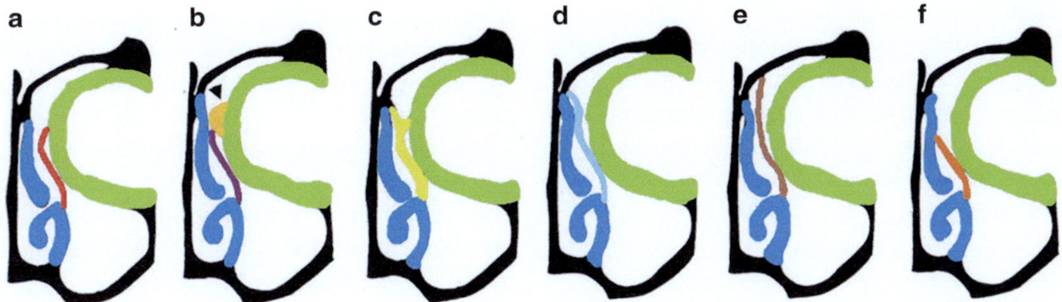

Fig. 17.1 Landsberg-Friedman classification [7]: anatomical variations of the uncinate process. Green: orbit; blue: inferior and middle turbinate; red-purple-yellow-light blue-brown-orange: anatomic variations of the uncinate process. The uncinate process can insert into: (**a**) the lamina papyrace; (**b**) the posterior wall of agger nasi cell; (**c**) the lamina papyracea and junction of the middle turbinate with the cribriform plate; (**d**) the junction of the middle turbinate with the cribriform plate; (**e**) the skull base or (**f**) the middle turbinate

17.4 Signs and Symptoms

Due to its slow growth, the mucocele may remain asymptomatic for a long time up to the sudden appearance of severe ocular or intracranial complications. Erosion of the orbit and skull can occur in up to 83.3% and 55.5% of cases, respectively [6]. The most common symptoms include facial pain, facial edema, headache, maxillofacial pressure, nasal obstruction, diplopia, periorbital pain, displacement of the eyeball, proptosis, decreased visual acuity, epiphora, meningitis, and signs of central nervous system inflammation. Acute infection of mucoceles (mucopyocele) increases the risk of intracranial or orbital complications such as brain abscess, epidural abscess, and subdural empyema.

The mucoceles extending to the orbit can cause proptosis. Those arising from the fronto-ethmoid complex push the eyeball forward, laterally, and downward, while those located near the orbital apex push the globe forward [10]. Fronto-ethmoidal mucoceles typically present with inferior globe displacement, palpable mass in the upper inner quadrant, diplopia. Visual loss is uncommon but may occur if management is delayed or if a secondary infection occurs. Posterior ethmoid and sphenoid mucoceles more often cause decrease of visual acuity and impaired ocular motility due to the close proximity to the cranial nerves II to VI and pituitary gland. These anatomical relations explain other possible symptoms, such as retro-orbital headache, anosmia, visual loss (sudden or gradual, binocular or monocular), oculomotor, trochlear or abducent nerve palsy, and rarely hypopituitarism. An Onodi cell is the most posterior ethmoid air cell that pneumatizes lateral and superior to the sphenoid sinus, occurring in 8–14% of the population. Due to its close proximity to the optic nerve, which often runs within its cavity, an Onodi cell mucopyelocele may lead to a dramatic loss of vision.

17.5 Pathologic Features

Many studies demonstrated that the mucocele keeps the characteristics of the respiratory epithelium with a preserved mucociliary clearance, once marsupialized. The macroscopic aspect is characterized by a cyst filled with a mucoid/gelatinous secretion. Recent mucoceles contain mucus material rich in water. During surgery, these lesions are of a fluid consistency and can easily be drained or suctioned out. In later phases, the mucus content dehydrates and the concentration of proteins and blood products increases. These mucoceles contain a solid, greenish-brown component, corresponding to hard dehydrated mucoid material. Microscopically, the cysts are lined with pseudostratified ciliated columnar epithelium, associated to fibrosis, granulation tissue, recent and remote hemorrhage, and cholesterol granulomas. In some instances, the epithelium may present foci of squamous metaplasia and may be associated with inflammatory cell infiltration, bone resorption, and new bone formation. Sinus mucoceles have been divided into internal and external types. The first type is characterized by the cystic herniation into the submucosal tissues of the bony wall, whereas the external type shows the cranial cavity or subcutaneous tissue extension [11].

17.6 Diagnostics

Computed tomography (CT) and magnetic resonance imaging (MRI) are the methods of choice for the diagnosis of paranasal sinus diseases. Mucoceles are generally isodense to the brain parenchyma (10–40 HU depending on the hydration and the protein concentration) (Fig. 17.2). The older the lesion, the higher is its attenuation value; multiple fine calcifications reflect thickened, dehydrated mucocele content. Contrast enhanced CT scan is unnecessary and reserved to

patients who have contraindications to MRI. The 3D reconstruction of the CT scan is very useful for assessing the entity of the bony erosion (Fig. 17.3).

MRI is the gold standard in differentiating a mucocele from a tumor and for excluding an underlying tumor causing ostium obstruction, and dura involvement by the mucocele membrane. T1-weighted signal is determined by protein concentration and mucus viscosity, while T2-weighted intensity is determined by the water content. Usually, mucoceles have high T2 signal and low to high T1 signal [2] (Fig. 17.4). As the mucocele progresses, the hydration decreases and proteins concentration increases leading to signal intensity changes. Enhancement within the center of the lesion or nodular peripheral enhancement should raise the suspect of a coexisting tumor. MRI signal intensity drops out in the following cases: allergic Aspergillus sinusitis, Charcot-Leyden crystals, and fungal hypha.

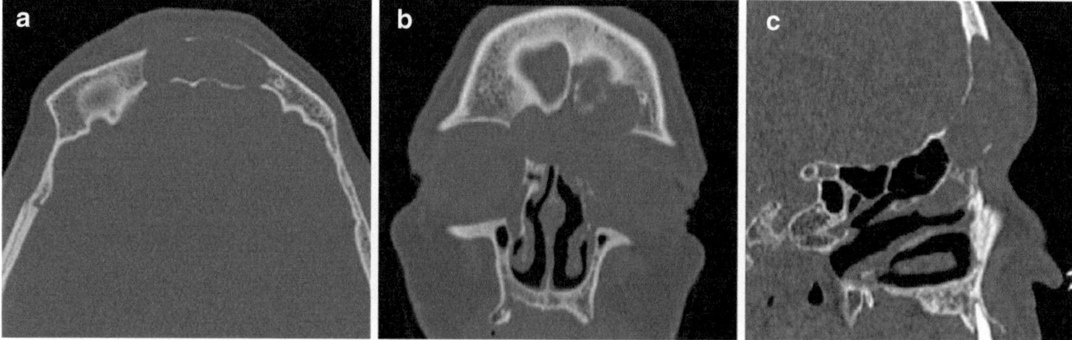

Fig. 17.2 CT scan of frontal sinus mucocele. (**a**) Axial view showing bilateral erosion of anterior and posterior frontal sinus walls; (**b**) Coronal view: the cystic lesion erodes the left frontal sinus recess and the medial portion of the roof of both orbits leading to bilateral intra-orbital invasion; (**c**) Sagittal view confirms the erosion of posterior and anterior wall of the frontal sinus and shows an intimate relation between the mucocele and forehead subcutaneous tissues

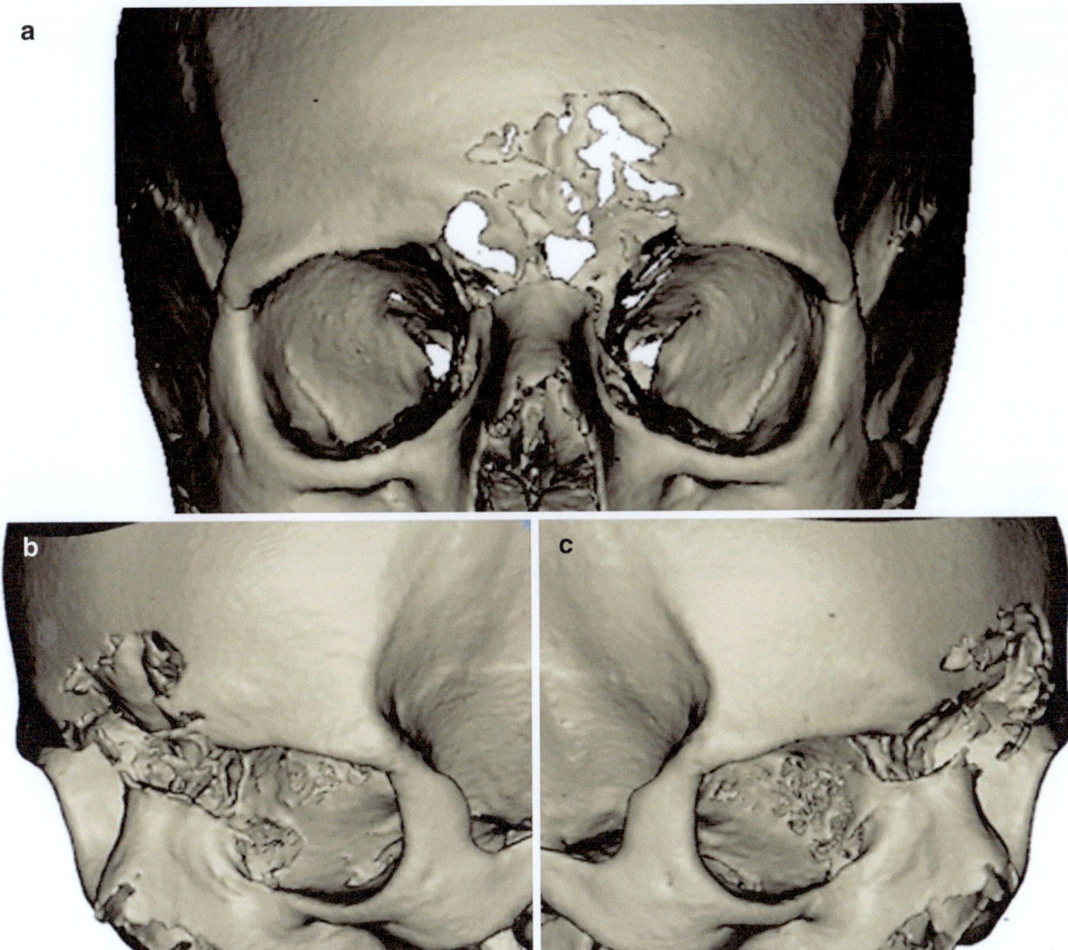

Fig. 17.3 3D reconstruction of CT scan of Fig. 17.2 assessing the entity of the mucocele extension. (**a**) The frontal view shows erosion of both the anterior and posterior walls of the frontal sinus; (**b**) Left and (**c**) Right three quarter views show bilateral erosion of the superomedial corner of the orbit as well as erosion of the anterior wall of the frontal sinus with the complete loss of the bony glabella

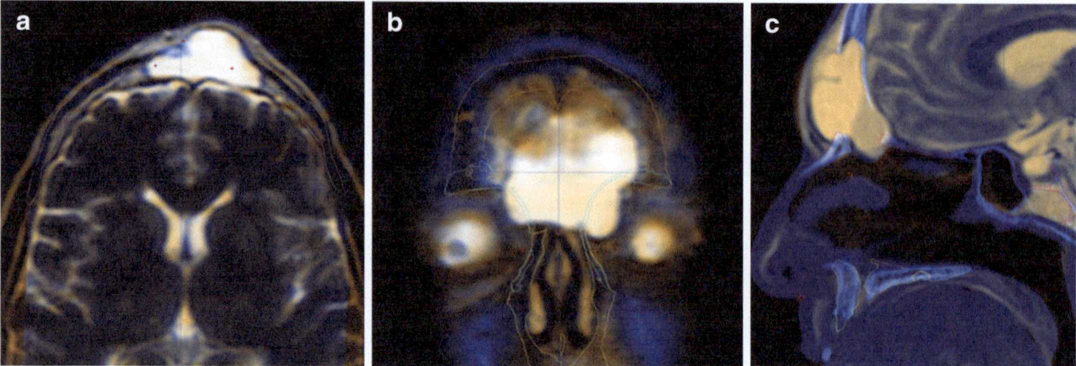

Fig. 17.4 T2-weighterd MRI sequences. (**a**) Axial view: anterior projection of the mucocele toward the forehead subcutaneous tissue with cleavable plane. It is also possible to appreciate, on the interface between the mucocele and the left frontal lobe, a small area with higher intensity suggesting a possible infiltration of the dura. (**b**) Coronal view confirms the bilateral invasion of the orbit through the medial portion of the orbital roofs; (**c**) Sagittal view shows the craniocaudal extension of the cystic lesion that appears not to extend over the frontal recess; expansion of the mucocele anteriorly, to the subcutaneous tissue, and posteriorly, to the anterior cranial fossa, is evident

17.7 Differential Diagnosis

The differential diagnosis of mucocele must include cholesterol granuloma, fungal and tubercular granulomas, encephalocele, epidermoid cyst, odontogenic cyst, chondroma, meningioma, salivary adenoma, paraganglioma, neurofibroma, and malignant neoplasms such as squamous cell carcinoma, adenocarcinoma, minor salivary gland tumors, osteosarcoma, chondrosarcoma, rhabdomyosarcoma esthesioneuroblastoma, and metastases (from melanoma, lymphoma, plasmatocytoma). Mucocele causing unilateral proptosis must be distinguished from inflammatory pseudotumour, dysthyroid eye disease, sinus tumor, retrobulbar orbital tumor, and metastatic lesions.

17.8 Treatment

The surgery is the gold standard treatment for paranasal sinuses mucoceles. The goal of the treatment is to eradicate the mucocele, ventilate the sinuses, solving any predisposing pathology, with the aim of decreasing morbidity and recurrence rate [12]. In case of infection, adjuvant antibiotic treatment is indicated. Several parameters must be considered: location, extension and size of the mucocele, anatomy of the frontal recess. The concomitant pathologies may imply distortion of the critical anatomical landmarks and neo-osteogenesis of the frontal recess which may hinder the endoscopic treatment. The frontal recess can become scarred with hard new bone in response to drilling; it may require to open the outflow tract leaving circumferential areas of denuded bone.

The paranasal sinuses are in close relationship with critical structures, such as orbit, optic nerve, carotid artery, and skull base. The proximity to these structures must be taken in account when approaching the paranasal sinus pathologies, especially mucoceles in which the bone erosion can lead to accidental injury to these structures.

The surgical navigation systems have significantly improved the approach to the sinus lesions. The navigated endoscopic endonasal surgery allows to achieve more complete resection in 81% of cases and to work more confidently with less stress in 95.2% [13]. Intra-operative navigation gives the opportunity to know exactly during the whole surgical procedure the instrument position in relationship with the anatomical structures and the lesion. It is mainly useful in cases of small and asymmetric frontal sinuses and to iden-

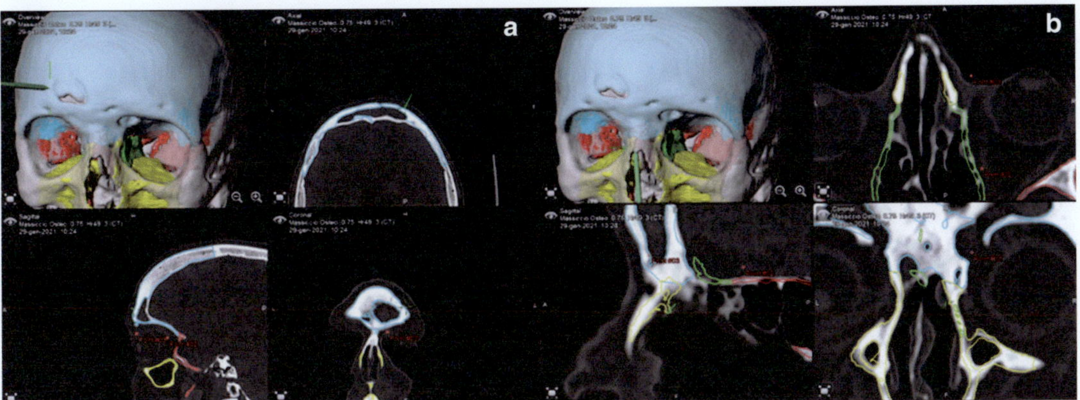

Fig. 17.5 Intraoperative navigation system. During the planning phase, it is possible to calibrate the CT or MRI scan setting some reference points and also to automatically detect the bony contours to ease the visualization of the anatomical limits and landmarks in the operating field. Intraoperative screenshots: touching a spot on the patient with the probe that area will be indicated on the CT and the 3D reconstruction: (**a**) the probe is touching the anterior wall of the frontal sinus in correspondence of an erosion; (**b**) the probe, inserted in the nose, is indicating the right frontonasal recess that is interested by inflammatory tissue

tify the inter-sinus septum in order to detach it from the frontal bony flap to avoid accidental fractures (Fig. 17.5).

When planning a surgical intervention, the preoperative visual acuity has prognostic value and may indicate the urgency of the treatment, especially in mucoceles arising from the posterior ethmoid or sphenoid sinuses and Onodi cells due to their close proximity with the optic nerve. It has recently been shown that even extreme vision loss may improve after surgical treatment of paranasal sinus mucoceles. The greatest improvement of the vision outcome occurs among patients with preoperative visual acuity ≥ 1.52 logMAR who underwent surgery within 6 days from the manifestation of the visual loss [10].

Surgical intervention can be achieved via endonasal endoscopic approach, external approach, or a combination of both. The first surgical open approaches were the anterior wall perforation (Ogston and Luck, 1884), the anterior wall ablation (Kuhnt, 1891), and the frontal osteoplastic flap procedure by Schonborn and Brieger in 1895 [14]. In 1920s, Lynch [15] described the external fronto-ethmoidectomy to treat frontal sinusitis, and Howarth [16] described an endonasal approach for drainage of mucoceles and pyoceles. However, these two approaches had the great disadvantage to promoting abundant scar reaction predisposing for a secondary mucocele. The osteoplastic flap is not free of adverse events; for this reason, in the years its use was limited to selected cases. With the introduction of the endoscopic technology in the 1980s, the treatment of paranasal sinuses pathology radically changed. In 1989, Kennedy et al. [17] introduced the endoscopic marsupialization, a conservative and minimally invasive procedure with decreased morbidity that preserves the sinus architecture avoiding external incisions and scarring [18]. Endoscopy offers several advantages, including better visualization of anatomic structures with no skin incisions and scarring, no osteotomies, preservation of the physiological mucociliary drainage, reduced blood loss, lesser postoperative morbidity, and shorter hospitalization time. It allows to continue endoscopic and radiographic control of the operated sinus cavity (Fig. 17.6).

According to the literature, poor anatomical visualization and large intracranial expansion of the mucocele are relative contraindications to endoscopic surgery. Absolute contraindications for the endonasal approach in the management of mucoceles include: far lateral localization of frontal sinus mucoceles; revision surgery after a Lynch-Howarth or Caldwell-Luc procedure that caused severe scars; maxillary sinus mucoceles located within the zygomatic bone; presence of a

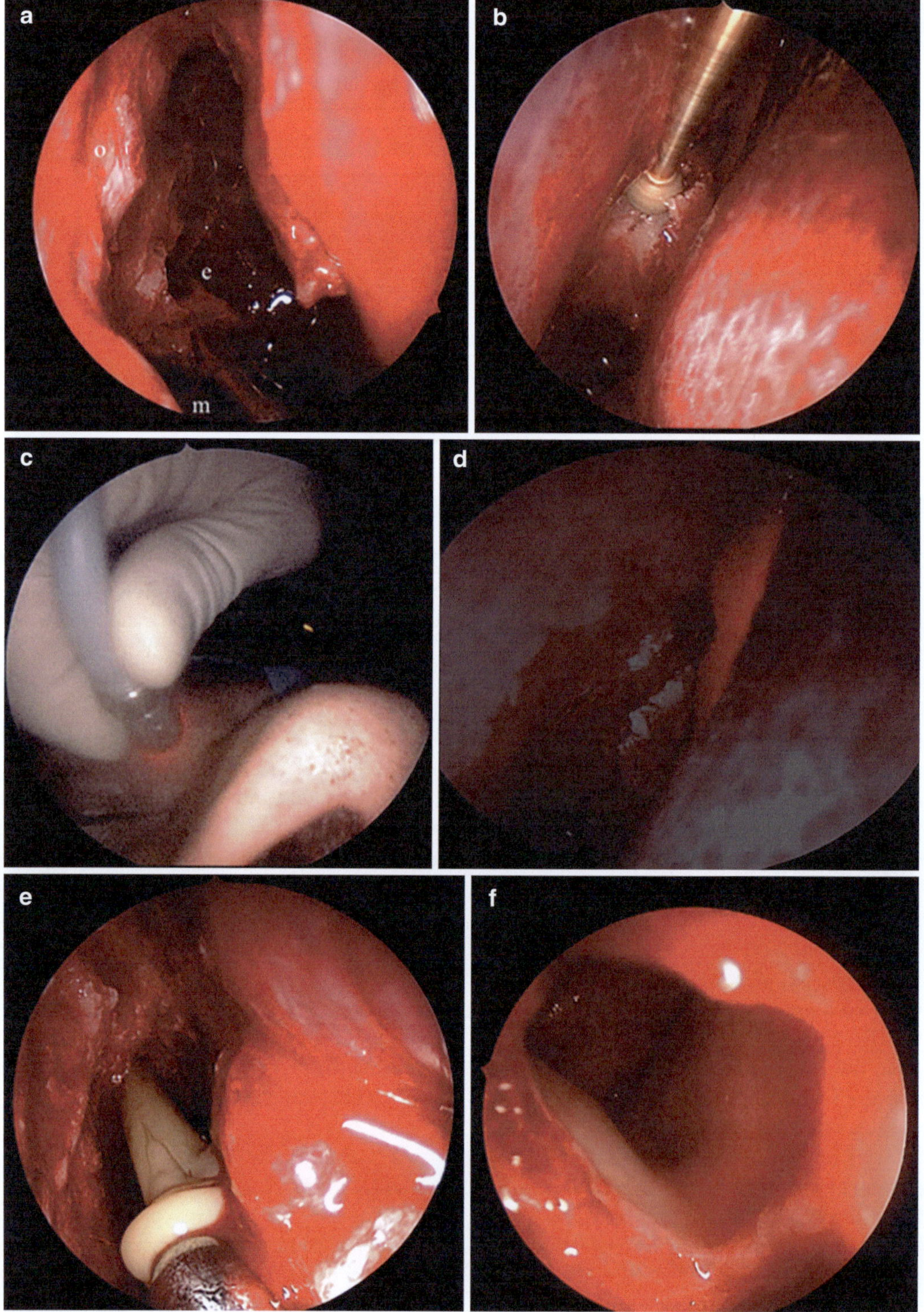

Fig. 17.6 Endoscopic marsupialization of a frontal sinus mucocele. (**a**) Right nasal fossa after maxillary sinus antrostomy and etmoidectomy; (**b**) Drilling of the frontal sinus recess; (**c**) Transillumination of the frontal recess; (**d**) Endonasal view of the transilluminated recess; (**e**) Leakage of mucus from the frontal sinus; (**f**) Insight of the empty frontal sinus following the marsupialization. *e* ethmoid sinus, *o* orbit, *t* turbinate, *m* maxillary sinus

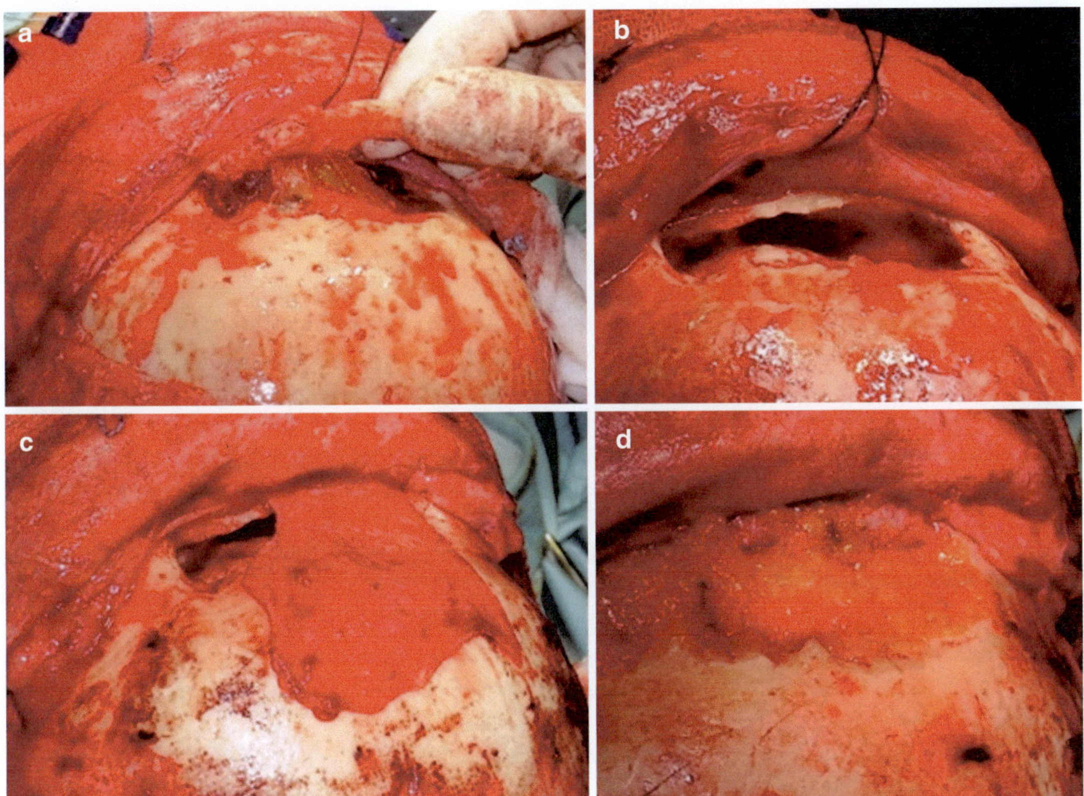

Fig. 17.7 Osteoplastic flap procedure and frontal sinus obliteration for a frontal sinus mucocele. (**a**) Lifting the frontal bone flap: the mucocele shows up as filled of thick green mucus; (**b**) The mucocele is eradicated, the mucosa of the frontal recess and of the sinus is removed as much as possible to avoid recurrences; (**c**) Harvesting of a galea flap to exclude the frontal sinus from the outflow tract; (**d**) Obliteration of the sinus with abdominal fat graft

cutaneous fistula that needs to be excised; mucoceles caused by malignancies that needs to be treated in one stage operation.

Nowadays, thanks to technical advancements of endoscopic surgery, the osteoplastic flap represents the final treatment strategy for refractory pathologies or inaccessible to the endoscopic approach; frontal sinus obliteration is usually the last resort once all other attempts have failed (Fig. 17.7). The open surgery offers several advantages including a wide surgical field that allows more radical excision and better control of bleeding or cerebrospinal fluid leak. On the other hand, open surgery is burdened by greater operatory stress, longer hospitalization time, greater blood loss, possibility of unaesthetic scarring [19]. In the latter years, many authors investigated the role of osteoplastic flap technique in the endoscopic era. These studies have shown that the open surgery is mandatory in several cases: inflammatory disease with osteitis that requires wide bone resection; difficult anatomy (narrowed frontal recesses, infrafrontal cells, or small frontal sinuses); mucoceles of the lateral wall of the maxillary sinus or too small to make endonasal marsupialization effective with high risk of synechia and recurrence; lateral frontal involvement which often requires an external (brow or coronal) or combined approach.

For mucoceles involving the lateral frontal sinus and invading the orbit, it is important to ensure marsupialization and a good frontal outflow to avoid accumulation of the mucocele contents. Every outflow obstruction must be treated via a standard endoscopic frontal sinusotomy together with the external approach. In 2010, Moe [20] described the endoscopic transorbital technique which, through different accesses (precaruncular, upper blepharoplasty, transconjunctival, or lateral retrocanthal), and depending on the target localization, creates a direct pathway to the frontal sinus and anterior cranial fossa [20, 21]. This approach provides a favorable path-to-target trajectory, otherwise inaccessible via endoscopic approach [22]. The mucocele is then decompressed and marsupialized under endoscopic visualization. Main adverse events of this approach are postoperative diplopia that may last for several weeks and temporary forehead paresthesia, typically lasting 3–6 months.

The treatment of giant mucoceles developing from the frontal and/or ethmoid sinuses and invading the cranial cavity is debated. According to a recent review, an endoscopic approach with wide marsupialization is safe and effective. However, 66% of giant lesions with significant brain and orbital compression are managed through external approaches. The open approach seems to be preferred because it allows rapid decompression of the brain thus avoiding potential neurologic complications, CSF leak, pneumocephalus, and residual mucocele lining. However, the morbidity associated with complete resection of the mucosal lining seems to outweigh the benefits; therefore, the marsupialization is favored. The mucosal lining of mucoceles may firmly adhere to the dura or the periorbita; thus the attempts for a complete removal may cause dural or periorbital breach. Since it has been shown that the mucocele does not lose normal respiratory epithelium, many authors agree that the stripping is not necessary and marsupialization is better than frontal sinus obliteration.

Beside endoscopic and external approaches, an in-office marsupialization procedure has been recently described for the frontal sinus mucocele with the Baloon technology under endoscopic visualization under local anesthesia. It seems to be a feasible alternative to the conventional surgery in selected patients (young, compliant, not anxious, and with no comorbidities). However, this technique is not indicated in mucoceles with multiple compartments within a mucocele and difficult bony architecture near the frontal sinus recess.

In 2014, Sama et al. [23] described a new algorithm for surgical management of frontal sinus mucoceles based on radiographic evidences of the mucocele position. The algorithm considers: position of the mucocele (medial/intermediate/lateral); maximum AP/LM dimensions (<1 cm) of the frontal ostium; presence of Type III/IV fronto-ethmoidal cells; degree of neo-osteogenesis (>50% of the frontal recess); presence of contralateral frontal sinus disease and other concurrent pathologies. Using this positional classification, they were able to plan the appropriate surgical intervention using the surgical algorithm. (Table 17.1) In most cases, the treatment is accomplished with the Draf's techniques: Type I (ethmoidectomy including cell septa removal in the region of the frontal recess); Type IIa (resection of the frontal sinus floor between the lamina papyracea and middle turbinate); Type IIb (resection of the frontal sinus floor to the nasal septum, anterior to the olfactory fossa); Type III (opening of the frontal sinus floor from the ipsilateral to contralateral lamina papyracea and removal of the upper nasal septum and frontal inter-sinus septum) [24]. According to this algorithm, the osteoplastic flap must be reserved to cases where: there is poor access to the supra-orbital cell or there are multiple (>3) co-existent complicating factors and malignant or notable second pathologies.

Table 17.1 Sama treatment algorithm [23]. Crossing the anatomical variations (lines) with the mucocele position (columns) it is possible to choose the better surgical management of the frontal sinus mucoceles

Complicating variable	Medial	Intermediate	Lateral
No complicating factors	I/IIa	IIa/IIb	III
AP/LM dimension, <1cmType III/IV FE cell	IIb	III	III/OPF
>50% neo-osteogenesis	III	III/OPF	OPF

17.9 Follow-Up

The follow-up consists of endoscopy control and MRI monitoring every 6 months for the first 2 years. Later, an annual MRI is sufficient, apart for complications [25]. According to the literature, the follow-up time must be of at least 6–7 years [1].

References

1. Dzhambazov KB, Kitov BD, Zhelyazkov HB, Traykova NI, Kehayov II, Kitova TT. Mucocele of the paranasal sinuses–retrospective analysis of a series of seven cases. Folia Med. 2018;60:147–53. https://doi.org/10.1515/folmed-2017-0077.
2. Bakshi. Image diagnosis: frontoethmoidal mucocele. Perm J. 2019;23:1. https://doi.org/10.7812/TPP/18-288.
3. De Paris SW, Goldberg AN, Indaram M, Grumbine FL, Kersten RC, Vagefi MR. Paranasal sinus Mucocele as a late complication of Dacryocystorhinostomy. Ophthalmic Plast Reconstr Surg. 2017;33:S23–4. https://doi.org/10.1097/IOP.0000000000000538.
4. Har-El G. Transnasal endoscopic management of frontal mucoceles. Otolaryngol Clin N Am. 2001;34:243–51. https://doi.org/10.1016/s0030-6665(05)70309-1.
5. Rodriguez DP, Orscheln ES, Koch BL. Masses of the nose, nasal cavity, and nasopharynx in children. Radiographics. 2017;37:1704–30. https://doi.org/10.1148/rg.2017170064.
6. Plantier D, Neto D, Pinna F, Mucocele VR. Clinical characteristics and outcomes in 46 operated patients. Int. Arch Otorhinolaryngol. 2019;23:088–91. https://doi.org/10.1055/s-0038-1668126.
7. Landsberg R, Friedman M. A computer-assisted anatomical study of the Nasofrontal region. Laryngoscope. 2001;111:2125–30. https://doi.org/10.1097/00005537-200112000-00008.
8. Barroso MS, Araújo BC, Jacinto J, Marques C, Gama I, Barros E. Association between the insertion type of the uncinate process and the development of frontal sinus mucoceles—is there a relationship? Acta Otorrinolaringol Esp. 2021;72:246–51. https://doi.org/10.1016/j.otoeng.2020.06.005.
9. Maldjian C. Giant mucocele secondary to cocaine abuse. Radiol Case Rep. 2021;16:589–92. https://doi.org/10.1016/j.radcr.2020.12.025.
10. Zukin LM, Hink EM, Liao S, Getz AE, Kingdom TT. Ramakrishnan VR endoscopic management of paranasal sinus mucoceles: meta-analysis of visual outcomes. Otolaryngol Head Neck Surg. 2017;157:760–6. https://doi.org/10.1177/0194599817717674.
11. Gnepp DR, Bishop JA. Gnepp's diagnostic surgical pathology of the head and neck. 3rd ed. Philadelphia, PA: Elsevier; 2020. ISBN: 9780323547802.
12. Alaraifi AK, Alrusayyis DF, Alzuwayed A, Alobaid F, AlRajeh M, Alhedaithy R. Endoscopic transorbital management of frontal sinus mucocele: a case report and review of the literature. J Surg Case Rep. 2021;2021:rjab491. https://doi.org/10.1093/jscr/rjab491.
13. Vicaut E, Bertrand B, Betton J-L, et al. Use of a navigation system in endonasal surgery: impact on surgical strategy and surgeon satisfaction. A prospective multicenter study. Eur Ann Otorhinolaryngol Head Neck Dis. 2019;136:461–4. https://doi.org/10.1016/j.anorl.2019.08.002.
14. McLaughlin RB. History of surgical approaches to the frontal sinus. Otolaryngol Clin N Am. 2001;34:49–58. https://doi.org/10.1016/s0030-6665(05)70294-2.
15. Lynch RC. The technique of a radical frontal sinus operation which has given me the best results. Laryngoscope. 1921;31:1–5. https://doi.org/10.1288/00005537-192101000-00001.
16. Howarth WG. Operations on the frontal sinus. J Laryngol Otol. 1921;36:417–21. https://doi.org/10.1017/S0022215100022398.
17. Kennedy DW, Josephson JS, Zinreich SJ, Mattox DE. Goldsmith MM endoscopic sinus surgery for mucoceles: a viable alternative. Laryngoscope. 1989;99:885–95. https://doi.org/10.1288/00005537-198909000-00002.
18. Ahmed T, Ahmed S, Kaushal N. Minimally invasive endoscopic approach towards management of frontoethmoidal mucocoele with lateral displacement of eyeball and proptosis—a case report. Ann Maxillofac Surg. 2021;11:129. https://doi.org/10.4103/ams.ams_420_20.
19. Stokken J, Wali E, Woodard T, Recinos PF, Sindwani R. Considerations in the management of giant frontal mucoceles with significant intracranial extension: a systematic review. Am J Rhinol Allergy. 2016;30:301–5. https://doi.org/10.2500/ajra.2016.30.4323.
20. Moe KS, Bergeron CM, Ellenbogen RG. Transorbital neuroendoscopic surgery. Neurosurgery. 2010;67:ons16–28. https://doi.org/10.1227/01.NEU.0000373431.08464.43.
21. Miller C, Berens A, Patel SA, Humphreys IM, Moe KS. Transorbital approach for improved access in the management of paranasal sinus Mucoceles. J Neurol Surg B. 2019;80:593–8. https://doi.org/10.1055/s-0038-1676982.
22. Romano A, Audino G, Abbate V, Dell'Aversana Orabona G, Salzano G, Seidita F, Sani L, Iaconetta G, Califano L. Combined Endonasal endoscopic and sub-brow Orbitotomy access to manage a lateral extending frontal sinus inverting papilloma with endo-orbital invasion: a case report. Indian J Otolaryngol Head Neck Surg. 2021;74:1510. https://doi.org/10.1007/s12070-021-02640-7.
23. Sama A, McClelland L, Constable J. Frontal sinus mucocoeles: new algorithm for surgical management. Rhinology. 2014;52:267–75. https://doi.org/10.4193/Rhino13.103.

24. Draf W. Endonasal micro-endoscopic frontal sinus surgery: the fulda concept. Oper Tech Otolaryngol Head Neck Surg. 1991;2:234–40. https://doi.org/10.1016/S1043-1810(10)80087-9.

25. Bouatay R, Aouf L, Hmida B, Korbi AE, Kolsi N, Harrathi K, Koubaa J. The role of imaging in the management of sinonasal mucoceles. Pan Afr Med J. 2019;34:3. https://doi.org/10.11604/pamj.2019.34.3.18677.

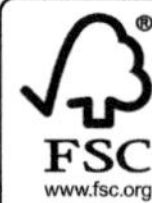